Handbook of Clinical Alcoholism Treatment

Handbook of Clinical Alcoholism Treatment

EDITORS

Bankole A. Johnson, M.D., Ph.D.

Wurzbach Distinguished Professor of Psychiatry and Pharmacology
Deputy Chairman for Research
Department of Psychiatry
The University of Texas Health Science Center at San Antonio
The South Texas Addiction Research and Technology (START) Center
San Antonio, Texas

Pedro Ruiz, M.D.

Professor and Vice Chairman
Department of Psychiatry and Behavioral Sciences
The University of Texas Medical School
Houston, Texas

Marc Galanter, M.D.

Professor of Psychiatry
Director, Division of Alcoholism and Drug Abuse
New York University School of Medicine
New York, New York

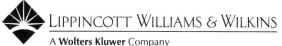

LIPPINCOTT WILLIAMS & WILKINS
A **Wolters Kluwer** Company
Philadelphia · Baltimore · New York · London
Buenos Aires · Hong Kong · Sydney · Tokyo

Acquisitions Editor: Charles W. Mitchell
Managing Editor: Joyce A. Murphy
Production Editor: Jennifer Jett
Cover Designer: Diana Andrews
Compositor: Maryland Composition Inc.
Printer: R.R. Donnelley

351 West Camden Street
Baltimore, Maryland 21201-2436 USA

530 Walnut Street
Philadelphia, PA 19106

Printed in the United States of America

Library of Congress Cataloging-in-Publication Data

Handbook of clinical alcoholism treatment / [edited by] Bankole Johnson,
Pedro Ruiz, Marc Galanter.
    p. ; cm.
Includes bibliographical references and index.
    ISBN: 0-7817-4158-0
    1.   Alcoholism—Treatment—Handbooks, manuals, etc. 2.
Alcoholics—Counseling of—Handbooks, manuals, etc.
    [DNLM: 1.   Alcoholism—therapy. 2.   Alcoholism—diagnosis. WM 274
H2363 2003] I. Johnson, Bankole A. II. Ruiz, Pedro, 1936– III.
Galanter, Marc.
    RC565.H265 2003
    616.86′1—dc22

                                                            2003017282

To purchase additional copies of this book, call our customer service
department at **(800) 638-3030** or fax orders to **(301) 824-7390**.
International customers should call **(301) 714-2324**.

Visit Lippincott Williams & Wilkins on the Internet: http://
www.LWW.com. Lippincott Williams & Wilkins customer service

representatives are available from 8:30 am to 6:00 pm, EST.03 04 05 06 07

                                   1 2 3 4 5 6 7 8 9 10

We wish to dedicate this handbook to Lyn, to Angela, and to the memory of Wynne. This handbook could not have been possible without the dedication, sacrifice, and support of our spouses. Lyn, Angela, and Wynne know quite well how important our careers are for us and how dedicated and committed we are to those who suffer directly or indirectly from alcoholism.

Bankole, Pedro, and Marc

Contents

Section I. Foundations of Alcoholism

Section II. Diagnostic Tools

Section III. Treatment Modalities

Section IV. Treatment Settings

Section V. Special Issues

Appendix

Contributing Authors

Nassima Ait-Daoud, M.D.
Assistant Professor of Psychiatry
The University of Texas Health Science Center at San Antonio
The South Texas Addiction Research and Technology (START)
Center
San Antonio, Texas

Raymond F. Anton, M.D.
Professor of Psychiatry and Behavioral Sciences
Institute of Psychiatry
Medical University of South Carolina
Charleston, South Carolina

Roland M. Atkinson, M.D.
Professor of Psychiatry
Oregon Health and Science University
Portland, Oregon

Pamela Bean, PhD, MBA
Executive Director of Research
Rogers Memorial Hospital
Madison, Wisconsin

Sheila B. Blume, M.D.
Clinical Professor of Psychiatry
State University of New York at Stony Brook
School of Medicine
Stony Brook, New York

James W. Cornish, M.D.
Associate Professor of Psychiatry
Department of Psychiatry
University of Pennsylvania
and Veterans Affairs Medical Center
Philadelphia, Pennsylvania

Patricia Culliton, M.A., L.Ac.
Director, Alternative Medicine Division
Department of Medicine
Hennepin County Medical Center
Adjunct Faculty
Center for Spirituality and Healing
University of Minnesota
Minneapolis, Minnesota

Katherine A. DeLaune, Ph.D.
Fellow
Substance Abuse Research Center
Department of Psychiatry and Behavioral Sciences
University of Texas Mental Sciences Institute
Houston, Texas

Sylvia J. Dennison, M.D.
Associate Professor
Department of Psychiatry
Chief, Division of Addiction Services
University of Illinois at Chicago
Chicago, Illinois

Carlo C. DiClemente, Ph.D., ABPP
Professor and Chairman
Department of Psychology
University of Maryland, Baltimore County
Baltimore, Maryland

Dennis M. Donovan, Ph.D.
Professor
Department of Psychiatry and Behavioral Sciences
University of Washington
Alcohol and Drug Abuse Institute
Seattle, Washington

Francisco Fernandez, M.D.
Professor and Chairman
Department of Psychiatry
University of South Florida
Tampa, Florida

David A Fiellin, M.D.
Associate Professor
Department of Internal Medicine
Yale University School of Medicine
New Haven, Connecticut

Kim Fromme, Ph.D.
Associate Professor
Department of Psychology
The University of Texas at Austin
Austin, Texas

Marc Galanter, M.D.
Professor of Psychiatry
Director, Division of Alcoholism and Drug Abuse
New York University School of Medicine
New York, New York

Gantt P. Galloway, Pharm.D.
Chief of Pharmacologic Research
Haight Ashbury Free Clinics
San Francisco, California

David Gastfriend, M.D.
Associate Professor of Psychiatry
Harvard Medical School
Director, Addiction Research Program
Department of Psychiatry
Massachusetts General Hospital
Boston, Massachusetts

Mark S. George, M.D.
Distinguished Professor of Psychiatry, Radiology, and Neurology
Director, Center for Advanced Imaging Research
Director, Brain Stimulation Laboratory
Department of Psychiatry
Charleston Alcohol Research Center
Medical University of South Carolina
and the Mental Health Service
Ralph H. Johnson VA Medical Center
Charleston, South Carolina

Stuart Gitlow, M.D., M.P.H.
Medical Director
Nantucket Family and Children's Service
Nantucket, Massachusetts

Harold W. Goforth, M.D.
Resident Physician
Department of Psychiatry
Stritch School of Medicine
Loyola University Medical Center
Maywood, Illinois

Sarah H. Heil, Ph.D.
Research Assistant Professor
Department of Psychiatry
University of Vermont
Burlington, Vermont

Scott E. Hemby, Ph.D.
Research Assistant Professor
Department of Pharmacology and Psychiatry/Behavioral Sciences
Yerkes National Primate Research Center, Neuroscience Division
Emory University School of Medicine
Atlanta, Georgia

Stephen T. Higgins, Ph.D.
Professor
Department of Psychiatry
University of Vermont
Burlington, Vermont

Martin A. Javors, Ph.D.
Professor
Departments of Psychiatry and Pharmacology
The University of Texas Health Science Center at San Antonio
San Antonio, Texas

Bankole A. Johnson, M.D., Ph.D.
Wurzbach Distinguished Professor of Psychiatry and Pharmacology
Deputy Chairman for Research
Department of Psychiatry
The University of Texas Health Science Center at San Antonio
The South Texas Addiction Research and Technology (START) Center
San Antonio, Texas

Lisa Jordan, Ph.D.
Assistant Professor
Department of Psychology
University of Maryland, Baltimore County
Baltimore, Maryland

Shimi K. Kang, M.D.
Clinical Research Fellow
Addiction Research Program
Department of Psychiatry
Massachusetts General Hospital
Harvard Medical School
Boston, Massachusetts
Resident in Psychiatry
University of British Columbia School of Medicine
Vancouver, British Columbia, Canada

Thomas S. King, Ph.D.
Associate Professor
Department of Cellular and Structural Biology
The University of Texas Health Science Center at San Antonio
San Antonio, Texas

Marc I. Kruse, M.A.
Graduate Student
Department of Psychology
The University of Texas at Austin
Austin, Texas

William B. Lawson, M.D., Ph.D.
Professor and Chairman
Department of Psychiatry
Howard University College of Medicine
Washington, DC

Xingbao Li, M.D.
Postdoctoral Fellow of Research Science
Department of Psychiatry
Charleston Alcohol Research Center
Medical University of South Carolina
Charleston, South Carolina

Julie Madaras, B.A.
Research Technician
University of Pennsylvania
Treatment Research Center
Philadelphia, Pennsylvania

Patricia Marinelli-Casey, Ph.D.
Assistant Research Psychologist
University of California Los Angeles
Department of Psychiatry and Biobehavioral Sciences
David Geffen School of Medicine
Los Angeles, California

Angela Marinilli, M.A.
Graduate Student
Department of Psychology
University of Maryland, Baltimore County
Baltimore, Maryland

Douglas B. Marlowe, J.D., Ph.D.
Director of Law & Ethics Research
Treatment Research Institute
Adjunct Associate Professor of Psychiatry
University of Pennsylvania School of Medicine
Philadelphia, Pennsylvania

Sarah N. Mattson, Ph.D.
Assistant Professor
Center for Behavioral Teratology
Department of Psychology
San Diego State University
San Diego, California

Robert Mickey, M.D.
Assistant Professor
Department of Psychiatry
Howard University College of Medicine
Washington, DC

Hugh Myrick, M.D.
Assistant Professor of Psychiatry
Department of Psychiatry
Charleston Alcohol Research Center
Medical University of South Carolina
and the Mental Health Service
Ralph H. Johnson VA Medical Center
Charleston, South Carolina

Melissa Nidecker, M.A.
Graduate Student
Department of Psychology
University of Maryland, Baltimore County
Baltimore, Maryland

Patrick G. O'Connor, M.D., M.P.H.
Professor
Chief, Section of General Internal Medicine
Department of Internal Medicine
Yale University School of Medicine
New Haven, Connecticut

Helen M. Pettinati, Ph.D.
Professor
Department of Psychiatry
University of Pennsylvania
Treatment Research Center
Philadelphia, Pennsylvania

Douglas Polcin, Ed.D.
Research Psychologist
Haight Ashbury Free Clinics
San Francisco, California

Margaret Primeau, Ph.D.
Associate Professor
Department of Psychiatry
Stritch School of Medicine
Loyola University Medical Center
Maywood, Illinois

Richard A. Rawson, Ph.D.
Adjunct Associate Professor
University of California Los Angeles
Department of Psychiatry and Biobehavioral Sciences
David Geffen School of Medicine
Los Angeles, California

Pedro Ruiz, M.D.
Professor and Vice Chairman
Department of Psychiatry and Behavioral Sciences
The University of Texas Medical School
Houston, Texas

Joy M. Schmitz, Ph.D.
Professor
Substance Abuse Research Center
Department of Psychiatry and Behavioral Sciences
University of Texas Mental Sciences Institute
Houston, Texas

Kenneth Silverman, Ph.D.
Associate Professor
Department of Psychiatry
Johns Hopkins University School of Medicine
Center for Learning and Health
Baltimore, Maryland

Michael O. Smith, M.D.
Assistant Clinical Professor of Psychiatry
Cornell-Weill Medical College
Director, Lincoln Hospital Recovery Center
New York, New York

Ruthlyn Sodano, B.A.
Research Associate
University of California Los Angeles
Department of Psychiatry and Biobehavioral Sciences
David Geffen School of Medicine
Los Angeles, California

Robert Swift, M.D., Ph.D.
Professor, Department of Psychiatry and Human Behavior
Brown University Medical School
Associate Chief of Staff for Research and Education
Providence VA Medical Center
Providence, Rhode Island

Claudia A. Voyles, M.A.O.M., L.Ac.
Training Chairperson for the National Acupuncture
Detoxification Association
Austin, Texas

Roger D. Weiss, M.D.
Associate Professor of Psychiatry
Alcohol and Drug Abuse Treatment Center
Department of Psychiatry
Harvard Medical School
McLean Hospital
Boston, Massachusetts

Foreword

I am pleased to accept the editors' request to write a foreword to *Handbook of Clinical Alcoholism Treatment*. The authors and editors aim at a comprehensive review, delineating epidemiological, biological, psychological, and sociocultural factors underlying the development of alcoholism. In addition, they present current developments on diagnostic and assessment tools and pharmacological and behavioral interventions for alcohol use disorders. Special populations and different treatment settings are also highlighted, and the clinical issues specific for each population and setting are discussed.

Alcoholism is an intractable, devastating disease responsible for a host of medical, economic, social, and personal afflictions worldwide. Due to the complex nature of alcoholism, it is unlikely that one type of treatment will cure all alcoholics. Instead, it is more practical to develop a menu of treatments that address the biological, psychological, social, and cultural elements of alcoholism. Fortunately, during the past decade, significant progress has been made in research to develop and rigorously test a variety of new pharmacological and behavioral treatments.

Advances in medications development have been highlighted by two promising medications, naltrexone and acamprosate. Naltrexone, an opioid antagonist, was approved by the Food and Drug Administration in 1994; it was the first medication approved for alcoholism treatment in over 50 years since the introduction of disulfiram. It also represents the first agent approved that reduces craving or the urge to drink. Acamprosate, an agent that interacts with the glutamate system, is approved and available in 24 countries around the world for alcoholism treatment, although at this time it has not been approved in the United States. Since naltrexone and acamprosate produce small to medium effects in reducing or preventing drinking, efforts are being made to develop new, more potent medications as well as to explore combinations of medications for enhanced effects. Also, since these medications do not work for everyone, research is under way to identify patients' characteristics predictive of a favorable treatment outcome (e.g., pharmacogenetics).

Advances have also been made in developing and testing an assortment of behavioral therapies. Efficacious interventions include cognitive behavioral therapy, motivation enhancement therapy, brief interventions, 12-step facilitation therapy, and couples therapy. Still, many alcoholics do not respond adequately to currently available behavioral therapies. Additional research is required to increase the overall effectiveness of behavioral interventions for the engagement, retention, adherence, and outcome of alcoholism treatment across various populations. In developing new behavioral therapies or modifying existing ones, it is important to understand their mechanisms of action (active components), that is, why and how they have their effects (mediators) and for whom and under what circumstances they are effective (moderators). New approaches may require the translation of basic behavioral science, cognitive science, social science, affective science, and neuroscience into behavioral therapy development.

Another strategy to enhance treatment outcome is to explore optimal combinations of behavioral therapies and medications. The National Institute on Alcohol Abuse and Alcoholism is currently supporting an 11-site trial, named COMBINE, to investigate the combination of naltrexone and acamprosate with two different types of behavioral therapies, Medication Management and a more intensive Combined Behavioral Intervention.

Developing effective therapies for special populations is another high priority. For example, many alcoholics suffer from a co-occurring psychiatric and/or substance use disorder. Research in this area, however, is in the early stages. Several fundamental clinical questions surrounding the treatment of psychiatric and substance use comorbidity remain. For instance, how does the treatment of one disorder improve or affect outcome for the other disorder? Also, does the treatment strategy differ for each type of psychiatric/substance abuse comorbidity as well as for subpopulations within a comorbidity (e.g., severity, gender, and primary versus secondary)?

New studies are under way in adolescents to evaluate various behavioral and pharmacological interventions in a variety of settings. New interventions involve tailoring to the developmental, psychological, and social needs of adolescents. Studies are also needed for other special populations including minority groups, those at risk or suffering from HIV/AIDS, children with fetal alcohol syndrome or alcohol-related neurodevelopment disorder, the elderly, those in the criminal justice system, and professional health care personnel.

In order to develop more effective strategies to treat or prevent alcoholism, it is essential to understand the factors leading up to the development of alcoholism as well as the processes involved in alcohol relapse and recovery. Identifying the biological, cognitive, behavioral, social, and cultural determinants that promote initial drinking, continuation of drinking, and cessation of drinking will provide a better opportunity to develop interventions that have a strong theoretical basis.

Finally, in recent years the methodology of alcohol clinical trials has been significantly advanced. State-of-the-art alcohol trials, such as Project MATCH and COMBINE, have significantly raised the standard of conducting clinical trials. Efforts are being made to standardize core assessment instruments and outcome measures across different studies. New research directions include developing and clinically evaluating alcohol-sensitive biomarkers to measure levels of drinking, determine relapse, measure alcohol-induced organ damage, and identify individuals who are predisposed to alcoholism.

This handbook was created in recognition of the need for pulling together the many aspects of alcoholism treatment described above in a coherent, comprehensive manner. It offers alcohol researchers a compendium of the most recent advances in the field and assistance with selecting the latest treatment options. We hope that sources of this kind will be used to move the field forward.

Raye Z. Litten, Ph.D.
Chief, Treatment Research Branch
Division of Clinical and Prevention Research
National Institute on Alcohol Abuse and Alcoholism
National Institutes of Health
Bethesda, Maryland

Preface

This book, the Handbook of Clinical Alcoholism Treatment, represents our attempt to address the growing concern in the health care field and in society at large over the prevalence and seriousness of alcohol abuse and dependence. Alcoholism is an illness that impacts on every aspect of the health and mental health care system, whether it is the psychiatric and mental health field, or the neurological, digestive, cardiovascular, and other subspecialized areas. Ongoing use of high amounts of alcohol clearly affects every organ and body system.

Alcoholism claims about 100,000 lives every year; approximately 6 million people in the United States currently abuse alcohol, and about 9 million are alcohol dependent. Additionally, the Epidemiological Catchment Area Study (ECA) noted that approximately 13.8% of Americans will experience an alcohol-related substance use disorder over the course of their lifetime. It has also been estimated that during the 1990s the annual direct and indirect cost attributed to alcohol/alcoholism was about $166 million. In general, close to 40% of all deaths in this country are related to alcohol. Alcoholism has a significant impact in all stages of the life cycle in this country, particularly adolescence. About 10 million youths between the ages of 12 and 20 years are current drinkers. The association between alcoholism and other substances of abuse as well as accidents, crime, and suicide is also very high. The impact of alcoholism on health care can be easily illustrated by the fact that suicide is the eighth leading cause of death in this country and liver-related disorders are the tenth leading cause of death.

Culture, race, and ethnicity also have a major influence on how alcohol is consumed, its impact on the organism, and how society responds to its use. Family traditions, religious beliefs and practices, and social setting characteristics are all very relevant and important in understanding alcohol use, abuse, and dependence. Thus, it is also important that we give attention to these very relevant factors. Genetic considerations are also key in this regard. In this respect, the pharmacogenetic, pharmacokinetic, and pharmacodynamic considerations with respect to alcoholism are crucial to understanding its biological underpinnings, and to its impact on different organ systems.

Taking all these essential factors into consideration, we conceptualized the design and creation of this handbook. In essence, we decided to address the crucial issues in the understanding of alcoholism and in the diagnosis and treatment of its related disorders and conditions. In so doing, we put together a group of the leading experts in the field and asked them to address the epidemiological, neurobiological, psychological, and sociocultural underpinnings of alcoholism, and to review all major diagnostic and treatment considerations related to alcoholism. Finally, we requested that they focus on preventive issues as well as specific issues related to gender, the life cycle, and special populations.

We are enormously grateful to the distinguished group of collaborators selected for this task. They have fully satisfied our expectations. We hope, however, that our handbook will satisfy and meet the expectations and needs of our readers as well.

Bankole A. Johnson, M.D., Ph.D.
Pedro Ruiz, M.D.
Marc Galanter, M.D.

Acknowledgments

We wish to express our gratitude and recognition to our executive editor/publisher, Charles W. Mitchell, whose encouragement, guidance, and confidence were essential for the conceptualization and creation of this handbook. Also, we owe a debt of appreciation to our managing editor, Joyce A. Murphy, whose assistance in the coordination of this volume was crucial. Finally, we want to thank Robert Cormier, Jr., whose editorial assistance was instrumental in completing this project.

Foundations of Alcoholism

EPIDEMIOLOGY OF ALCOHOLISM

Bankole A. Johnson

Alcoholism is a major cause of morbidity and mortality in the United States. It is a tremendous burden to the families of those who suffer from the disease, and it is associated with a huge societal cost. About 44% of the adult population over the age of 18 years is made up of drinkers who have consumed more than 12 drinks in the preceding year. Eight million U.S. citizens are dependent upon alcohol, and an additional 5.6 million abuse alcohol. Alcoholism tends to run in families. Over 50% of the adult Americans have a past history or a close relative with alcoholism, and up to one quarter of minors under the age of 18 years have been exposed to familial alcoholism or alcohol abuse. Alcohol use is implicated in up to one quarter of violent crimes and more than 16,000 fatal car accidents each year. Alcohol abuse costs the nation $185 billion per annum—over $600 for every man, woman, and child living in the United States.

This chapter will first appraise the health benefits and potential risks of alcohol, then how alcohol manifests over the life span (especially among youth and the elderly), then evaluate the relationship of age, gender, and other socio-demographic factors with drinking, and finally conclude with an evaluation of the association between alcohol use, drunk driving, and violence.

WHAT ARE THE HEALTH BENEFITS AND RISKS OF ALCOHOL CONSUMPTION?

Potential Benefits

Perhaps the most publicized potential health benefit of alcohol consumption is the reduced risk of coronary heart disease—the most common cause of death in the U.S. Studies conducted in Europe and the United States all show that moderate levels of drinking are associated with reduced risk of coronary heart disease in both men and women. However, there are important differences due to the different nomenclatures that have been used to describe drinking behavior. For example, the U.S. Department of Agriculture, the U.S. Department of Health and Human Services, and the National Institute on Alcohol Abuse and Alcoholism all differ in their definition as to what constitutes moderate drinking in the United States. Generally, drinking in the range of fewer than 1 to 3 standard drinks* per week and no more than 1 and 2 standard drinks per day for women and men, respectively, may be associated with reduced risk of death from coronary heart disease. Interestingly, the incidence of coronary heart disease is actually slightly higher among abstainers than those who drink moderately. Further, it is clear that alcohol's protective

---

* One standard drink is defined as 12 oz. of beer, 5 oz. of wine, or 1.5 oz. of 80 proof liquor.

effects on the heart are lost when men and women drink more than 5 and 2 drinks per day, respectively. It cannot, however, be assumed that the relationship between drinking and reduced mortality from coronary heart disease in moderate drinkers compared with abstainers is simply causal; indeed, many factors confound the explanation for this relationship, e.g., lifestyle, use of other abused substances (such as tobacco), and socioeconomic status.

The exact mechanism by which alcohol use may be protective against morbidity in those with coronary heart disease has not been elucidated fully. However, some authorities have pointed to the disparate benefits of different types of alcoholic beverages as providing some important clues. The evidence regarding the relationship between the type of alcoholic beverage and the risk of death from coronary heart disease is mixed. While the evidence has tended to favor wines (particularly red wines, which are high in tannins) as conferring the best protection by lowering blood lipids and fats and by increasing the body's concentration of antioxidants, it also may be the case that an equally critical factor is the pattern of drinking. For instance, wines appear to be more typically consumed in modest amounts, especially with meals, when compared with beers and spirits, and are therefore more likely to be ingested more slowly. In contrast, binge drinking of all types of beverages increases the risk of mortality from coronary heart disease.

Evidence concerning the potential protective effects of alcohol on other types of vascular disease is somewhat equivocal. While the preponderance of the literature would suggest a slight reduction in the risk of stroke in men consuming no more than a few drinks each day, it also must be acknowledged that heavy drinking is an important risk factor for stroke, especially among women and youth. It is doubtful whether low to moderate drinking is associated with lowered risk for hypertension. Nevertheless, it appears relatively well established that heavy drinking increases hypertension; correspondingly, alcohol abusers who reduce their heavy drinking to social drinking levels experience beneficial reductions in blood pressure. It is doubtful, and indeed controversial, as to whether alcohol use reduces the risk of peripheral vascular disease; this is because even when some benefits have been demonstrated, these have mostly been seen in heavy drinkers (i.e., those consuming more than 5 drinks/day)—just the type of individual who would be prone to experiencing other important adverse health consequences at these consumption levels.

There is a large body of literature suggesting that moderate alcohol intake may be associated with reduced stress in social drinkers. Nevertheless, those with stress-related psychiatric disorders do not tend to report much relief from drinking; indeed, among these individuals, attempts at "stress relief" drinking tend to simply increase the risk of alcohol dependence.

Potential Risks

The link between alcohol consumption and liver cirrhosis has been established firmly. Up to 900,000 U.S. citizens have liver cirrhosis, and more than 20,000 die each year. Of these, more than one third of the cases of cirrhosis are attributable to excessive alcohol consumption. For all age groups, and among blacks and whites, the risk of cirrhosis increases with rising alcohol consumption levels;

however, women may be especially vulnerable to this disease. Importantly, intermediate types of hepatocellular disease, such as fatty infiltration, often precede the development of cirrhosis.

Alcohol use (even in mouthwash) has been associated with several types of cancers—notably, cancers of the oropharynx. Rates of cancer appear to be linked with both the amount and concentration of the alcoholic beverage, presumably because this is associated with local tissue damage. When combined with smoking, alcohol's ability to cause oropharyngeal cancer is increased markedly. Most authorities would agree that alcohol intake is associated with chronic gastritis and the later development of carcinoma, as well as increased risk for pancreatic and rectal cancer. The case for increased breast cancer risk in drinkers appears to be most compelling among those receiving hormone replacement therapy. There is little evidence that alcohol intake is associated with prostate or endometrial cancers.

Those who consume more than 29 standard drinks per week, compared with abstainers, have double the risk of mental disease. Individuals with psychiatric disorders (particularly those associated with affective and anxiety states) tend to have relatively high rates of alcohol dependence. For example, some studies report alcohol abuse rates of up to 60% among those with bipolar disorder. While acute alcohol intake reduces cognitive function, the relationship between alcohol intake and dementia is less well understood. While high levels of prolonged drinking appear to predispose to dementia, some controversy exists as to whether this is due to the exacerbation of underlying Alzheimer's disease or to multi-infarct dementia rather than pure alcohol dementia *per se.*

Alcohol consumption, particularly drinking to intoxication and binge drinking, increases the risk of injury from a variety of sources—use of heavy machinery, vehicular accidents, falls, and fires. These injuries also are correlated with the magnitude of alcohol-induced performance deterioration. There is no level of drinking at which there is no risk; instead, risk rises steadily with consumption. This relates even to over-learned tasks in most adults, such as driving an automobile. Interestingly, older adults appear to exhibit a U-shaped relationship between alcohol intake and occupational injury, with abstainers and heavy drinkers being the most likely to be injured. This may imply that elderly abstainers may be doing so because of co-occurring medical illness, which may itself be associated with the risk of injury.

The likelihood of aggression also is increased by drinking. However, this relationship is complex, and the disinhibiting effects of alcohol may manifest most among those with underlying impulse dyscontrol or frank anti-social personality disorder. Traumatic injuries associated with violent behavior also become more likely the greater the amount of alcohol that has been consumed up to 6 hours before the event.

Overall mortality rates due to alcohol consumption have been studied extensively in most developed countries, including Europe and the United States. In an illustrative study conducted in 25 European countries, an increase of 1 liter per capita per year in alcohol consumption was associated with a 1% rise in all causes of morbidity; the converse was true for drinking reductions. Interestingly, such studies also show a U-shaped relationship between morbidity and drinking, with abstainers and heavy drinkers appearing to be the most vulnerable. This is presumed to be due to the protective effects of alcohol on the risk of death from coronary heart disease in light to moderate drinkers. Thus, for those drinking 6 or more drinks/day, the mortality rate due to alcohol was over 130 and over 145 deaths per 100,000 for women and men, respectively. In developing countries where the prevalence of coronary heart disease is relatively low, the relationship between alcohol consumption and overall mortality rate is relatively linear. In the Global Burden of Disease study, combined examination of the years of life lost and of the years lived with disability revealed that alcohol use accounts for about 3.5% of the global burden of disease—1.5% of all deaths, 2.1% of all life years lost, with 6% attributed to the amount of time the individual survived with disability. Indeed, a recent survey by the World Health Organization places alcoholism fifth on its list of the global burdens of disease and injury, the first being malnutrition. The global burden of disease due to alcohol use was greatest in countries with the highest per-capita consumption, such as in Latin America, and lowest in nations with much less alcohol intake, such as in the Middle East.

DO RATES OF ALCOHOLISM VARY ACCORDING TO AGE?

Over the last century, statistics have been collected on drinking behavior across cohorts born in the same year or range of years. These data show a leftward shift in the cumulative probabilities of alcohol abuse and dependence among alcohol users; that is, alcohol abuse and dependence are greatest in the cohort of those born between 1968 and 1974, decrease with birth date cohorts, and are smallest for the 1894–1937 group. Basically, these data show that the cumulative probabilities of alcohol abuse and of dependence among alcohol users are 0.75 and above 0.40, respectively. These data indicate that individuals have been starting to use alcohol and to develop alcohol-related problems at an increasingly earlier age over the last century. Since the data from cohorts born within the last 35 years are still being collected over their life spans, the peak age of developing alcohol dependence, thought to be about 40 years, has had to be estimated from the cohort of those born between 1940 and 1957, or earlier. Two populations do, however, merit special attention: underage and elderly drinkers.

Rising rates of underage drinking have been the cause of much public concern. Although there has been a decrease over the last two decades in alcohol use among those over the age of 12 years, from 72.9% in 1979 to 63.7% in 2001, there has been little or no change in underage drinking patterns for the last decade. More than one half of 14 year olds and three quarters of high school aged children have sampled alcohol, and greater than 5 million (30%) binge drink at least once a month. Data from the 2000 National Household Survey on Drug Abuse show that the average age of drinking initiation among those aged between 12 years and 20 years is 14 years. Individuals who start to drink before their fifteenth birthday, compared with those who initiate drinking after the age of 21 years, are 4 times more likely to develop alcohol dependence—higher still for those who commence drinking at an even earlier age. Thus, the postponement of drinking until adulthood reduces the risk of lifetime alcohol dependence. In a recently published U.S.-based study, it was estimated that drinkers constituted 50% and 52.8% of 12 to 20 year olds and those over 21 years, respectively. Further, of the 4.21 billion drinks consumed per month, underage drinkers consumed 19.7% of the total and spent approximately $22.5 billion obtaining alcoholic beverages. Indeed, the age of drinking onset is an important predictor of the risk of later development of alcohol dependence. Basically, the earlier the onset of drinking, the greater is the risk for developing alcohol dependence. Earlier rates of problem drinking onset also are associated with a greater frequency of delinquency and a range of antisocial behaviors. Thus, this crisis of underage drinking is particularly telling on society since this cohort is over-represented in costs due to alcohol-related consequences such as delinquency and crime, unwanted pregnancies, injuries due to violence or accidents, and death. Among male youth of varying race and ethnicity, whites and Hispanics, compared with blacks, have the highest rates of binge drinking; for females, whites have the highest rate, with blacks and Hispanics having similar drinking frequencies.

The proportion of elderly (i.e., individuals over the age of 65 years) Americans in the population is rising. It is estimated that there will be a greater than 73% rise in the proportion of elderly in the population over the next two decades. In 1994, about 12.5% of Americans were elderly, and this is projected to rise to 20% by 2030. Striking differences in drinking between elderly men and women are often obscured by the general statistic of a trend toward a slight reduction in alcohol sales and reported drinking over the last 20 years. In particular, the proportion of drinking among elderly men has risen by about 10%; in contrast, the proportion of elderly women who drink has gone down by about 12%. The prevalence of alcohol-related complications also has risen. This finding is, however, not simply due to the increased drinking but is the result of the interaction between drinking and other socio-environmental factors. For instance, elderly men are living longer and are, therefore, having more chronic health-related problems and life events. Thus, even among the elderly with low to moderate drinking levels, the related health consequences have continued to increase as the individual gets older. This appears to be particularly pertinent for elderly white men, who, by virtue of lifestyle and socioeconomic advantage, can be expected to continue with low to moderate drinking even as they get older. A more disturbing trend appears to be the expected growth in alcohol-related problems among elderly Hispanics. Over the next decade and beyond, the growth in the elderly population will be greatest among Hispanics when compared with other racial and ethnic groups. Since Hispanics, compared with other racial or ethnic groups, are more likely to maintain chronic heavy drinking patterns, and are presently more socioeconomically disadvantaged than whites, this subgroup may soon exert the heaviest burden of care on the health system for the treatment of alcohol-related problems.

DOES ALCOHOL CONSUMPTION VARY BY ETHNICITY, GENDER, PLACE OF RESIDENCE, OR RELIGION?

Drinking patterns vary between racial and ethnic groups and also between men and women. Generally, as part of the typical drinking life cycle, as adults grow older their drinking tends to lessen; however, this does not hold true for all racial or ethnic groups. White males peak earlier in their drinking, between the ages of 18 and 25 years, followed by Hispanic and black men, who achieve their maximum drinking between the ages of 26 and 30 years. However, Hispanic males do not appear to undergo age-related drinking reductions over time; instead, they are more likely to persist with chronic and elevated drinking levels across the life span. This has led to the suggestion that the persistence of alcohol-related psychosocial problems, such as partner abuse, is especially high among Hispanics. Generally, whites still have the highest consumption of alcohol, followed by Hispanics and blacks. While a lot has been made of reportedly high rates among Native Americans, this is not universally the case, as there are marked differences among tribes.

Over the last 50 years, women have been catching up with men in their alcohol consumption rates. In the 1940s, men were about 2.4 times more likely than women to have a lifetime diagnosis of alcohol dependence. Nowadays, the lifetime prevalence rate is only slightly higher in men. Men are, however, more likely than women to maintain a diagnosis of alcohol dependence once it has been established. When women develop problem drinking, the trajectory toward dependence is shorter than that of men. Attitudes toward drinking also may play a role in the alcohol consumption behavior of women. For instance, black women, compared with their white counterparts, apparently live in a social environment that is more accepting of drinking.

City dwellers and those in suburbs have higher rates of alcohol dependence when compared with individuals who live in rural areas or small towns. Low drinking rates appear to be typical for Jews, Episcopalians, and rural Baptists.

WHAT ARE THE MOST HARMFUL ASSOCIATIONS BETWEEN DRINKING AND SOCIAL BEHAVIOR? FOCUS ON DRUNK DRIVING AND VIOLENCE

Of the psychosocial consequences that can be associated with problem drinking, those related to the potential for violence and driving while impaired have received the most focused attention. Data compiled in 1997 show that more than 16,000 individuals died in alcohol-related vehicular accidents—about one death every half-hour—and another million are injured each year. The highest rates of impaired driving are seen in white men (4.4%), compared with Hispanic (3.1%) and black (2.8%) males. Among alcohol-related vehicular fatalities, 40% of the deaths involve someone other than the driver. Indeed, one in three Americans will be involved in an alcohol-related vehicular accident in their lifetime. Among various age groups, the highest rates of driving while impaired are seen in males between the ages of 21 and 34 years. Alcohol-related vehicular accidents cost the United States over $45 million per annum in rehabilitation and hospital costs, as well as lost productivity.

Over one quarter of the 11 million violent crimes committed in the United States each year are associated with recent alcohol use. Alcohol use is implicated in over two thirds of partner abuse. Further, levels of domestic violence decrease when a drinking partner is treated without relapsing from alcohol dependence. According to data from the National Crime Victimization Survey (1992–1995), alcohol was the most common abused substance associated with violent incidents either alone or in combination with other drugs; in contrast, crimes associated with abused drugs alone were relatively infrequent—5% in all. The most violent of crimes appear to have the highest associations with drinking. For instance, alcohol use was implicated in 47% of homicides committed in New York between 1984 and the end of 1988. Also, murderers in state prison report that alcohol was involved in over half the number of the homicides that they committed. While alcohol use does not appear to affect the incidence of rape, prior drinking appears to enhance the risk of concomitant physical injury during the sexual assault. Interestingly, alcohol use also increases the propensity of being the victim of a violent crime, particularly with respect to female victims of sexual assault. Binge drinking rather than steady consumption appears to be a particularly important risk factor for all types of alcohol-related violence.

SUMMARY

Alcoholism is a major cause of morbidity and mortality in the United States. While low drinking levels may be associated with some cardiovascular benefits, intemperate alcohol consumption is associated with important health-related risks. Problem drinking is associated with increased rates of mental disorder, injuries, and a variety of organic diseases, particularly liver cirrhosis and breast cancer. Underage drinking has reached almost epidemic levels in the United States. The age at which drinking is initiated appears to be getting earlier. The earlier the age of drinking onset, the greater is the risk of alcohol dependence. Indeed, an early onset of problem drinking also increases the risk of a range of antisocial behaviors, including delinquency and crime. Over the last 50 years, the drinking pattern of women has become increasingly similar to that of men. Nevertheless, women who drink heavily appear to have a shorter trajectory toward alcohol dependence than do men. While there is a general trend for adults to drink less as they grow older, drinking problems among the elderly also are on the increase, partly because individuals are living longer and are, therefore, experiencing health problems that can be exacerbated by alcohol. Particularly, white and Hispanic elderly men, albeit for different reasons, appear to be at increasing risk for developing alcohol-related problems. Nevertheless, whites still drink more than Hispanics, who in turn consume less alcohol than blacks. Among the various racial and ethnic groups, heavy drinking behavior among male Hispanics has shown the steepest rise, and this has been associated with increasing rates of violence, particularly partner abuse, within this subgroup. Alcohol use, either alone or in combination with another abused drug, is often associated with violent acts; the more violent the act, the greater is the association with drinking. In comparison, drug-taking alone is infrequently associated with violent acts—less than 5% in all. Individuals who are close to the scenes of binge drinking are more likely to be the victims of violent crime; this is particularly true of women, who are most prone to sexual assault. Since young adults are most likely to be involved in alcohol-related vehicular accidents, the impact on society is particularly striking. Driving while impaired costs the nation over $45 million per annum in rehabilitation and hospital costs, as well as lost productivity. Finally, further research is needed to understand the rapidly changing pattern of alcohol use and its associated problems, particularly as they relate to providing new tools for prevention, early intervention, and treatment.

SUGGESTED READINGS

Caetano R, Kaskutas LA: Changes in drinking patterns among whites, blacks and Hispanics, 1984–1992. J Stud Alcohol 56:558–565, 1995.

Dawson DA, Grant BF, Chou SP, Pickering RP: Subgroup variation in U.S. drinking patterns: results of the 1992 National Longitudinal Alcohol Epidemiologic Study. J Subst Abuse 7:331–344, 1995.

Foster SE, Vaughan RD, Foster WH, Califano JAJ: Alcohol consumption and expenditures for underage drinking and adult excessive drinking. JAMA 289:989–995, 2003.

Grant BF: Prevalence and correlates of alcohol use and DSM-IV alcohol dependence in the United States: results of the National Longitudinal Alcohol Epidemiologic Survey. J Stud Alcohol 58:464–473, 1997.

Grunbaum JA, Kann L, Kinchen SA, et al: Youth risk behavior surveillance—United States, 2001. MMWR Surveill Summ 51:1–62, 2002.

Martin SE, Bachman R: Contribution of alcohol to the likelihood of completion and severity of injury in rape incidents. Violence Women 4:694–712, 1998.

Thun MJ, Peto R, Lopez AD, et al: Alcohol consumption and mortality among middle-aged and elderly U.S. adults. N Engl J Med 337:1705–1714, 1997.

U.S. Department of Health and Human Services. 10th Special Report to the U.S. Congress on Alcohol and Health. NIH and NIAAA, June 2000.

NEUROBIOLOGY OF ALCOHOLISM

Scott E. Hemby

Research related to the behavioral actions of abused drugs, including ethanol, has established that these compounds can serve as reinforcers. The relationship of reinforcement with brain neurochemistry has been the objective of recent research, and while significant advances have occurred in identifying some of the basic neurobiological processes involved in the behavioral effects of abused drugs, the field remains in its infancy. For example, while significant advances have been made in the technology used to assess neurotransmitter activity during or following drug intake, it has not been as easy to discern how these observed changes are directly related to behaviors that are engendered and maintained by ethanol. That is, few experiments have provided concurrent measures of reinforced behavior (e.g., self-administration) and neurotransmitter release or function. Studies evaluating the neurochemical effects of response-independent drug administration (e.g., place conditioning) have provided data related to the pharmacologic actions of abused drugs; however, response-independent drug administration does not reliably produce reinforcing effects and, therefore, may not reflect the magnitude or quality of biological activity observed with drug self-administration.

A driving hypothesis in drug abuse research has been the psychomotor stimulant theory of addiction—an attempt to provide a unifying theory of the mechanisms that mediate drug (including alcohol) abuse. According to this theory, all addictive drugs have psychomotor stimulant properties and exert reinforcing effects on behavior, both of which are mediated by the mesocorticolimbic dopamine system. The mesocorticolimbic dopamine pathway has received considerable attention as a critical substrate for the reinforcing effects of a variety of events including feeding, drinking, sexual behavior, electrical brain stimulation, and drug self-administration. Results from several studies suggest that specific loci in the mesocorticolimbic pathway play an important role in the reinforcing effects of ethanol, cocaine, and heroin.

BEHAVIOR AND BIOANALYTICAL PROCEDURES

Two of the most widely used procedures in drug abuse research are the conditioned place preference and self-administration procedures. Generally, conditioned place preference is considered to be a reliable indicator of the abuse liability of drugs and is commonly used to approximate affective states associated with abused drugs. Generally, drug administration is paired with environmental stimuli distinctive from those paired with vehicle administration. Following training, subjects are tested for preference or aversion for the drug-paired environment in the absence of the drug. Advantages of conditioned place preference include the ability to assess the rewarding or aversive effects of drugs, the ability to test subjects in a drug-free state, the minimal number of drug exposures required to produce conditioned place preference, and the general concordance between drugs which produce conditioned place preference and those that are self-administered by laboratory animals and humans. Two important shortcomings of the conditioned place preference paradigm are, however, the lack of dose dependency and the response-independent nature of drug administration. Therefore, a strict interpretation of the definition of reinforcement indicates that conditioned place preference is simply not a measure of the reinforcing effects of drugs, but instead a measure of the conditioned stimulus effects of abused compounds.

Self-administration is a useful model for investigating the manner in which neurochemical and neuropharmacologic processes influence behaviors related to drug reinforcement. In general, a particular behavior or class of behaviors (lever press, alley running, nose poke) emitted by the experimental subject is maintained by drug administration (e.g., oral, intravenous, or intracranial) and is therefore considered a measure of reinforcement in the sense proposed by B. F. Skinner. Principal advantages of the self-administration procedure include the following: (1) drugs abused by humans are self-administered by animals in the laboratory; (2) a number of species have been shown to readily acquire and maintain self-administration of a variety of drugs; (3) dose-dependency of drug intake can be measured; and (4) the ability to study both the primary and secondary (conditioned) reinforcing effects of drugs is provided. However, it is important to note that reinforcement does not explain ethanol abuse or addiction; simply, it allows for quantification of the initiation and maintenance of a response occurring in the presence of specific stimuli that results in the presentation of the reinforcing stimulus. Other factors, such as learning, memory, and performance, may alter both the acquisition and expression of reinforcement.

NEUROTRANSMITTER SYSTEMS

Dopamine

Dopamine neurons of the ventral mesencephalon have been categorized into A8, A9, and A10 cell groups. The A9 group corresponds to the substantia nigra and the A10 region the ventral tegmental area. The A9 group contains the cell bodies of the nigrostriatal dopamine system that project predominantly, although not exclusively, to the caudate nucleus (striatum). Likewise, the cell bodies of the ventral tegmental area project to several basal forebrain areas including the nucleus accumbens/ventral anterior striatum, bed nucleus of the stria terminalis, diagonal band of Broca and olfactory tubercles, the prefrontal and anterior cingulate cortices, the hippocampus, and the amygdala. The term *mesotelencephalic dopamine system* is commonly used to refer to both pathways because of the close proximity of the A9 and A10 cell bodies and the considerable overlap of the projection fields. The effects of dopamine were originally considered to be mediated by activation of either D_1 or D_2 receptors. While both receptors are coupled to G proteins, D_1 stimulates Gs protein, activating adenylate cyclase and, in turn, stimulating cyclic adenosine monophosphate production. In contrast, the D_2 receptor interacts with Gi protein to inhibit adenylate cyclase activity. With the advent of recombinant DNA technology, three variants of these receptors were cloned, and dopamine receptors are now categorized into two subfamilies: D_1-like (D_1 and D_5 [D_{1b} in rats]) and D_2-like (D_2, D_3, and D_4).

Serotonin

It is important to stress that the mesolimbic dopamine system does not mediate reinforcement in isolation. Indeed, there is strong evidence that midbrain dopamine is itself modulated, primarily by γ-aminobutyric acid (GABA), serotonin (5-HT), endogenous opioids, and excitatory amino acids. Of the nine serotonin nuclei, the dorsal and median raphe and the centralis superior nuclei provide the most extensive serotonin innervation of the ventral tegmental area, substantia nigra, hippocampus and septal areas, cortical and striatal areas including the nucleus accumbens. The $5-HT_1$ class (divided into an additional four subclasses, A-D) contains both presynaptic and postsynaptic receptors, and subclasses A, B, and D of the $5-HT_1$ receptor exert their effects by increasing cyclic adenosine monophosphate turnover, whereas $5-HT_{1c}$ (and $5-HT_2$) receptors are linked to phosphatidyl inositol. The $5-HT_{1a}$ receptor serves as an autoreceptor and also postsynaptic receptor. Receptors in the subclasses $5-HT_2$ and $5-HT_3$ are all postsynaptic receptors. Of note, the $5-HT_3$ receptor exerts its effects via the ligand-gated ion channel and has been shown to be a positive modulator of dopamine release, particularly in the nucleus accumbens. Recent studies indicate that $5-HT_3$ receptors may augment the activities of GABA and cholecystokinin in the central nervous system. The $5-HT_2$ receptor manifests activity by increasing the turnover of phosphatidyl inositol.

Opioids

Opiate receptors are found in high levels in the nucleus accumbens and moderate levels in most cortical areas, the amygdala, parts of the hippocampus, olfactory tubercles, striatum septum, diagonal band of Broca, and the stria terminalis. In the ventral tegmental area, only μ and κ receptors are found at moderate and low levels, respectively. The localization of opiate receptors in the regions of the cell bodies and terminal field projections of the mesocorticolimbic dopamine pathway suggest considerable opportunity for interaction. Like D_2 receptors, opiate receptors are coupled to G proteins that inhibit adenylate cyclase activity and/or affect ion channel conductance. The net result of opiate receptor activation is membrane hyperpolarization either by increased K^- conductance (μ and δ) or inhibition of Ca^{2+} channels, resulting in inhibition of transmitter release.

GABA

GABA is the most extensively distributed neurotransmitter in the central nervous system. GABA-containing neurons are the main efferent pathway of the mesolimbic dopamine system. Importantly, GABA efferents innervate connections from the nucleus accumbens to the substantia innominata and ventral pallidum. GABA receptors are arranged in complexes, and the main subtypes are $GABA_A$ and $GABA_B$. $GABA_A$ receptors exert their effect via ion channels that result in increased chloride conductance, while the $GABA_B$ receptors are coupled to G proteins. Activity at the $GABA_A$ receptor is potentiated by sedatives such as barbiturates, benzodiazepines, and ethanol. Also, benzodiazepines and barbiturates have potent anxiolytic activity that might be related to their reinforcing effects and abuse liability.

MECHANISMS OF ETHANOL REINFORCEMENT

Consistent with the psychostimulant theory of addiction, considerable attention has focused on both direct and indirect ways in which dopaminergic mechanisms mediate ethanol reinforcement. Data from metabolic imaging studies indicate an important role for dopamine and a variety of other neurotransmitter systems in the reinforcing effects of ethanol. For example, ethanol self-administration increases cerebral metabolism in rats, as measured by 2-deoxyglucose, in the midbrain dopamine cell body regions (ventral tegmental area and substantia nigra) and axonal targets of these cell populations (rostrum and shell of nucleus accumbens, medial prefrontal cortex, lateral septum, basolateral and central nucleus of amygdala). Interestingly, the dopamine receptor antagonist α-flupenthixol blocked glucose utilization in the mesolimbic and nigrostriatal structures at low ethanol doses but was less efficacious at higher ethanol doses, suggesting involvement of additional neurotransmitter systems. The most firmly established self-administration studies that demonstrate neurotransmitter involvement remain those based on the effects of systemic and central administration of antagonists as well as lesions studies.

Dopamine

One way in which to identify involvement of discrete neuroanatomical substrates in drug reinforcement is via intracranial self-administration. In this procedure, drug self-administration is maintained by the direct application of the drug into discrete neuroanatomical loci. So far, the ventral tegmental area is the only brain region that appears to support the intracranial self-administration of ethanol. Alcohol-preferring rats will self-administer ethanol directly into the ventral tegmental area, as will outbred rat strains, albeit at higher ethanol concentrations. *In vivo* microdialysis studies have shown that ethanol self-administration in nondependent rats is associated with an increase in nucleus accumbens baseline extracellular dopamine concentrations ($[DA]_e$), and this dopamine elevation is exaggerated in animals selectively bred for alcohol preference. Furthermore, both nucleus accumbens $[DA]_e$ and the percent increase in $[DA]_e$ in response to ethanol administration are predictors of ethanol preference in rats. Furthermore, $[DA]_e$ in the nucleus accumbens are significantly elevated during ethanol self-administration sessions. These studies provide correlative evidence of a role for mesolimbic dopamine in ethanol reinforcement. More direct evidence of dopaminergic involvement is derived from pharmacologic manipulations. The literature indicates the involvement of D1, D2, or D3 receptor subtypes in ethanol self-administration and place conditioning, and their antagonists have been shown to reduce the salience of ethanol-related contextual stimuli in rodents—a point of particular interest in light of treatment aimed at craving and relapse. These experiments have been paralleled by studies assessing the role of dopamine within particular brain regions in ethanol reinforcement. D2 antagonist administration into the nucleus accumbens or D2/D3 receptor antagonism in the ventral tegmental area reduces ethanol self-administration. The apparent discrepancy in these data can be reconciled when one understands that D2 agonist administration in the ventral tegmental area activates autoreceptors, thereby decreasing release, whereas D2 antagonism in the nucleus accumbens blocks dopamine activity in that region—the net effect being decreased dopaminergic neurotransmission. It is interesting that D2 knockout mice do not self-administer ethanol; however, the lack of effect may be due to decreases in general reinforcement mechanisms, as other reinforcers were also affected.

In addition to the application of antagonists into discrete brain regions, a fundamental understanding of specific neurotransmitter involvement in drug reinforcement also relies on the use of neurotoxins injected into those regions. The excitotoxin ibotenic acid, which destroys cell bodies in the area of injection, has been shown to increase ethanol consumption when injected into the nucleus accumbens. Application of the dopamine selective neurotoxin 6-hydroxydopamine into the mesolimbic pathway results in significant decreases of dopamine content in several terminal regions, including the nucleus accumbens. Such lesions appear to alter the quality of ethanol self-administration but do not affect the quantity of reinforcers, suggesting that the dopamine neurons themselves may not be the only substrate involved in ethanol reinforcement. In summary, these studies suggest that the functional integrity of the mesolimbic dopamine system is important but not necessary for ethanol self-administration. Future studies should explore the involvement of more selective ligands in other brain regions.

Serotonin

There is a growing body of evidence of serotonin's involvement in ethanol reinforcement. Systemic administration of ethanol at moderate to high doses results in increased $[5\text{-}HT]_e$ in the nucleus accumbens, caudate-putamen, and ventral hippocampus of rats, while decreasing firing rates of dorsal raphe nucleus cells. Ethanol intake in adult rats is decreased by central administration of the selective serotonergic neurotoxin 5,7-dihydroxytryptamine. In adult rats, specific 5,7-dihydroxytryptamine lesions of the prefrontal cortex lead to significant depletion of monoamines and decreased ethanol intake, whereas similar lesions of the amygdala or median/dorsal raphe nucleus do not affect ethanol consumption. These studies have driven research aimed at identifying specific mechanisms that contribute to ethanol reinforcement. The selective serotonin reuptake inhibitor fluoxetine decreases ethanol self-administration in a dose-dependent manner. However, if pharmacologic inhibition of ethanol-reinforced responding is due to attenuation of the reinforcing effects of ethanol, then classical extinction patterns of behavior should be associated with such pharmacologic treatments. One study showed that fluoxetine administered to rats in single daily injections produced a significant decrease in ethanol-reinforced responding beginning on the first day of treatment, which increased on subsequent days of the treatment regimen. Responding returned to pretreatment levels following cessation of fluoxetine treatment. Food intake, while somewhat suppressed initially, appeared to return to baseline levels on subsequent treatment days. These results are consistent with an initial fluoxetine-induced suppression, the further reduction in responding for ethanol, and an eventual return to baseline for food and water intake, suggesting that fluoxetine reduces ethanol reinforcement by both specific reduction of its reinforcing effects and early nonspecific decreases in appetitive behavior. Similarly, dexfenfluramine, an indirect agonist, decreases ethanol intake, an effect that is reversed by the 5-HT$_{2C}$ antagonist SB242,084. The 5-HT$_{2C}$ agonist Ro60–0175 also decreases ethanol self-administration, which can be reversed by the aforementioned 5-HT$_{2C}$ antagonist, indicating a critical role for this receptor subtype in ethanol reinforcement. However, other subtypes are likely to contribute to ethanol reinforcement. The 5-HT$_2$ receptor antagonist ritanserin and a 5-HT$_{2A}$ antagonist (MDL100,797) both decrease alcohol intake in rats, suggesting that general activation of the 5-HT$_2$ receptors mediates ethanol reinforcement, at least in part. 5-HT$_3$ antagonists (e.g., ICS 205–930, MDL72222) also block ethanol consumption and self-administration in rats. Extension of this work into humans has suggested that the 5-HT$_3$ antagonist ondansetron may decrease the urge to drink alcohol and alcohol consumption in biological alcoholics. Additionally, 5-HT$_3$ antagonists (except zacopride) have been shown to attenuate alcohol-related behaviors in other paradigms, such as drug discrimination, which may be critically involved in the expression of alcohol-seeking behavior. The lack of efficacy of zacopride may be related to nonspecific effects, particularly those at the 5-HT$_4$ receptor. Region-specific overexpression of the 5-HT$_3$ receptor in the rodent forebrain also leads to decreased ethanol self-administration. Further dose-response self-administration studies across animal species are needed to establish these promising results in identifying a role for the 5-HT$_3$ receptor in ethanol reinforcement. Information on the 5-HT$_1$ family subtype on ethanol reinforcement is limited and equivocal. 5-HT$_{1A}$ receptor antagonism can increase preference for an environment associated with ethanol administration; 5-HT$_{1B}$ activation has been shown to decrease ethanol self-administration, and 5-HT$_{1b}$ knockout mice do not differ from wild types in their consumption of ethanol. Interestingly, fenfluramine, fluoxetine, 5-HT$_{1A}$ agonists (e.g., 8-OH-(R)-(+)-2-dipropylamino-8-hydroxy-1,2,3,4-tetrahydronaphthalene and buspirone), and 5-HT$_{1B/2C}$ agonists (N-[3-(trifluoromethyl)phenyl]-piperazine), but not 5-HT$_{2A/2C}$ agonists, decrease responding maintained by a conditioned stimulus associated with ethanol, suggesting possible leads for treatments aimed at craving and relapse.

Ionotropic Mechanisms

The behavioral effects of several drugs of abuse have been associated with various other neurotransmitter systems, including the inhibitory and excitatory amino acids. For example, chloride channel blockers, such as picrotoxin, decrease ethanol self-administration in alcohol-preferring rats and outbred rat strains. GABA receptor function is considered to be involved in the reinforcing effects of ethanol, particularly the benzodiazepine receptor site. Ethanol self-administration is attenuated by systemic administration of the benzodiazepine inverse agonist RO 15–4513, the benzodiazepine antagonist RO 15–1788, and the picrotoxin ligand isopropylbicyclophosphate. In addition, the GABA$_A$ antagonist SR 95531 has been reported to decrease self-administration in rats when administered directly into the central nucleus of the amygdala, bed nucleus of the stria terminalis, or nucleus accumbens. Similarly, intra-ventral tegmental area injections of picrotoxin or the benzodiazepine inverse agonist Ru 34000 and intra-nucleus accumbens injections of the benzodiazepine partial inverse agonist RO 19–4603 attenuate the reinforcing effects of ethanol. In contrast, bicuculline and picrotoxin administration increase the amount of time rats spend in an environment previously paired with ethanol. RO 15-4513, which reduced ethanol self-administration, does not alter ethanol-induced conditioned place preference.

N-methyl-D-aspartate receptors also appear to be involved in ethanol reinforcement, whereas non-N-methyl-D-aspartate glutamate receptors do not appear to have a specific role. Administration of N-methyl-D-aspartate receptor antagonists phencyclidine, (e)-4-(3-phosphonoprop-2-enyl)piperazine-2-carboxylic acid, and MRZ-21579 or intra-accumbens administration of ($\pm$)-2-amino-5-phosphonopentanoic acid (AP-5) decreases ethanol self-administration; however, acamprosate failed to alter ethanol self-administration except when administered systemically at high doses. MRZ-21579 did not alter responding maintained by water, but substituted for some of the stimulus properties of ethanol. In contrast, phencyclidine and (e)-4-(3-phosphonoprop-2-enyl)piperazine-2-carboxylic acid affect responding maintained by other reinforcers. Interestingly, ethanol administration either decreases or has no effect on extracellular glutamate concentrations in the nucleus accumbens, suggesting a post-synaptic mechanism of action that may be specific to the binding site of MRZ-21579.

Conventional wisdom suggests that calcium channel blockers exert an inhibitory effect on midbrain dopamine and thus have been considered potential treatment approaches. Using a free-choice paradigm in rats and monkeys, calcium channel blockers have been shown to decrease ethanol consumption. Nifedipine decreases self-administration of low doses of ethanol, whereas verapamil is without effect. Furthermore, neither nifedipine, nimodipine, verapamil, nor isradipine block the effects of ethanol in humans, drawing into question their potential application in ethanol abuse management.

Opiate Receptors

Opiate receptor systems also have been implicated in the reinforcing effects of alcohol. For example, ethanol alters opiate binding to μ and δ receptors and increases β-endorphin levels of alcohol-preferring rats with a history of alcohol self-administration. Additionally, morphine increases consumption of low doses of ethanol and decreases consumption of moderate to high doses. In μ knockout mice, ethanol intake is abolished, whereas ethanol intake is increased in δ knockout mice—probably due to the inherent anxiety-like expression in the strain. A specific role of μ opiate receptors is further supported by the finding that the opiate antagonists naloxone and naltrexone and the μ receptor antagonist D-Phe-Cys-Tyr-D-Trp-Orn-Thr-Pen-Thr-NH$_2$ decrease ethanol consumption in rodents, while the δ antagonist ICI 174,864 has no effect. Consistent with these results, recent clinical trials have demonstrated that naltrexone treatment decreases alcohol drinking in dependent individuals, suggesting that selective μ receptor antagonists may be an important avenue for further investigation in the treatment of ethanol abuse.

SUMMARY

The previous review of the role of various neurotransmitter systems in ethanol reinforcement is intended to be illustrative and not exhaustive. More likely, several neurotransmitters in various brain regions are probably involved in the complex phenomenon of ethanol reinforcement. However, the relevance of studies investigating single neurotransmitter/single receptor types/single brain regions should not be minimized. Instead, the reader should keep in mind that a more complete understanding of drug reinforcement will require a multidimensional analysis of brain function. We propose the following set of criteria for establishing that a neurotransmitter is critical to the reinforcing effects of drugs:

1. The neurotransmitter of interest, compounds that alter the availability of the neurotransmitter, or compounds that selectively activate respective neurotransmitter receptors should be self-administered directly into brain regions involved in drug reinforcement. Furthermore, these effects should be blocked by receptor-specific antagonists.
2. Unspecified increases in neurotransmitter concentrations, locomotor activity, or the induction of stereotypical behavior may not predict reinforcing effects. Furthermore, global effects on general performance or cognitive functioning may not be related to the reinforcing process.
3. The extracellular level of the neurotransmitter of interest should parallel self-administration behavior, and this relationship should be dose-dependent.
4. Selective neurotoxic lesions that alter the functional integrity of the neurotransmitter pathway should alter the self-administration of the drug. The pattern of attenuated responding should be extinction-like if a complete blockade has been obtained.
5. Selective breeding or genetic cloning to alter the availability of the neurotransmitter or neurotransmitter receptors should result in changes in response-contingent behavior compared to wild-type strains.

An essential facet of abused drugs is their ability to serve as reinforcers. While the last decade has witnessed a rapid expansion of research implicating various neurotransmitter systems and receptor classes as substrates of ethanol reinforcement, it is becoming evident that the interaction between several neurotransmitters offers a more fundamental explanation. Combinations, staging of medications, and an understanding of not only the effect of the neurobiological process on behavior but the converse may be necessary. Clearly, integration of the biologic and psychosocial aspects of reinforcement will provide some potential solutions. A greater integration of neuroscience disciplines will play a strong role in the development of the field. Of note is the need to develop a better understanding of the internal principles that govern reinforcement itself, and how this accommodates biological and individual differences as well as the impact of contextual situations. Essential to this understanding is the use of appropriate behavioral models, namely procedures that rely on the response-dependent administration of alcohol. Moreover, procedures to evaluate relative reinforcing efficacy and alcohol withdrawal/relapse need to be further developed. Of increasing importance is the need to apply what is learned from alcohol studies to the more complex issue of comorbid alcohol and drug use, the most frequently encountered pattern in the human condition. Of equal importance is the need for the preclinical researcher to more closely approximate human alcohol intake patterns and drug usage in the laboratory, thereby providing a useful framework for testing putative therapeutic agents for treating alcoholism.

SUGGESTED READINGS

Chester JA, Cunningham CL: GABA(A) receptor modulation of the rewarding and aversive effects of ethanol. Alcohol 26:131–143, 2002.

Hemby SE, Johnson BA, Dworkin SI: Neurobiological basis of drug reinforcement. In: Johnson BA, Roache JD (eds.), Drug Addiction and Its Treatment: Nexus of Neuroscience and Behavior. Philadelphia: Lippincott-Raven, 1997, pp. 137–169.

McBride WJ, Li TK: Animal models of alcoholism: neurobiology of high alcohol-drinking behavior in rodents. Crit Rev Neurobiol 12:339–369, 1998.

McBride WJ, Murphy JM, Ikemoto S: Localization of brain reinforcement mechanisms: intracranial self-administration and intracranial place-conditioning studies. Behav Brain Res 101:129–152, 1999.

Weiss F, Porrino L J: Behavioral neurobiology of alcohol addiction: recent advances and challenges. J Neurosci 22:3332–3337, 2002.

PSYCHOLOGICAL FOUNDATIONS

Joy M. Schmitz
Katherine A. DeLaune

Alcohol problems and the individuals who have them are diverse. The notion of a single cause or model that explains problem drinking and alcoholism has been largely replaced by the contemporary view of the disease as a multifaceted phenomenon emerging from biological, pharmacological, psychological, and social factors. Whereas this chapter focuses on psychological concepts explaining alcohol-related behavior, the reader is encouraged to consider this information in relation to the ultimate goal of developing a broader and more comprehensive theory.

Psychological theories of alcoholism are numerous and vary in their explanatory power. Some older explanations about the nature of alcohol problems have been discarded because of their limited support and utility. For example, the longstanding "moral" model viewed alcoholism as willful misconduct for which the individual was accountable and capable of making other choices. This model emphasized personal choice as the primary causal factor of the disorder, but paid little attention to other factors. In contrast, the popular "disease" model of alcoholism viewed the disorder as a distinct condition characterized by loss of control over alcohol. Understood as irreversible and incurable, the disease was best treated by total and lifelong abstention from alcohol. The implication of this model is that alcoholism is caused by some inherent physical and psychological abnormalities of the individual rather than being related to alcohol itself or to environmental factors. Whereas few of these older psychological theories have disappeared completely, newer theories have come along to expand upon and modify original foundations on the basis of additional empirical information. As a result, theories evolve, mature, and facilitate progress in the field.

Rather than detail the historical development of psychological theories of drinking and alcoholism, a discussion that goes beyond the scope of this chapter and has been presented in depth elsewhere (see Suggested Readings), this chapter reviews four psychological theories that are current, explanatory (as opposed to descriptive), empirically supported, and influential in predicting, preventing, or reducing alcohol problems. Learning theory, presented first, has played a key role in explaining how environmental stimuli associated with alcohol consumption can come to maintain drinking behavior via conditioned responding. The next section summarizes cognitive theory that focuses on the constructs of urges and craving in relation to alcohol use and relapse. The third section on alcohol expectancy theory builds upon learning and cognitive principles in explaining how attitudes and beliefs come to direct behavior, either through personal direct experience or observation. Finally, the social learning theory is presented as a more all-encompassing model that emphasizes the role of the social environment, cognitions, and outcome expectancies.

LEARNING THEORY

Behavioral models of alcoholism emphasize the role that learning plays in the development of the disorder. Through both classical and operant conditioning, associations are formed between events, and information learned about these associations serves to reinforce the behavior of drinking. Consider that the consumption of alcohol takes place in the presence of numerous different stimuli in the drinking environment. The smell and taste of an alcoholic beverage represent one obvious type. More subtle stimuli may include the setting (e.g., at a bar) or context (e.g., during a celebration) in which alcohol is consumed, or the individual's internal state at the time of consumption (e.g., happy, depressed, lonely). Through repeated pairings of alcohol with particular environmental cues, the cues become conditioned stimuli that elicit drinking behavior. These learned associations then lead to the expectancy that alcohol will be consumed in certain types of situations. Thus, simply smelling alcohol, driving past the neighborhood bar, or feeling sad may serve as a cue that triggers alcohol consumption.

The pharmacological effects of alcohol can include stress reduction and disinhibition, which serve to further reinforce the behavior of drinking. For example, having a few drinks may help an individual "loosen up" and feel more comfortable at a party. The individual initially finds drinking reinforcing for this tension-relieving quality, and as repeated occasions of stress reduction due to alcohol are experienced, the drinking habit is strengthened. The expectancy may then develop that alcohol is a useful coping mechanism, and drinking behaviors are maintained by anticipation of this positive outcome. However, with too much drinking, negative consequences begin to arise (e.g., feelings of guilt, inability to discharge responsibilities, withdrawal symptoms upon cessation). These consequences act as further incentives to drink, in order to relieve the anxiety or physical discomfort that they inspire. At this point drinking becomes negatively reinforced by the termination of these effects.

Levels of impairment due to alcohol consumption vary among individuals, and research has demonstrated that this is due to more than individual physiological differences. Instead, expectations about the consequences of impairment are important mediating factors in the behavior exhibited after alcohol consumption. For example, studies have shown that when drinkers are trained to expect positive reinforcement for unimpaired (i.e., sober) behavior, they are able to consume greater amounts of alcohol without exhibiting impairment than are control subjects. Such tolerance disappears fairly quickly if the reward is then withheld.

In summary, learning theory posits that associations between events are central to the development and maintenance of alcoholism. Conditioned responses are established through pairings of environmental cues and alcohol consumption; between alcohol consumption and its pharmacological effects; and between alcohol's effects and environmental consequences. These learned associations lead to the formation of expectancies related to drinking, its impact on behavior, and its consequences. These expectancies, in turn, mediate drinking behavior and are central to understanding an individual's response to alcohol use.

COGNITIVE THEORY

Cognitive theories of alcoholism represent a shift towards an information-processing approach to explaining the disorder. This corresponds to movement away from a purely behavioral perspective, as well as recognition of the fact that individual differences in the effects of alcohol on behavior and affect cannot be fully explained by its pharmacological impact on physiology.

Early cognitive models emphasized the content of alcohol-related mental processes in relation to the pharmacological effects of alcohol on cognitive processes. For example, the self-awareness model posits that alcohol consumption decreases self-awareness, thereby reducing self-evaluation of one's performance and thus decreasing anxiety. This in turn increases the probability of drinking. Such conceptualizations have evolved and shifted in focus, with more recent approaches emphasizing the construct of craving.

A number of cognitive models of craving have been proposed, all sharing the view that cravings arise as products of information-processing systems, rather than as instinctual urges. The outcome expectancy model suggests that craving occurs after exposure to alcohol-related cues. These cues, which are based on past drinking experiences, trigger expectations regarding alcohol's effects, and these positive expectations influence subsequent behavior. The model makes a distinction between cravings and urges, both of which are important antecedents to drinking. Cravings trigger urges and represent desire for the positive outcomes related to alcohol consumption. Urges, the intent to engage in drinking behaviors, then lead to drinking. Thus, in this model, unlike some others, craving alone is insufficient to cause drinking.

The dual-affect model describes mutually inhibitory positive-affect and negative-affect craving systems. Negative-affect craving is triggered by events such as negative emotional states, aversive experiences, or recognition that alcohol is not accessible. Activation of the system leads to cravings, negative affect, alcohol-seeking behavior, and physiological responses similar to withdrawal. In contrast, positive-affect craving may be activated by positive emotions, consumption of small amounts of alcohol, or knowledge that alcohol is available. Activation of this system leads to cravings, positive affect, alcohol-seeking behavior, and physiological responses reflecting alcohol's stimulating effects. In either system, the intensity of the craving is dependent upon the degree to which environmental cues match and activate relevant information stored in memory networks.

The cognitive processing model of craving, in contrast to those described above, suggests that craving and alcohol use are not necessarily directly linked. This model emphasizes the difference between automatic and nonautomatic processes related to drinking behaviors. In an alcoholic who is not trying to quit, alcohol use is controlled by automatic cognitive processes; environmental cues trigger drinking behaviors that have become routine and automatized, and craving plays no role. However, if automatic behaviors are blocked (e.g., the liquor store is closed), nonautomatic cognitive processes must be activated to solve the problem. Similarly, in an alcoholic who encounters environmental cues but is trying to abstain, nonautomatic processes must be invoked to interrupt and prevent what are typically automatic sequences of drinking behavior. It is these more effortful nonautomatic processes that produce cravings. Situations such as these that induce cravings represent problems that need to be solved, and the amount of cognitive effort they require determines the intensity of the craving.

Despite conceptual differences among the various cognitive models, all share the assumption that alcohol effects are cognitively mediated. How one responds to the effect of alcohol depends, in part, on the cognitive structures and processes activated in the presence of certain stimuli.

EXPECTANCY THEORY

Expectancy theory incorporates both cognitive and pharmacological processes into an explanation of abusive and nonabusive drinking patterns. This model suggests – and a vast body of research demonstrates – that the anticipated consequences of alcohol use can influence not only the amount of alcohol consumed, but also its behavioral effects on the drinker.

An expectancy is a learned relationship between a stimulus, a response, and the outcome of that response. This relationship can be learned through direct experience or vicariously, through observing others. In addition, the information learned may generalize from the original stimulus to others that are similar in nature. In the most general sense, an alcohol expectancy refers to a specific anticipated consequence of drinking, and six expectancies originally were identified: that alcohol (1) transforms experiences in a positive way; (2) enhances social and physical pleasure; (3) enhances sexual performance and experience; (4) increases power and aggression; (5) increases social assertiveness; and (6) reduces tension. Anticipation of these positive outcomes leads to increased alcohol consumption, and as drinking experience increases, these expectancies become more elaborate and consolidated for the individual.

More recent conceptualizations emphasize a network, process-oriented approach. Rather than viewing an expectancy as a unitary construct (e.g., the belief that drinking will enhance social pleasure), the term is broadened to include an array of neurocognitive functions, such as memory and habit learning mechanisms and memory aspects of emotion. Thus it is an expectancy system that influences the processing of new information and prepares the individual to respond to future circumstances based on their similarity to past experiences.

When an individual encounters a situation similar to a past experience in which drinking occurred, an alcohol expectancy memory system is activated. This can then activate an affective state, which in turn can activate a sequence of behaviors related to that affective state. Subsequent affect and behavior is influenced by whichever associations are activated first. For example, one observation has been that heavier drinkers may be more likely to first activate positive associations related to arousal, such as feeling happy and disinhibited, whereas lighter drinkers first activate positive associations related to relaxation, such as feeling calm and content. Activation of these expectancy systems leads to activation of behavior and affect consistent with them, so that heavier drinkers drink more as they become more active, and lighter drinkers drink less as they slow down in general.

One point of controversy is the exact function that expectancies serve in impacting drinking behaviors. Some researchers view expectancies as moderators of behavior; for example, anxiety predicts alcohol consumption, but only for those who believe that alcohol will reduce anxiety. In contrast, others argue that expectancies exert a more direct causal influence on behavior and as such must be viewed as mediators. For example, feelings of anxiety activate an expectancy system comprised of memories of behavior and affect related to past experience with anxiety. Drinking is likely to occur if the system activated includes positive associations to alcohol consumption.

Although a significant body of research supports the fact that an alcohol expectancy memory system is part of the causal pathway leading to alcohol use and alcoholism, the question remains as to exactly what its structure is.

SOCIAL LEARNING THEORY

Social learning theory incorporates elements of each of the theories described above. From a social learning perspective, addictive behaviors, including problem drinking, represent a category of learned habits that have been acquired and are governed by basic classical and operant learning principles. However, emphasis is also placed on the social context in which these behaviors are learned. Key to understanding problem drinking is identifying its determinants, including situational/environmental factors, alcohol expectancies, and learning history related to alcohol. Also important is an examination of the consequences of alcohol consumption, including both positive and negative effects. Self-efficacy and coping skills are two additional constructs that play a major role.

As discussed in the section on learning theory, drinking behaviors can be learned through direct experience or vicariously, by observing others. Youth grow up in a particular culture in which norms related to drinking are learned from the media and by observing adults. Initial drinking experiences are seen as part of the socialization process that has been modeled by these sources. In fact, the attitudes and behaviors of parents regarding alcohol appear to be among the best predictors of adolescent drinking. For example, the child who associates their parents' relaxation time with drinking may come to value alcohol for its stress-reducing qualities.

The social environment in which drinking occurs is also significant. This includes the physical setting (e.g., a bar, a friend's living room) as well as others who are present. For example, studies have demonstrated that heavier drinking is likely to occur when the drinker is with a group rather than alone or with just one individual. Other situational determinants of drinking are the social context (e.g., a party) and the internal state (e.g., happy, bored) of the drinker. As alcohol consumption is paired repeatedly with any of these factors, they become conditioned cues that elicit a drinking response.

Expectancies are an important cognitive component of the social learning model. As described in an earlier section, alcohol expectancy memory systems develop based on an individual's past experiences with alcohol, and factors such as characteristics of the social environment in which drinking occurs are key components. Expectancies impact drinking behaviors when environmental cues activate expectancy systems, which in turn activate affect and behaviors consistent with them. An individual who has experienced stress reduction from drinking alcohol in the past may be more likely to do so again because feelings of stress activate an expectancy system that includes positive associations with drinking.

Another cognitive component of social learning theory is self-efficacy, or an individual's sense that she/he can cope successfully in a particular situation. "Coping" may be defined as an attempt to adapt to stress. Depending on an individual's social learning history, alcohol use or other addictive behaviors may come to serve as maladaptive coping strategies, particularly if the individual lacks other, more adaptive skills. For example, the adolescent who never learns ways to handle anxiety without alcohol is likely to rely on drinking as a means of decreasing anxiety or stress, and, as a result, to feel less capable of managing problem situations without alcohol.

Research has demonstrated a fairly consistent relationship between the constructs of coping and self-efficacy, with those who possess a larger repertoire of coping responses tending also to have higher self-efficacy. As discussed, this is important in the development and maintenance of alcoholism, but it also has significant implications for recovery and relapse. A high-risk situation is one in which there is an increased likelihood that drinking will occur (e.g., home alone feeling depressed or bored). When confronted with a high-risk situation, individuals with adequate coping skills and/or confidence in their ability to cope successfully are more likely to remain abstinent, whereas those lacking in skills or self-efficacy are more likely to use drinking as a means to cope. Therefore a critical component of recovery is the acquisition and improvement of coping skills. Through repeated practice in dealing with high-risk situations, skill levels and self-efficacy are increased, and the potential for abusive drinking is reduced.

SUMMARY

A psychological theory is valued not only for its ability to explain a phenomenon of interest, but also for its ability to inform clinical practice. In general, each of the theories described above has associated treatment applications. Consider, for example, the approach used by a therapist trained to treat clients with alcohol problems from a learning theory perspective versus a therapist who ascribes to social learning theory. For the former, interventions such as counterconditioning, extinction, and contingency management are seen as most appropriate. The social learning therapist, on the other hand, is likely to apply interventions such as coping skills training and problem-solving. Unfortunately, treatment providers tend to hold narrow views of what works, based on their affiliation or commitment to a particular theory. The reality is that there is no single superior theory, nor are the different theories equally valid. Rather, the current psychology literature on alcoholism offers an array of empirically supported treatments based on the theories presented above.

Ultimately, the various psychological concepts of drinking and alcoholism must be incorporated into integrative, multivariate models that recognize other processes, including biological, genetic, and pharmacological factors. Advances toward integration have been made. For example, social learning theory recognizes that genetic and psychosocial factors interact to produce coping skills deficits. Accordingly, individuals at high risk can alter the course of alcoholism by learning new behaviors and skills to better manage their genetic and social learning vulnerabilities. While we are far from understanding the neurological substrates associated with drinking excessively in the presence of conditioned environmental stimuli, some connections have been established. For example, it is now possible to identify brain regions activated during craving versus those activated during states of intoxication. Having a better understanding of how biological actions underlie behavioral and psychological processes is likely to speed up the development of theoretically based treatment interventions.

In conclusion, this selective review illustrates the important role of psychological processes involved in the development, maintenance, and treatment of drinking and alcoholism. For the most part, current psychological theories rest on a solid empirical base for support. Nevertheless, gradual theoretical change is inevitable as rival hypotheses are put to the test. Remaining open to discoveries in other disciplines and other areas of psychopathology is likely to lead to more powerful and influential psychological approaches to drinking and alcoholism.

ACKNOWLEDGMENT

Preparation of this chapter was supported in part by a grant from the National Institute on Alcohol Abuse and Alcoholism (No. AA11216–03).

SUGGESTED READINGS

Baker TB (ed.): Special issue: Models of addiction. J Abnorm Psychol 97(2):113–245, 1988.

Leonard KE, Blane HT: Psychological Theories of Drinking and Alcoholism. Second Edition. New York: Guilford Press, 1999.

Marlatt GA, Gordon JR (eds.): Relapse Prevention: Maintenance Strategies in the Treatment of Addictive Behaviors. New York: Guilford Press, 1985.

Miller WR, Hester RK: Treatment for alcohol problems: toward an informed eclecticism. In: Hester RK, Miller WR (eds.), Handbook of Alcoholism Treatment Approaches: Effective Alternatives. Second Edition. Boston: Allyn and Bacon, 1995.

Tiffany ST: Cognitive concepts of craving. Alcohol Res Health 23(3): 215–224, 1999.

SOCIO-CULTURAL AND INDIVIDUAL INFLUENCES ON ALCOHOL USE AND ABUSE BY ADOLESCENTS AND YOUNG ADULTS

Kim Fromme
Marc I. Kruse

It is clear that alcohol use does not typically originate at the age of 21 (the legal age for drinking in the United States), but rather is initiated during adolescence. In fact, experimentation with alcohol begins on average at the age of 13 years, and by the time adolescents are in the eighth grade, over 50% have consumed alcohol, and nearly 1 in 4 has been drunk. By the time adolescents reach their senior year in high school, nearly 80% report having consumed alcohol and over 60% admit to getting drunk, with 50% drinking and 1 in 3 becoming intoxicated at least once within the previous 30 days. It is, however, commonly recognized that young adults (ages 18–24 years) exhibit the highest rates of alcohol consumption of all age groups, with nearly 1 in 5 of these individuals meeting diagnostic criteria for alcohol abuse or dependence.

Although it has been argued that heavy drinking behavior is often a transitory phenomenon for most youth, the lives of many of these individuals are permanently affected by the negative consequences of alcohol consumption. Adolescents and young adults are at an increased risk for suffering a number of adverse behavioral problems associated with their drinking, many with potentially lifelong negative consequences (e.g., driving while under the influence, committing and/or being the victim of violent behaviors including sexual assault, suffering injuries, engaging in unplanned and/or unprotected sex). Alcohol is a major factor in the four leading causes of death for adolescents and young adults: motor vehicle crashes, unintentional accidents (e.g., drowning, alcohol poisoning), homicide, and suicide. For example, in 2000, more than one third of all adolescent (36.6%) and young adult (42.4%) motor vehicle fatalities were alcohol-related. In addition, recent estimates from national studies reveal that 1,400 college students between the ages of 18 years and 24 years die annually in alcohol-related incidents. Given these facts, it is imperative to develop an understanding of the socio-cultural and individual factors that influence alcohol use and abuse by this large subset of the population.

FACTORS THAT INFLUENCE ADOLESCENT AND YOUNG ADULT DRINKING

Alcohol use by adolescents and young adults is governed by a dynamic interplay of background factors, personality traits, expectancies, perceived norms, and personal motivations that occur within a social context and physical environment that frequently supports and values drinking.

Background Factors

Gender, age, ethnicity, academic performance, and family history of alcoholism have all been associated with different patterns of alcohol use and negative consequences. Young adult men consistently drink at higher levels than their female counterparts, and peak alcohol use occurs among individuals 19 to 21 years of age. Ethnicity has been consistently associated with different patterns of alcohol use, with Caucasians drinking at the highest levels. For youth who are attending school, a linear inverse association also has been observed between grade point average and the amount of alcohol consumed, with heavy drinkers reporting not only lower grades, but also missing more classes and admitting to not studying for exams more frequently as a result of their drinking.

There is increasing evidence that genetic factors significantly contribute to the development of alcohol abuse and dependence as well as the experience of alcohol-related problems in the children of alcoholics. It is estimated that the children of alcoholics are four times more likely to develop alcoholism than children without an alcoholic parent, and that more than 50% of alcoholics are themselves the child of at least one alcoholic parent. A number of genetically based predispositions to alcohol abuse have been hypothesized, including a reduced sensitivity to the effects of alcohol. Sons of alcoholics who demonstrated lower subjective intoxication in response to an alcohol challenge were more likely to develop alcohol-related problems or dependence 15 years later.

In addition to being at an increased risk for developing alcoholism, children of alcoholics are more likely to report lower self-esteem, have an increased risk of experiencing depression, anxiety, academic, and social problems, and are more likely to demonstrate externalizing behavior disorders and select peer groups supportive of substance use than their peers without an alcoholic parent. Although the exact genetic mechanisms have yet to be fully identified, parental modeling, transmission of alcohol expectancies, and decreased monitoring or supervision are environmental factors that may mediate the effects of parental alcoholism on the development of alcohol use and abuse in the children of alcoholics.

Personality Traits

Although the search for a single "addictive personality" has not been successful, a number of biologically based temperament and personality traits have a clear association with both the onset of alcohol use and the development of subsequent abuse and dependence. Traits of sensation-seeking, impulsivity, and low social conformity are related to earlier onset and heavier alcohol use in adolescents and young adults. Sensation-seeking most generally refers to a personality trait characterized by the willingness to engage in risky behaviors for the novelty or excitement of the experience. High sensation seekers are more likely to drink heavily and to use illicit drugs than low sensation seekers. Impulsivity, a trait characterized by a lack of forethought and behavioral under-control, has been consistently associated with both drinking patterns and alcohol-related problems. For example, adolescents and young adults (aged 16–21 years) who were diagnosed with an Alcohol Use Disorder scored significantly higher on several measures of impulsivity than adolescents without an Alcohol Use Disorder.

Problem Behavior Theory suggests that a single dimension of unconventionality in personality characteristics underlies adolescent involvement in socially proscribed activities, including alcohol and other substance use. Low social conformity, reflecting a tendency toward non-traditionalism, is also associated with both the initiation and continuation of alcohol and drug use. The relation between social conformity and alcohol use or problems is stronger for males than females, perhaps because of a stronger link with social deviancy among men. Social deviancy generally includes a history of conduct problems, fearlessness, and reckless disregard for others, and there is a high correspondence between a diagnosis of Conduct Disorder in childhood or adolescence and the development of an Alcohol Use Disorder.

In addition to their direct effects on the initiation and maintenance of alcohol use, personality traits also appear to moderate alcohol's effect on behavior. Adolescents and young adults who score high on measures of sensation-seeking, impulsivity, and social deviancy experience more negative consequences from drinking than peers who score lower on these personality traits. High sensation-seeking and impulsive youth may choose to combine alcohol with potentially dangerous activities (e.g., driving) or fail to take appropriate behavioral precautions (e.g., use condoms) when they drink.

Alcohol Expectancies

Social learning theory provides a framework within which alcohol consumption can be explained, in part, by expectations about the effects of drinking alcohol. An individual's alcohol expectancies can be either "positive" (benefits people expect from drinking alcohol) or "negative" (unappealing consequences people expect from drinking). Alcohol expectancies originate prior to actual alcohol consumption, with children as young as five years old holding quite clear beliefs about the effects of alcohol. Positive expectancies increase and become more homogenous through adolescence, and by about age 17, the expectancies of adolescents and young adults are remarkably similar. Alcohol expectancies remain relatively stable until the early 20's, when they have been found to decrease during the junior and senior years of college.

Alcohol expectancies have consistently predicted the initiation of drinking among adolescents, the onset of problem drinking, and the quantity and frequency of alcohol use among both adolescents and young adults. Although debate continues on the relative importance of positive versus negative expectancies in the prediction of drinking and related consequences, there is substantial evidence for a positive correlation between positive alcohol outcome expectancies and level of alcohol consumption. In a recent study of adolescents and young adults, the heaviest drinkers held more generalized and extreme beliefs about the positive effects of alcohol including expectancies that alcohol would enhance social behavior, improve cognitive functioning, increase arousal, reduce tension, and lead to sexual excitement. Additionally, youth expect more positive effects from alcohol intoxication than from moderate doses of alcohol — a finding that offers insight into a possible motivation for heavy drinking among adolescents and young adults.

Alcohol expectancies also mediate the association between personality traits and heavy drinking. For example, individuals high in sensation-seeking who believe that alcohol enhances positive experiences consume more alcohol in social and sexual situations than high sensation-seeking individuals who do not believe that alcohol enhances such experiences.

Perceived Peer Norms

Perceived peer support for drinking is thought to underlie the initiation and maintenance of adolescent and young adult drinking. Indeed, drinking is both an accepted and often expected behavior among these age groups, with occasional intoxication viewed as normal. A number of traditions, such as high school proms, post-exam celebrations, tailgate parties at football games, and drinking games and contests further promote heavy drinking among youth. A significant discrepancy has been observed, however, between the actual amount of alcohol consumed by adolescents and young adults and their beliefs about drinking among their peers. Youth consistently believe they drink less than their peers, and overestimate both the amount of alcohol their peers consume and the proportion of their peers who are heavy drinkers.

The overestimation of peer drinking provides a plausible explanation for the initiation and continuation of heavy, problematic drinking among adolescents and young adults. As they perceive heavy drinking as being typical, these individuals may drink heavily to "keep up" or fit in. In fact, one of the best predictors of adolescents' or young adults' drinking is their perception of their peers' alcohol consumption.

These distortions in the perception of normative peer drinking also may offer insights into why heavy-drinking youth are notoriously resistant to change. Compared to their perceptions of normative drinking, heavy drinkers view themselves as consuming less than their average peer, and are, therefore, not likely to consider their drinking pattern as problematic. For example, when asked to describe their drinking behavior relative to their average peer, 63% of college-aged binge drinkers said they considered themselves to be moderate drinkers, whereas an additional 29% identified themselves as light drinkers. Similarly, 66% of those identified as abusing alcohol reported that they considered themselves to be moderate drinkers, whereas an additional 19% felt they were light drinkers compared to the average student.

Perceived peer norms also have been shown to mediate the effects of personality traits on alcohol consumption. Adolescents and young adults who score high on personality measures of social affiliation place increased importance on social interactions and acceptance by their peers. Relative to those low in the trait of social affiliation, youth high in social affiliation have a greater tendency to match the perceived alcohol use of their peers, perhaps in their attempts to gain acceptance and fit in with a desired peer group.

Personal Motivations

Adolescence and young adulthood are times of increased personal freedom and opportunities to establish independence from parents or guardians. The development of close interpersonal relationships, with same and opposite gender peers, and the achievement of academic or career success are the two primary goals of most adolescents and young adults. For the majority of youth, the initial focus is on establishing interpersonal relationships and being accepted into a peer group. The desire for social affiliation, support, and acceptance from same and opposite gender peers is a powerful motivational force for adolescents and young adults. In this context, underage drinking may be viewed as a developmentally normative behavior that helps fulfill important social functions by facilitating the formation of friendships. By placing drinking into this developmental perspective, alcohol consumption has been viewed as goal-directed action in which adolescents and young adults shape their own development through purposeful action.

As youth begin to satisfy their primary goal of developing friendships and establishing a peer group, their focus may, naturally, shift toward achieving academic and career success. The development of a life plan often brings a sense of direction and purpose that may be a protective factor for adolescents and young adults by reducing the likelihood that they will engage in a variety of problem behaviors, including heavy drinking. Additional responsibilities, including organized athletics, employment, or involvement in religious or civic activities, may serve a similar role, with those individuals who are involved in these activities being less likely to drink heavily. What is traditionally labeled the "maturing out" process might better be understood as a change in primary goal orientation from interpersonal relationships to academic and career success. In fact, for nondependent drinkers, alcohol use dramatically decreases as individuals accept traditional adult responsibilities such as full-time employment, marriage, or parenthood.

Social Context and Environmental Influences

The social context and physical environment play critical roles in determining alcohol use by adolescents and young adults. The amount and quality of adult supervision or monitoring has often been implicated as a major contributor to underage drinking. Parental monitoring is clearly related to the development of childhood problem behaviors, adolescent substance use, and academic achievement. In one longitudinal study, parental monitoring both discouraged the initiation of drug and alcohol use and reduced heavy substance use. Conversely, low parental monitoring predicted the onset of both regular and heavy drinking (defined as five or more drinks at one time) over a 3-year period among adolescents (aged 12–16 years at the year 1 assessment).

An additional environmental risk factor is the ease with which adolescents and young adults can obtain alcohol. The most prevalent source of alcohol for underage drinkers is private social events, although accessibility of alcohol is also enhanced by the ease with which underage drinkers can obtain fake identification cards, become aware of outlets that sell to minors, or have older friends who are willing to provide them with alcohol. Despite increased pressure to discourage outlets from selling alcohol to minors, evidence suggests that underage drinkers are still able to purchase alcohol with no questions asked more than 50% of the time. Such accessibility is likely to increase with age and peaks when the individual reaches the age of 21 years and alcohol is legally available.

Peer and Parental Influence

As important socializing agents, parents and peers are thought to influence the alcohol use of adolescents and young adults through both passive and active means. Passive influences include the modeling of alcohol use as well as perceived attitudes about drinking, whereas active influences include direct offers or encouragement to drink. Observation of parental drinking is clearly more influential for adolescents who tend to live at home with their parents than for young adults who have moved out of their parents' house. In fact, the relative influence of parents and peers shifts across time, with parental factors playing a more critical role in younger adolescents, but peers having a greater impact over time and with increasing age. Parental disapproval of drinking has been shown to deter the onset of adolescent drinking, but the strongest predictor of regular or heavy drinking is the alcohol use of friends. Offers of alcohol and the modeling of alcohol use are two mechanisms through which peer influence is also exerted. Not surprisingly, time spent with peers is a reliable predictor of different trajectories of heavy drinking, with greater peer involvement contributing to more frequent heavy drinking.

It has been questioned whether friendships change behaviors or behaviors change friendships. Social selection theory suggests that adolescents and young adults actively create their peer groups by selecting similar others with whom to associate and deselecting, or effectively ending friendships with, peers as differences develop. Selection processes may exaggerate the effect of peer influence on behavior by misattributing similarities between youth and their peers to peer influence and discounting the importance of peer selection. Efforts to disentangle the effects of peer influence and selection on adolescents and young adults indicate that the importance of each effect varies depending on the prevalence of the behavior. Specifically, peer selection is a stronger predictor of behaviors that are relatively rare within a particular population, and peer influence is a stronger determinant of behaviors that are more prevalent. Accordingly, peer selection is a more powerful determinant of early adolescent drinking, whereas peer influence more strongly predicts the drinking behavior of older adolescents and young adults, for whom alcohol consumption is prevalent.

Cultural Attitudes and the Influence of Mass Media

Published in 1969, the classic cross-cultural studies of MacAndrew and Edgerton clearly demonstrated both the existence and importance of cultural attitudes or beliefs about the effects of drinking alcohol. Their studies showed that people from diverse cultures exhibited whatever intoxicated behavior was deemed acceptable and expected within their culture. For example, if a culture endorsed the belief that one could attribute responsibility for one's behavior to alcohol, alcohol intoxication led to drunken disinhibition. When such an attribution was not endorsed by the culture at large, alcohol did not lead to disinhibited behavior.

In modern societies, cultural attitudes are often reflected, and perhaps shaped, by mass media. Awareness of alcohol advertising has been associated with increased knowledge of brands and drinking slogans (e.g., "Miller Time"), positive beliefs about drinking, and adolescents' intentions to drink as adults. Content analyses of alcohol commercials and portrayals of alcohol consumption on television and in movies reveal that drinkers are typically characterized as attractive, sociable, and members of higher socioeconomic classes. Not surprisingly, positive alcohol expectancies mediate the association between alcohol advertising and intentions to drink among adolescents. This pattern of media influence is likely to continue given the fact that the beer industry spent $800 million on advertising in 1999 alone, or over three times the $243 million budget of the National Institute on Alcohol Abuse and Addiction (NIAAA) for that same fiscal year.

COLLEGE ATTENDANCE AS AN ADDITIONAL RISK FACTOR

College-bound high school seniors report fewer occasions of heavy drinking than their non-college-bound peers, but this pattern reverses when collegiate and non-collegiate drinking rates are compared. Rates of heavy alcohol use are higher for both men and women who are full-time undergraduates compared to others aged 18 to 22 years. Seventy percent of college-enrolled youth report drinking alcohol on a monthly basis, and 40% to 50% report binge drinking (defined as the consumption of four or more drinks for women and five or more drinks for men during a single drinking occasion) at least once during the previous two-week period.

Although high school seniors have shown a net decrease in occasions of heavy drinking since 1980, college students have maintained a high rate of heavy episodic alcohol use. Over the past 20 years there have been substantial increases in the frequency of drinking, drunkenness, drinking to get drunk, and alcohol-related problems among college students who use alcohol. Consequently, recent statistics indicate that 31% of college students meet the criteria for a diagnosis of alcohol abuse and 6% meet the criteria for a diagnosis for alcohol dependence.

The college experience may facilitate the consumption of alcohol in at least four important ways. First, when college students move away from their parents' home and into an on-campus dormitory (or the equivalent), they find themselves in an environment with markedly less direct supervision of their behavior. In contrast to the linear increase in privacy throughout the college years, adult supervision typically decreases across college, with parental supervision replaced by Resident Assistants in dormitories or by no supervision in apartments. The absence of parental supervision may provide a partial explanation for the increase in alcohol consumption among college students. Second, for most students, college provides an increase in the availability of alcohol, reflected in increased opportunities to consume alcohol and diversity of social settings where alcohol is available. Third, alcohol consumption is viewed as a socially normative and peer-approved behavior in college, providing students with an environment supportive of alcohol consumption. Finally, post-secondary education traditionally provides a reprieve from adult responsibilities that are known to decrease alcohol consumption, such as work and parenthood, and allows for an extended period of opportunity for personal growth and involvement in risky patterns of behavior.

EFFORTS TO REDUCE ADOLESCENT AND YOUNG ADULT DRINKING

In response to increased awareness of heavy adolescent and young adult alcohol use and abuse, a variety of prevention programs have been developed and implemented in recent years. General educational interventions or values clarification programs are by far the most common prevention effort used, despite the fact that they are remarkably ineffective. The Drug Abuse and Resistance Education program is one of the largest nationwide prevention programs for youth, yet it has consistently been found to be ineffective in reducing drug and alcohol use. There is, in fact, evidence that Drug Abuse and Resistance Education may be iatrogenic to participants by promoting experimentation with drugs and alcohol at a younger age.

In contrast, motivational enhancement, cognitive-behavioral skills training, and expectancy challenge interventions have yielded significant reductions in alcohol use and associated problems among adolescents and young adults. Such programs focus on the benefits of moderation (rather than exclusively on abstinence) and attempt to increase motivation and behavioral skills to reduce drinking, while decreasing misperceptions about peer norms and positive alcohol expectancies. Experiential expectancy procedures also have been used to challenge individual alcohol expectancies by providing beverages containing either alcohol or a placebo in a controlled setting. Participants are asked to guess who in their group consumed alcohol and who did not. When they have difficulty making this distinction, the roles of alcohol expectancies versus the pharmacological effects of alcohol are discussed. These programs have demonstrated short-term changes in alcohol expectancies and drinking behaviors in specific groups of college students.

Targeted programs for high-risk groups and programs that include families of the adolescent or young adult have shown substantial promise in reducing problematic alcohol use. High-risk college freshmen who participated in a 45-minute in-person motivational feedback session reduced their alcohol consumption and negative consequences, with these reductions maintained through a 2-year follow-up. This intervention was replicated with first-year members of fraternities (who are known to be heavier drinkers) and showed reductions in overall alcohol consumption and a decrease in estimated peak blood alcohol levels from 0.12 mg% to 0.08 mg%. Further, when parents were taught about binge drinking and encouraged to talk with their sons and daughters before they left for college, the students reported lower drinking rates and associated negative consequences during their first semester of college.

Large-scale social norms prevention programs have attempted to counteract misperceptions of heavy adolescent and young adult drinking by providing more accurate information. A number of academic institutions have implemented campus-wide social-norms campaigns with the hope of decreasing alcohol use by correcting misperceived norms. In at least one instance, a five-year program

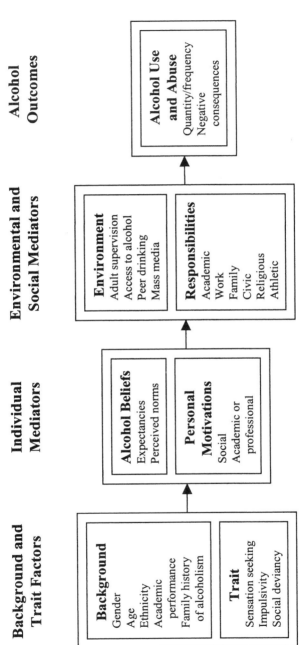

Fig. 4.1.   Socio-cultural model of adolescent and young adult alcohol use and abuse.

designed to change perceptions of normative college drinking resulted in a 19% (70% to 51%) decrease in the number of students who perceived college binge drinking as normative and a corresponding 9% (43% to 34%) reduction in self-reported binge drinking. Moreover, changes in normative perceptions were among the strongest factors in discriminating college students who changed their drinking behaviors from those who did not.

A MODEL FOR THE ETIOLOGY AND PREVENTION OF ADOLESCENT AND YOUNG ADULT ALCOHOL USE

This chapter has reviewed many of the individual and socio-cultural influences that contribute to alcohol use and abuse among adolescents and young adults and the prevention strategies which have been implemented to address them. We now propose a conceptual model (see Fig. 4.1) whereby background and personality traits influence individual factors, such as alcohol expectancies and perceived peer norms, which in turn contribute to particular types of environments that may either facilitate or discourage drinking. Inherent to this model is the idea that personal motivations, expectancies, and perceived norms change along a development trajectory during the transition from adolescence to young adulthood and on to the attainment of full adult status. As individuals solidify a peer group and transition into new responsibilities (e.g., employment), their emphasis on social activities is expected to decrease. Then, as they make career choices and face decisions about secondary and post-graduate education, motivations regarding academic achievement or career success are likely to increase and time spent in recreational activities may decrease. Furthermore, with additional drinking experience, positive alcohol expectancies may be challenged and perceived peer norms should become more accurate. Thus, this conceptual model supports the finding that most young adults will "mature out" of heavy drinking patterns over time.

The proposed model also provides a framework for developing more effective interventions for adolescent and young adult alcohol use and abuse. Such programs would address the proposed causal factors that both occur earlier in the developmental chain of events leading to alcohol-related problems (e.g., parental monitoring) and may be most amenable to change. Obviously, it would be difficult to change the individual's personality, whereas changes in alcohol expectancies and perceived peer norms are quite feasible. Interventions which take a developmental perspective and capitalize on the dynamics of personal motivations may also yield an increased probability of success in reducing problematic alcohol use by adolescents and young adults.

SUGGESTED READINGS

Bachman JG, O'Malley PM, Schulenberg JE, Johnston LD, Bryant AL, Merline AC: The Decline of Substance Use in Young Adulthood: Changes in Social Activities, Roles, and Beliefs. Mahwah, NJ: Lawrence Erlbaum Associates, 2002.

Borsari B, Carey KB: Peer influences on college drinking: A review of the research. J Subst Abuse 13:391-424, 2001.

Jones BT, Corbin W, Fromme K: A review of expectancy theory and alcohol consumption. Addiction 96:57–72, 2001.

Leonard K, Blaine H: Psychological Theories of Drinking and Alcoholism, 2nd Ed. New York: Guilford Press, 1999.

Wechsler H, Lee JE, Kuo M, Seibring M, Nelson TF, Lee H: Trends in college binge drinking during a period of increased prevention efforts: Findings from 4 Harvard School of Public Health College Alcohol Study Surveys: 1993–2001. J Am Coll Health 50(5):203–217, 2002.

Diagnostic Tools

ALCOHOLISM: DIAGNOSTIC CONSIDERATIONS

Pedro Ruiz

In the United States, alcohol is used by as much as 90% of the adult population during their lives. Additionally, 60% of males and 30% of females have at least one alcohol-related adverse episode during their life span. Also, the per capita average of alcohol consumption is approximately 2.31 gallons over the age of 14 years. Furthermore, the decrease in the consumption of alcohol observed since the beginning of the 1980s is perhaps due to the increase in the drinking age, educational efforts, and health-related factors.

Across cultures, alcohol is the most frequently used central nervous system depressant, and also the cause for a substantial morbidity and mortality. For instance, alcohol produces an increased risk of accidents, violence, and suicide. Alcohol use is associated with over 50% of highway fatalities (drivers or pedestrians). Additionally, over 50% of murderers and/or their victims were intoxicated at the time of the violent/criminal act. In the work setting, alcohol causes accidents, absenteeism, and low productivity. Alcoholism is also commonly seen among the homeless population. Fortunately, most people moderate their drinking and never develop abuse or dependence. Additionally, most adults drink infrequently or are light drinkers. Also, 11% of the adult population only drink, on average, about one ounce per day.

With respect to heavy drinking (two or more drinks per day), there are some notable ethnic differences. The rate for African Americans is 4.8%, for whites - 6.4%, and for Hispanic Americans - 7.3%. In terms of gender, about 13% of men and 3% of women are heavy drinkers. Frequent intoxication appears to be more common in youth (especially in high school and college dropouts) and among the lower socioeconomic groups. Usually, the first episode of intoxication is seen in the mid teens, and dependence in the mid 20s and mid 30s.

Among the factors that contribute to alcoholism are: price, availability, stress, culture, expectations, personal experiences, interpersonal problems, environmental issues, and hereditary conditions. With respect to hereditary factors, alcohol dependence is present in families, with familial patterns being 3–4 times higher among monozygotic twins than dizygotic twins. Also, 3–4 fold increases in alcoholism are observed in children whose biological parents are alcoholics compared with those raised by non-alcoholic, adopted parents.

In general, 5% of the adult population tend to suffer from alcohol abuse, and 8% of the adult population have alcohol dependence. Alcohol abuse and alcohol dependence are more often seen in males than in females, at a ratio of 2.5 to 1. Whites and African Americans have similar rates of alcohol abuse and alcohol dependence, while Hispanic Americans have a higher rate. Among Asians, the rate of consumption is low, especially among Japanese, Chinese, and Koreans. In these Asian groups, 50% of the population have a deficiency of the enzyme aldehyde dehydrogenase. Due to the lack of this enzyme, the metabolism of alcohol is impaired, leading to palpitations and facial flushing from high levels of acetaldehyde in the blood. Thus, the Asian population tend to avoid alcohol or to drink smaller amounts.

DIAGNOSTIC CATEGORIES

Alcohol Use Disorders and Alcohol-Induced Disorders include the following diagnostic categories*:

Alcohol Use Disorders
- Alcohol Dependence (303.90)
- Alcohol Abuse (305.00)

Alcohol-Induced Disorders
- Alcohol Intoxication (303.00)
- Alcohol Withdrawal (291.8)
- Alcohol Intoxication Delirium (291.0)
- Alcohol Withdrawal Delirium (291.0)
- Alcohol-Induced Persisting Dementia (291.2)
- Alcohol-Induced Persisting Amnestic Disorder (291.1)
- Alcohol-Induced Psychotic Disorder, With Delusions (291.5)
- Alcohol-Induced Psychotic Disorder, With Hallucinations (291.3)
- Alcohol-Induced Mood Disorder (291.8)
- Alcohol-Induced Anxiety Disorder (291.8)
- Alcohol-Induced Sexual Dysfunction (291.8)
- Alcohol-Induced Sleep Disorder (291.8)
- Alcohol-Related Disorder Not Otherwise Specified (291.9)

DIAGNOSTIC CRITERIA

Alcohol Dependence (303.90)

A maladaptive pattern of substance use, leading to clinically significant impairment or distress, as manifested by three (or more) of the following, occurring at any time in the same 12-month period:

(1) tolerance as defined by either of the following:
    (a) a need to markedly increase amounts of the substance (alcohol) to achieve intoxication or desired effect
    (b) markedly diminished effect with continued use of the same amount of the substance (alcohol)
(2) withdrawal, as manifested by either of the following:
    (a) the characteristic withdrawal syndrome for the substance (alcohol)
    (b) the same (or a closely related) substance (alcohol) is taken to relieve or avoid withdrawal symptoms
(3) the substance (alcohol) is often taken in larger amounts or over a longer period than was intended
(4) there is a persistent desire or unsuccessful effort to cut down or control substance (alcohol) use

*Reprinted with permission from the Diagnostic and Statistical Manual of Mental Disorders, Fourth Edition, Text Revision. Copyright 2000 American Psychiatric Association.

(5) a great deal of time is spent in activities necessary to obtain the substance, use the substance, or recover from its effects
(6) important social, occupational, or recreational activities are given up or reduced because of substance use
(7) the substance use is continued despite knowledge of having a persistent or recurrent physical or psychological problem that is likely to have been caused or exacerbated by the substance (alcohol) (e.g., continued drinking despite recognition that an ulcer was made worse by alcohol consumption)

Specify if:
• with physiological dependence: evidence of tolerance or withdrawal
• without physiological dependence: no evidence of tolerance or withdrawal

Course Specifiers:
• Early Full Remission: This specifier is used if, for at least 1 month but for less than 12 months, no criteria for dependence or abuse have been met
• Early Partial Remission: This specifier is used if, for at least 1 month but less than 12 months, one or more criteria for dependence or abuse have been met (but the full criteria for dependence have not been met)
• Sustained Full Remission: This specifier is used if none of the criteria for dependence or abuse have been met at any time during a period of 12 months or longer
• Sustained Partial Remission: This specifier is used if full criteria for dependence have not been met for a period of 12 months or longer; however, one or more criteria for dependence or abuse have been met
• On Agonist Therapy: This specifier is used if the individual is on a prescribed agonist medication, and no criteria for dependence or abuse have been met for that class of medication for at least the past month (except tolerance to, or withdrawal from, the agonist). This category also applies to those being treated for dependence using a partial agonist or an agonist/antagonist
• In a Controlled Environment: This specifier is used if the individual is in an environment where access to alcohol and controlled substances is restricted, and no criteria for dependence or abuse have been met for at least the past month. Examples of these environments are closely supervised and substance-free jails, therapeutic communities, or locked hospital units

Alcohol Abuse (305.00)

Based on DSM-IV criteria, alcohol abuse consists of:

A. a maladaptive pattern of substance use (alcohol) leading to clinically significant impairment or distress, as manifested by one (or more) of the following, occurring within a 12-month period:
   (1) recurrent alcohol use resulting in a failure to fulfill major role obligations at work, school, or home
   (2) recurrent alcohol use in situations in which it is physically hazardous (e.g., driving while intoxicated)
   (3) recurrent alcohol-related legal problems (e.g., arrests because of driving while intoxicated)

(4) continued alcohol use despite having persistent or recurrent social or interpersonal problems caused or exacerbated by the effects of alcohol (e.g., physical fights)

B. the symptoms have never met the criteria for alcohol dependence

Alcohol Intoxication (303.00)

A. recent ingestion of alcohol

B. clinically significant maladaptive behavior or psychological changes (e.g., inappropriate sexual or aggressive behavior) that develop during, or shortly after, alcohol ingestion

C. one (or more) of the following signs, developing during, or shortly after, alcohol use:
1. slurred speech
2. incoordination
3. unsteady gait
4. nystagmus
5. impairment in attention or memory
6. stupor or coma

D. the symptoms are not due to a general medical condition and are not better accounted for by another mental disorder

Alcohol Withdrawal (291.8)

A. cessation of (or reduction in) alcohol use that has been heavy and prolonged

B. two (or more) of the following, developing within several hours to a few days after Criterion A (above):
(1) autonomic hyperactivity (e.g., sweating or pulse rate greater than 100)
(2) increased hand tremor
(3) insomnia
(4) nausea or vomiting
(5) transient visual, tactile, or auditory hallucinations or illusions
(6) psychomotor agitation
(7) anxiety
(8) grand mal seizures

C. the symptoms in Criterion B (above) causing clinically significant distress or impairment in social, occupational, or other important areas of functioning

D. the symptoms are not due to a general medical condition and are not better accounted for by another mental disorder

Course Specifier:

With Perceptual Disturbances: This specifier applies when hallucinations occur with intact reality testing or when illusions occur in the absence of delirium. If hallucinations occur in the absence of intact reality testing, a diagnosis of Alcohol-Induced Psychotic Disorder, With Hallucinations should be considered

Alcohol Intoxication Delirium (291.0)

A. disturbance of consciousness (i.e., reduced clarity or awareness of the environment), with reduced ability to focus, sustain, or shift attention

B. a change in cognition (i.e., memory deficit, disorientation) or the development of a perceptual disturbance that is not better accounted for by a pre-existing, established, or evolving dementia

C. the disturbance develops over a short period of time (usually

hours to days) and tends to fluctuate during the course of the day
D. there is evidence from the history, physical examination, or laboratory findings of either (1) or (2):
   (1) the symptoms in Criteria A and B developed during Alcohol
       Intoxication
   (2) medication use is etiologically related to the disturbance

Note: This diagnosis should be made instead of a diagnosis of
Alcohol Intoxication only when the cognitive symptoms are in excess
of those usually associated with the intoxication (alcohol) syndrome,
and when the symptoms are sufficiently severe to warrant independent clinical attention.

Alcohol Withdrawal Delirium (291.0)

A. disturbance of consciousness (i.e., reduced clarity of awareness
   of the environment), with reduced ability to focus, sustain, or
   shift attention
B. a change in cognition (i.e., memory deficit, disorientation) or the
   development of a perceptual disturbance that is not better accounted for by a pre-existing, established, or evolving dementia
C. the disturbance develops over a short period of time (usually
   hours to days) and tends to fluctuate during the course of the
   day
D. there is evidence from the history, physical examination, or laboratory findings that the symptoms in Criteria A and B developed
   during, or shortly after, a withdrawal syndrome

Alcohol-Induced Persisting Dementia (291.2)

A. the development of multiple cognitive deficits manifested by both
   (1) memory impairment (impaired ability to learn new informa-
       tion or to recall previously learned information)
   (2) one (or more) of the following cognitive disturbances:
       (a) aphasia (language disturbance)
       (b) apraxia (impaired ability to carry out motor activities
           despite intact motor functioning)
       (c) agnosia (failure to recognize or identify objects despite
           intact sensory functioning)
       (d) disturbances in executive functioning (i.e., planning, or-
           ganizing, sequencing, abstracting)
B. the cognitive deficits in Criteria A-1 and A-2 each cause significant
   impairment in social or occupational functioning and represent
   a significant decline from a previous level of functioning
C. the deficits do not occur exclusively during the course of a delirium and persists beyond the usual duration of Alcohol Intoxication or Withdrawal
D. there is evidence from the history, physical examination, or laboratory findings that the deficits are etiologically related to the
   persisting effects of substance use (e.g., alcohol abuse, a medication)

Alcohol–Induced Persisting Amnestic Disorder (291.1)

A. the development of a memory impairment as manifested by impairment in the ability to learn new information or the inability
   to recall previously learned information
B. the memory disturbance causes significant impairment in social

or occupational functioning and represents a significant decline from a previous level of functioning

C. the memory disturbance does not occur exclusively during the course of a delirium or a dementia and persists beyond the usual duration of Alcohol Intoxication or Withdrawal

D. there is evidence from the history, physical examination, or laboratory findings that the memory disturbance is etiologically related to the persisting effects of substance use (e.g., alcohol abuse, a medication)

Alcohol-Induced Psychotic Disorder (291.5)

A. prominent hallucinations or delusions

   Note: Do not include hallucinations if the persons have insight that they are substance-induced

B. there is evidence from the history, physical examination, or laboratory findings of either (1) or (2):
   (1) the symptoms in Criterion A developed during, or within a month of, Alcohol Intoxication or Withdrawal
   (2) medication use is etiologically related to the disturbance

C. the disturbance is not better accounted for by a Psychotic Disorder that is not alcohol-induced. Evidence that the symptoms are better accounted for by a Psychotic Disorder that is not alcohol-induced might include the following: the symptoms precede the onset of the alcohol use (or medication use); the symptoms persist for a substantial period of time (e.g., about a month) after the cessation of acute withdrawal or severe intoxication, or are substantially in excess of what would be expected given the type or amount of the alcohol used or the duration of use; or there is other evidence that suggests the existence of an independent non-Alcohol-Induced Psychotic Disorder (e.g., a history of recurrent non-alcohol–related episodes)

D. the disturbance does not occur exclusively during the course of a delirium

   Note: This diagnosis should be made instead of a diagnosis of Alcohol Intoxication or Alcohol Withdrawal only when the symptoms are in excess of those usually associated with the intoxication or withdrawal syndrome, and when the symptoms are sufficiently severe to warrant independent clinical attention

Alcohol–Induced Mood Disorder (291.8)

A. a prominent and persistent disturbance in mood predominates in the clinical picture and is characterized by either (or both) of the following:
   (1) depressed mood or markedly diminished interest or pleasure in all, or almost all, activities
   (2) Elevated, expansive, or irritable mood

B. there is evidence from the history, physical examination, or laboratory findings of either (1) or (2):
   (1) the symptoms in Criterion A developed during, or within a month of, Alcohol Intoxication or Withdrawal
   (2) medication use is etiologically related to the disturbance

C. the disturbance is not better accounted for by a Mood Disorder that is not alcohol-induced. Evidence that the symptoms are better accounted for by a Mood Disorder that is not alcohol-induced might include the following: the symptoms preceded the onset of the alcohol use (or medication use); the symptoms persist for a substantial period of time (e.g., about a month) after the cessation of acute withdrawal or severe intoxication, or are substantially in excess of what could be expected given the type or amount of the alcohol used on the duration of use; or there is other evidence suggesting the existence of an independent non-Alcohol–Induced Mood Disorder (e.g., a history of recurrent Major Depressive Episodes)

D. the disturbance does not occur exclusively during the course of a delirium

E. the symptoms cause clinically significant distress or impairment in social, occupational, or other important areas of functioning

Note: The diagnosis should be made instead of a diagnosis of Alcohol Intoxication or Alcohol Withdrawal only when the mood symptoms are in excess of those usually associated with the intoxication or withdrawal syndrome, and when the symptoms are sufficiently severe to warrant independent clinical attention

Specify Types:

- With Depressive Features: if the predominant mood is depressed
- With Manic Features: if the predominant mood is elevated, euphoric, or irritable
- With Mixed Features: if symptoms of both mania and depression are present and neither predominates

Specify if:

- With Onset During Intoxication: if the criteria are met for intoxication with the alcohol and the symptoms develop during the intoxication
- With Onset During Withdrawal: if criteria are met for withdrawal from the alcohol and the symptoms develop during, or shortly after, an alcohol withdrawal syndrome

Alcohol–Induced Anxiety Disorder (291.8)

A. prominent anxiety, panic attacks, or obsessions or compulsions predominate in the clinical picture

B. there is evidence from the history, physical examination, or laboratory findings of either (1) or (2):
  - (1) the symptoms in Criterion A developed during, or within one month of, Alcohol Intoxication or Withdrawal
  - (2) medication use is etiologically related to the disturbance

C. the disturbance is not better accounted for by an Anxiety Disorder that is not alcohol-induced. Evidence that the symptoms are better accounted for by an Anxiety Disorder that is not alcohol-induced might include the following: the symptoms preceded the onset of the alcohol use (or medication use); the symptoms persist for a substantial period of time (e.g., about a month) after the cessation of acute withdrawal or severe intoxication, or are substantially in excess of what would be expected given the type or amount of alcohol used or the duration of use; or there is other evidence suggesting the existence of an independent non-Alcohol-Induced Anxiety Disorder (e.g., a history of recurrent alcohol-related episodes)

D. the disturbance does not occur exclusively during the course of a delirium

E. the disturbance causes clinically significant distress or impairment in social, occupational, or other important areas of functioning

Note: This diagnosis should be made instead of a diagnosis of Alcohol Intoxication or Alcohol Withdrawal only when the anxiety symptoms are in excess of those usually associated with the intoxication or withdrawal syndrome, and when the anxiety symptoms are sufficiently severe or warrant independent clinical attention

Specify if:
- With Generalized Anxiety: if excessive anxiety or worry about a number of events or activities predominates in the clinical presentation
- With Panic Attacks: if Panic Attacks predominate in the clinical presentation
- With Obsessive-Compulsive Symptoms: if obsessions or compulsions predominate in the clinical presentation
- With Phobic Symptoms: if phobic symptoms predominate in the clinical presentation

Specify if:
- With Onset During Intoxication: if the criteria are met for intoxication with the alcohol and the symptoms develop during the intoxication syndrome
- With Onset During Withdrawal: if criteria are met for withdrawal from alcohol and the symptoms develop during, or shortly after, an alcohol withdrawal syndrome

Alcohol–Induced Sexual Dysfunction (291.8)

A. clinically significant sexual dysfunction that results in marked distress or interpersonal difficulty predominates in the clinical picture
B. there is evidence from the history, physical examination, or laboratory findings that the sexual dysfunction is fully explained by alcohol use as manifested by either (1) or (2):
    (1) the symptoms in Criterion A developed during, or within a month of, Alcohol Intoxication
    (2) medication use is etiologically related to the disturbance
C. the disturbance is not better accounted for by a Sexual Dysfunction that is not alcohol-induced. Evidence that the symptoms are better accounted for by a Sexual Dysfunction that is not alcohol-induced might include the following: the symptoms preceded the onset of the alcohol use or dependence (or medication use); the symptoms persist for a substantial period of time (e.g., about a month) after the cessation of intoxication, or are substantially in excess of what would be expected given the type or amount of the alcohol use or the duration of use; or there is other evidence suggesting the existence of an independent non-Alcohol-Induced Sexual Dysfunction (e.g., a history of recurrent non-alcohol–related episodes)

Note: This diagnosis should be made instead of a diagnosis of Alcohol Intoxication only when the sexual dysfunction is in excess of that usually associated with the intoxication syndrome and when the dysfunction is sufficiently severe to warrant independent clinical attention

Specify if:

- With Impaired Desire: if deficient or absent sexual desire is the predominant feature
- With Impaired Arousal: if impaired sexual arousal (e.g., erectile dysfunction, impaired lubrication) is the predominant feature
- With Impaired Orgasm: if impaired orgasm is the predominant feature
- With Sexual Pain: if pain associated with intercourse is the predominant feature

Specify if:

- With Onset During Intoxication: if the criteria are met for intoxication with alcohol and the symptoms develop during the alcohol intoxication syndrome

Alcohol–Induced Sleep Disorder (291.8)

A. a predominant disturbance in sleep that is sufficiently severe to warrant independent clinical attention
B. there is evidence from the history, physical examination, or laboratory findings of either (1) or (2):
    (1) the symptoms in Criterion A developed during, or within a month of, Alcohol Intoxication or Withdrawal
    (2) medication use is etiologically related to the sleep disturbance
C. the disturbance is not better accounted for by a Sleep Disorder that is not alcohol-induced. Evidence that the symptoms are better accounted for by a Sleep Disorder that is not alcohol-induced might include the following: the symptoms precede the onset of alcohol use (or medication use); the symptoms persist for a substantial period of time (e.g., about a month) after the cessation of acute withdrawal or severe intoxication, or are substantially in excess of what would be expected given the type or amount of the alcohol used or the duration of use; or there is other evidence suggesting the existence of an independent non-Alcohol-Induced Sleep Disorder (e.g., a history of recurrent non-alcohol-related episodes)
D. the disturbance does not occur exclusively during the course of a delirium
E. the sleep disturbance causes clinically significant distress or impairment in social, occupational, or other important areas of functioning

Note: This diagnosis should be made instead of a diagnosis of Alcohol Intoxication or Alcohol Withdrawal only when the sleep symptoms are in excess of those usually associated with the alcohol intoxication or withdrawal syndrome, and when the symptoms are sufficiently severe to warrant independent clinical attention

Specify Types:

- Insomnia Type: if the predominant sleep disturbance is insomnia
- Hypersomnia Type: if the predominant sleep disturbance is hypersomnia

- Parasomnia Type: if the predominant sleep disturbance is Parasomnia
- Mixed Type: if more than one sleep disturbance is present and none predominates

Specify if:
- With Onset During Intoxication: if the criteria are met for intoxication with alcohol and the symptoms develop during the alcohol intoxication syndrome
- With Onset During Withdrawal: if criteria are met for withdrawal from alcohol and the symptoms develop during, or shortly after, an alcohol withdrawal syndrome

Alcohol–Related Disorder Not Otherwise Specified (291.9)

The Alcohol-Related Disorder Not Otherwise Specified category is for disorders associated with the use of alcohol that are not classifiable as Alcohol Dependence, Alcohol Abuse, Alcohol Intoxication, Alcohol Withdrawal, Alcohol Intoxication Delirium, Alcohol Withdrawal Delirium, Alcohol–Induced Persistent Dementia, Alcohol-Induced Persisting Amnestic Disorder, Alcohol-Induced Psychotic Disorder, Alcohol-Induced Mood Disorder, Alcohol-Induced Anxiety Disorder, Alcohol-Induced Sexual Dysfunction, or Alcohol-Induced Sleep Disorder.

COMORBIDITY CONSIDERATIONS

Alcohol-Related Disorders are conditions with high psychiatric and medical comorbidities. From a psychiatric point of view, Mood Disorders, Anxiety Disorders, Schizophrenia, Antisocial Personality Disorder, and Suicide are conditions that are frequently associated with Alcohol-Related Disorders. Among adolescents, Conduct Disorders and repetitive antisocial behavior are often associated with Alcohol Abuse and Alcohol Dependence.

Medically, Alcohol-Related Disorders co-occur with an extensive number of medical illnesses or conditions. For instance, among heavy drinkers, liver cirrhosis and pancreatitis are often observed. Likewise, a series of gastrointestinal conditions can co-occur with Alcohol-Related Disorders, such as dyspepsia, gastritis, hemorrhoids, stomach and duodenal ulcers, esophageal varices, and cancer, especially esophageal and stomach cancer. Cardiovascular conditions can also co-occur, such as increased low-density lipoprotein cholesterol and triglycerides as well as cardiomyopathy. Additionally, neurological conditions can co-occur, such as peripheral neuropathy, cognitive deficits, degenerative changes in the cerebellum, and Wernicke-Korsakoff syndrome, many of them due to vitamin deficiencies, particularly B vitamins, and especially thiamine. Blackouts and seizures, as well as fractures and subdural hematomas resulting from falls while intoxicated, often occur among heavy drinkers. Moreover, infections due to suppression of immune mechanisms, insomnia, peripheral edema, spontaneous abortions, erectile dysfunctions, fetal alcohol syndrome, and feminizing characteristics among males such as decreased testicular size due to decreased testosterone levels are among the conditions that can co-occur with Alcohol-Related Disorders.

Clinicians, especially primary care practitioners, should be aware of these comorbidity considerations and rule them out when diagnosing and treating patients who suffer from Alcohol-Related Disorders.

CONCLUSION

In this chapter, all relevant clinical manifestations of Alcohol-Related Disorders were addressed and discussed. The primary aim of this chapter was to make clinicians and practitioners, especially from primary care settings, quite familiar with all diagnostic aspects of Alcohol-Related Disorders. It is hoped that this clinically related information will also be of benefit to them when attempting to diagnose and treat Alcohol-Related Disorders in their day-to-day practice.

SUGGESTED READINGS

American Psychiatric Association: Diagnostic and Statistical Manual of Mental Disorders, Fourth Edition, Text Revision. Washington, D.C.: American Psychiatric Association, 2000.

American Psychiatric Association: Practice Guideline for Treatment of Patients with Substance Use Disorders: Alcohol, Cocaine, Opioids, 1995.

Group for the Advancement of Psychiatry: Alcoholism in the United States; Racial and Ethnic Considerations. Washington, D.C.: American Psychiatric Press, Inc., Report No. 141, 1996.

Lowinson JH, Ruiz P, Millman RB, Langrod JG (eds.): Substance Abuse: A Comprehensive Textbook, Third Edition. Baltimore, MD: Williams & Wilkins, 1997.

SELF-REPORT ASSESSMENT INSTRUMENTS

Dennis M. Donovan

The present chapter focuses on three broad domains of alcohol-related, self-report assessment instruments that would be included in a more thorough and comprehensive assessment to aid in treatment planning. The first includes variables related to *treatment entry and engagement*, such as the reasons for seeking treatment, barriers to entering treatment, and the individual's readiness to change. The second includes problems *related to alcohol use*, such as the severity of dependence, craving, and the experience of negative consequences. The third includes *alcohol-related cognitive–expectational variables* such as the outcomes that the individual anticipates receiving from drinking, the degree of confidence that he/she has to be in high-risk relapse settings without drinking, and the perceived risk of relapse associated with such settings relative to the individual's ability to cope. Measures useful in the assessment of these domains are found in Table 6.1; these represent exemplars of a larger number of instruments per domain.

The present chapter assumes that a diagnosis of alcohol use disorder has been established through structured or semi-structured diagnostic interview protocols. It also assumes that information about the quantity, frequency, and pattern of alcohol consumption has been derived by structured interview and/or self-report techniques. Clearly, a number of other dimensions are important to a comprehensive clinical assessment, such as personality function, psychopathology and comorbid Axis-I psychiatric disorders, Axis-II personality disorders, stress and coping, and social support. These other dimensions influence both treatment process and outcome and, as such, need to be taken into account in treatment planning. However, these domains are beyond the scope of the present chapter. A number of recent publications have discussed the conceptual, methodological, and practical aspects of assessment in addictive behaviors, while others have reviewed measures used in the assessment process. Readers seeking a more in-depth review of the assessment process and instruments are directed to these papers, the references for which are found at the end of this chapter.

VARIABLES RELATED TO TREATMENT ENTRY AND ENGAGEMENT

Treatment-Seeking

A number of questions arise as the clinician first meets an individual seeking treatment for alcohol problems. One of the first is "what brings you to treatment now, and how ready are you for treatment?" The underlying dimension of interest is the level of client motivation,

Table 6.1.   Assessment Domains and Examples of Self-Report Measures in the Assessment of Alcohol Use Disorders

Assessment Domains and Instruments	Authors/Citations
1. Variables Related to Treatment Entry and Engagement	
a. Treatment-Seeking	
Treatment Seeking Scale (TSS)	J. A. Cunningham, L. C. Sobell, M. B. Sobell, J. Gaskin, *Addict. Behav.* **19**, 691 (1994).
Alcohol and Drug Consequences Questionnaire (ADCQ)	J. A. Cunningham, L. C. Sobell, D. R. Gavin, M. B. Sobell, F. C. Breslin, *Psychol. Addict. Behav.* **11**, 107 (1997).
b. Barriers to Treatment	
Reasons for Delaying or Not Entering Treatment	J. A. Cunningham, L. C. Sobell, M. B. Sobell, S. Agrawal, T. Toneatto, *Addict. Behav.* **18**, 347 (1993).
Allen Barriers to Treatment	K. Allen, *Int. J. Addict.* **29**, 429 (1994).
c. Readiness to Change	
University of Rhode Island Readiness for Change Assessment (URICA)	E. A. McConnaughy, J. O. Prochaska, W. F. Velicer, *Psychother. Theory Res. Practice* **20**, 368 (1983).
Stages of Change Readiness and Treatment Eagerness Scale (SOCRATES)	W. R. Miller, J. S. Tonigan, *Psychol. Addict. Behav.* **10**, 81 (1996).
Readiness to Change Questionnaire (RCQ)	S. Rollnick, N. Heather, R. Gold, W. Hall, *Br. J. Addict.* **87**, 743 (1992).
Readiness to Change Questionnaire – Treatment Version (RCQ-TV)	N. Heather, A. Luce, D. Peck, B. Dunbar, I. James, *Addict. Res.* **7**, 63 (1999).
2. Problems Related to Alcohol Use	
a. Severity of Dependence	
Alcohol Dependence Scale (ADS)	H. A. Skinner, B. A. Allen, *J. Abnorm. Psychol.* **91**, 199 (1982).
Severity of Alcohol Dependence Questionnaire (SADQ)	N. Heather, S. Rollnick, M. Winton, *Br. J. Clin. Psychol.* **22**, 11 (1983).
Short Alcohol Dependence Data (SADD)	D. Raistrick, G. Dunbar, R. Davidson, *Br. J. Addict.* **78**, 89 (1983).
b. Craving	
Temptation and Restraint Inventory (TRI)	R. L. Collins, W. M. Lapp, *Br. J. Addict.* **87**, 62 (1992).
Preoccupation with Alcohol Scale (PAS)	K. E. Leonard, M. K. Harwood, H. T. Blane, *Alcohol. Clin. Exp. Res.* **12**, 394 (1988).

(Continued)

Table 6.1. Continued

Assessment Domains and Instruments	Authors/Citations
Obsessive Compulsive Drinking Scale (OCDS)	R. F. Anton, D. H. Moak, P. Latham, *Alcohol. Clin. Exp. Res.* **19**, 92 (1995).
Alcohol Urge Questionnaire (AUQ)	M. J. Bohn, D. D. Krahn, B. A. Staehler, *Alcohol. Clin. Exp. Res.* **19**, 600 (1995).
Penn Alcohol Craving Scale (PACS)	B. A. Flannery, J. R. Volpicelli, H. M. Pettinati, *Alcohol. Clin. Exp. Res.* **23**, 1289 (1999).
c. Negative Alcohol-Related Consequences	
Michigan Alcoholism Screening Test (MAST)	M. L. Selzer, *Am. J. Psychiatry* **127**, 1653 (1971).
Drinker Inventory of Consequences (DrInC)	W. R. Miller, J. S. Tonigan, R. Longabaugh, *Drinker Inventory of Consequences (DrInC): An instrument for assessing adverse consequences of alcohol abuse. Test manual* (National Institute on Alcohol Abuse and Alcoholism Project MATCH Monograph Series Volume 4, Rockville, MD, 1995).
Alcohol Use Inventory (AUI)	K. W. Wanberg, J. L. Horn, F. M. Foster, *J. Stud. Alcohol* **38**, 512 (1977).

3. Alcohol-Related Cognitive–Expectational Factors

a. Outcome Expectancies	
Alcohol Expectancy Questionnaire (AEQ)	S. A. Brown, B. A. Christiansen, M. S. Goldman, *J. Stud. Alcohol* **48**, 483 (1987).
Alcohol Effects Questionnaire (AEFQ)	D. J. Rohsenow, *J. Consult. Clin. Psychol.* **51**, 752 (1983).
Alcohol Expectancy Questionnaire – 3rd Revision (AEQ-3)	W. H. George, M. R. Frone, M. L. Cooper, M. Russell, J. B. Skinner, M. Windle, *J. Stud. Alcohol* **56**, 177 (1995).
Alcohol Beliefs Scale (ABS)	G. J. Connors, T. J. O'Farrell, H. S. G. Cutter, D. L. Thompson, *J. Stud. Alcohol* **48**, 461 (1987).
Drinking Expectancy Questionnaire (DEQ)	R. M. Young, R. G. Knight, *J. Psychopathol. Behav. Assessment* **11**, 99 (1989).
Comprehensive Effects of Alcohol scale (CEOA)	K. Fromme, E. A. Stroot, D. Kaplan, *Psychol. Assessment* **5**, 19 (1993).

(Continued)

Table 6.1.   Continued

Assessment Domains and Instruments	Authors/Citations
Effects of Drinking Alcohol (EDA)	B. C. Leigh, *J. Stud. Alcohol* **48**, 467 (1987).
Negative Alcohol Expectancy Questionnaire (NAEQ)	J. McMahon, B. T. Jones, *J. Assoc. Nurses Subst. Abuse* **12**, 17 (1993).
b. Efficacy Expectancies and Relapse Risk	
Inventory of Drinking Situations (IDS)	H. M. Annis, J. M. Graham, C. S. Davis, *Inventory of Drinking Situations (IDS) user's guide* (Addiction Research Foundation, Toronto, 1987).
Situational Confidence Questionnaire (SCQ)	H. M. Annis, J. M. Graham, *Situational Confidence Questionnaire user's guide* (Addiction Research Foundation of Ontario, Toronto, 1988).
Alcohol Abstinence Self-Efficacy Scale (AASE)	C. C. DiClemente, J. P. Carbonari, R. P. G. Montgomery, S. O. Hughes, *J. Stud. Alcohol* **55**, 141 (1994).
Drink Refusal Self-Efficacy Questionnaire (DRSEQ)	R. M. Young, T. P. S. Oei, C. M. Crook, *J. Psychopathol. Behav. Assessment* **13**, 1 (1991).
Reasons for Drinking Questionnaire (RFDQ)	W. H. Zywiak, G. J. Connors, S. A. Maisto, V. S. Westerberg, *Addiction* **91 (Suppl)**, S121 (1996).
Assessment of Warning-Signs of Relapse (AWARE)	W. R. Miller, R. J. Harris, *J. Stud. Alcohol* **61**, 759 (2000).

both for behavior change and for treatment involvement, which are not necessarily equivalent.

It has often been thought necessary to "hit bottom" before an individual seeks treatment. It has also been thought that individuals must be internally motivated before change will occur through treatment and that those individuals who seek treatment under some coercive pressure (e.g., legal requirement) will have poorer outcomes than those who seek and enter treatment voluntarily. However, it does not appear that these conditions apply universally to all who enter treatment. In many cases, individuals do not appear to "hit bottom" before initiating a change process, and those who are coerced into treatment often have outcomes comparable to, if not better than, those of individuals entering treatment voluntarily.

Many people appear able to stop their drinking and maintain abstinence without formal treatment. A number of factors contribute to the decision to seek treatment. While the severity of substance dependence is an important contributor, it is often the presence of significant problems in other areas such as employment, marital, and/or psychological functioning that propel the individual toward treatment. A number of self-report measures are helpful in assessing this underlying motivation. Cunningham and colleagues at the Centre for Addiction and Mental Health (formerly the Addiction Research Foundation), Toronto, have developed an integrated set of such measures. The Treatment Seeking Scale (TSS) asks clients to rate on a 5-point Likert scale (0 = Not at all affected or influenced, 4 = Extremely affected or influenced) the extent to which each of 10 factors influenced their decision to seek treatment. These factors include such things as "hitting bottom"; being warned to stop using by spouses, significant others, and/or physicians; knowing someone who quit; experiencing a major change in life situation or lifestyle; experiencing significant health problems and having had a significant religious experience.

The item on the Treatment Seeking Scale that was rated as having the greatest influence on seeking treatment was having weighed the "pros" and "cons" of continuing to use alcohol or drugs. That is, treatment seekers had engaged in a "decisional balance" in which they evaluated the costs of continuing drinking and the benefits of stopping. This finding led to the development of a related measure, the Alcohol and Drug Consequences Questionnaire *(ADCQ)*. Clients are asked to rate how important each of 29 variables would be for them if they stopped or cut down on their alcohol use. The items formed two factors. The first included items reflecting the costs involved in change and giving up their substance use (e.g., difficulty relaxing, feeling frustrated and anxious, difficulty having a good time). The second factor reflected positive benefits of change (e.g., feeling better physically, fewer problems with family and friends, more control in life). It was found that those who rated the benefits of change as more important also attached greater importance to their goal of stopping alcohol use. Furthermore, scores on the ADCQ were found to predict drinking behavior at a 12-month follow-up. Individuals who expected the costs of change to be greater drank more per drinking day, consumed more alcohol overall, and had a smaller proportion of abstinent days over the 12-month follow-up period.

Barriers to Treatment

Despite a desire to change their behavior and a willingness to seek treatment as a means to facilitate change, many individuals never make it into treatment. This might be due to the vacillation in the relative perceived value of the pros and cons being weighed, which often accompanies ambivalence as one approaches treatment. Another contributor may be the individual's running up against real or perceived barriers that make entering treatment difficult. A number of scales have been developed to assist the clinician in systematically assessing potential barriers to treatment entry. The work of Cunningham and colleagues again serves as an exemplar. They developed a brief measure, the Reasons for Delaying or Not Entering Treatment, to assess reasons why substance abusers delay or have chosen not to enter treatment. The reasons include psychological issues (e.g., embarrassment, pride, perceived stigma), attitudinal items (e.g., negative attitude toward treatment, wanting to handle problem on one's own), and practical barriers (e.g., monetary costs involved with treatment). The Allen Barriers to Treatment scale was developed specifically for use with female substance abusers. This is a group that often has difficulty in seeking and engaging in treatment, in part due to some gender-specific barriers. The scale covers perceived barriers in three general domains: characteristics of the treatment program (e.g., costs, availability of resources, insurance requirements), individual client characteristics (e.g., race, lack of insurance coverage, beliefs about alcohol, health, treatment, and recovery), and socioenvironmental factors (e.g., life events, current problems, lack of social support for sobriety). It is anticipated that identifying potential barriers during the intake assessment may allow discussion of possible problem-solving methods to overcome and/or adapt to so that they will not prevent treatment entry.

Readiness to Change

The person's motivation for behavior change, through either self-change or treatment, and the perceived impedance of barriers in the person's life will contribute to his/her readiness to change. The transtheoretical model of change, as developed by Prochaska and DiClemente, suggests that individuals go through a series of steps in deciding to change their substance use behavior. Initially the individual does not see that he/she has a problem with alcohol, even though others do consider his/her drinking to be problematic. This stage, described as *precontemplation*, involves what have traditionally been known as denial and minimization. As a result, individuals in this stage are unlikely to see a need for change and surely not for treatment. However, at some point the individual may begin to think more about his/her drinking and to consider it a potential problem that should be changed. This stage, *contemplation*, is one in which the person likely will engage in the decisional balance process, weighing the costs and benefits of continuing to drink at the current levels and also weighing the pros and cons of stopping or moderating drinking. This is a period noted for its ambivalence, as the individual vacillates between the desire to continue drinking, albeit with fewer negative consequences, and the perceived need to change. At some point, for some people, the perceived need for change outweighs the desire to continue drinking, and the individual makes a commitment, often making it public to significant others, to take concrete steps to facilitate the change. This stage is called *commitment*. It is most often followed by the *action* stage, in which the individual moves beyond just thinking about possible change strategies to actually implementing one or more such strategies. In the *maintenance* phase, the individual has made the desired changes and is working actively to reduce the likelihood of relapse.

A number of measures have been developed to assess the individual's stage of readiness. The original such measure is the University of Rhode Island Readiness for Change Assessment (URICA). The URICA consists of 32 items, with 8 items covering each of four stages (precontemplation, contemplation, action, and maintenance). It has been useful in developing motivational typologies among alcoholics seeking treatment and in outpatient treatment. It also appears that the severity of alcohol dependence has a direct positive effect on motivation, as assessed by the URICA, to change at treatment entry. Further, the cognitive, emotional, and behavioral processes of change used by the individual are predicted by his/her stage of readiness. The Stages of Change Readiness and Treatment Eagerness Scale (SOCRATES) was modeled on the URICA, except that its items are specific to alcohol and drinking behavior. Through the course of its development, the scale has been reduced from 40 items to the 19-item version now in use. Factor analyses identified three primary dimensions: ambivalence about change, recognition of substance-related problems, and taking steps to change.

A considerably briefer measure (12 items), the Readiness to Change Questionnaire (RCQ) was developed for use primarily in settings other than formal substance abuse treatment programs, such as general medical clinics and emergency rooms, as a companion to screening measures for alcohol problems. While found to be useful in such opportunistic screening contacts, the RCQ has a low level of reliability when used with substance abusers in treatment. This has led to the further development of the scale to make it appropriate for use in treatment settings, the Readiness to Change Questionnaire – Treatment Version (RCQ-TV). A major change in the RCQ-TV is its orientation toward abstinence rather than a focus on reduced drinking as in the original RCQ. The new treatment version consists of 15 items, with 5 items on each of three scales derived through factor analysis: precontemplation, contemplation, and action.

PROBLEMS RELATED TO ALCOHOL USE

Severity of Dependence

An important domain for assessment is the severity of the individual's alcohol dependence, since this factor may contribute to decisions about the type and intensity of treatment to recommend. This is particularly true with the increased use of criteria that incorporate elements of severity, craving, and relapse potential into patient placement decisions. In the mid-1980s, the World Health Organization (WHO) promoted the concept of the "dependence syndrome." This concept has been operationalized in the diagnostic formulations of both the American Psychiatric Association's *Diagnostic and Statistical Manual – 4th Edition* (DSM-IV) and the World Health Organization's *International Classification of Diseases – 10th Revision* (ICD-10), as well as the structured diagnostic interviews that have been developed to assess the syndrome.

The dependence syndrome consists of a cluster of interrelated physiological, behavioral, and cognitive phenomena. These include a strong desire or compulsion to drink alcohol, with a subjective awareness of this compulsion; difficulties in controlling alcohol-taking behavior in terms of its onset, termination, or levels of use (e.g., alcohol is consumed in larger amounts or over a longer period than was intended); a physiological withdrawal state when the person cuts down or stops drinking, including use of the alcohol to try to relieve or avoid withdrawal symptoms; evidence of tolerance, such as the need for increased amounts of alcohol in order to achieve effects originally produced by lower amounts; progressive neglect of alternative pleasures or interests because of alcohol use (e.g., drinking and preoccupation with acquiring alcohol take precedence over other activities); increased amount of time necessary to obtain or take alcohol or to recover from its effects; continued alcohol use despite clear evidence of overtly harmful consequences; unsuccessful attempts to stop alcohol use; and reinstatement of use patterns after an initial relapse following a period of abstinence. Not all of these features need to be present at all times or with the same degree of intensity across time for an individual or across individuals.

An important element of the dependence syndrome concept is that it views dependence as falling along a continuum of severity, rather than the more typical binary diagnostic categorization (e.g., alcohol dependence is either present or absent). One method that has been used in both clinical and research settings to assess severity is merely to count the number of alcohol dependence diagnostic criteria endorsed. However, this may not provide a good index since there is no intensity-rating dimension for these criteria. This has given rise to a number of self-report measures of alcohol dependence, most of which embody the dependence syndrome concept in the assessment. One of the earliest measures is the Alcohol Dependence Scale (ADS). It consists of 25 items that cover alcohol withdrawal symptoms, impaired control over drinking, awareness of a compulsion to drink, increased tolerance to alcohol, and salience of drink-seeking behavior. A number of other severity measures have also been used. The Severity of Alcohol Dependence Questionnaire (SADQ) consists of 20 items across five subscales that measure physical withdrawal, affective withdrawal, withdrawal relief drinking, alcohol consumption, and rapidity of reinstatement. The Short Alcohol Dependence Data (SADD) scale, consisting of 15 items, is appropriate to a broader range of drinkers, particularly those in the mild-to-moderate range of dependence.

Craving

In addition to these measures, which attempt to provide a comprehensive assessment of the multidimensional dependence syndrome, a number of other self-report instruments have been developed to assess narrower components of the syndrome. Examples of this include the Temptation and Restraint Inventory (TRI) and the Preoccupation with Alcohol Scale (PAS). The TRI assesses the individual's difficulty controlling alcohol intake, attempts to limit drinking, negative emotional states as a reason for drinking, concern about and plans to reduce drinking, and cognitive preoccupation or thoughts about drinking. The 15-item PAS assesses a cognitive-behavioral style characterized by excessive concern over the availability of alcohol, an active seeking out of drinking, and a gravitation of thoughts and behavior around alcohol.

Another more circumscribed element of the alcohol dependence syndrome for which measures have been developed is craving. Three measures have been used to assess craving. The first of these to be developed, and that which has the most empirical work on its research and clinical utility, is the Obsessive Compulsive Drinking Scale (OCDS). It is meant to assess obsessive thoughts about alcohol use and compulsive behaviors toward drinking. Results of factor analysis indicate that the 14 items of the OCDS form three distinct factors: resistance/control impairment (e.g., "How much of an effort do you make to resist these thoughts [about alcohol] or try to disregard or turn your attention away from these thoughts as they enter your mind when you're not drinking"?), obsession or thoughts about alcohol (e.g., "How much of your time when you're not drinking is occupied by ideas, thoughts, impulses, or images related to drinking?"), and interference (e.g., "How much do these ideas, thoughts, impulses, or images interfere with your social or work functioning?"). Two other brief measures of craving have been developed and used in both research and clinical settings. The Alcohol Urge Questionnaire (AUQ) was derived from a large pool of items that were thought to measure subjects' desire for a drink, expectations of positive effects following drinking, relief of withdrawal and negative affect following drinking, and intention to drink. However, the results of factor analyses suggested a single factor that is assessed by the 8 items comprising the AUQ. The Penn Alcohol Craving Scale (PACS) is a 5-item measure that assesses the frequency, intensity, and duration of craving, the ability to resist drinking, and an overall rating of craving for alcohol for the previous week. These three measures of craving are highly correlated, are related to severity of alcohol dependence, are responsive to change across treatment, and appear to predict treatment outcome.

NEGATIVE ALCOHOL-RELATED CONSEQUENCES

Another important contribution of the dependence syndrome concept is the distinction made between "dependence" and alcohol-related "disabilities," or the negative physical, psychological, and psychosocial consequences that accompany long-term, hazardous, or harmful drinking. One of the earliest measures of the consequences of drinking is the 25-item Michigan Alcoholism Screening Test (MAST) and its abbreviated versions, the 10-item Brief MAST (bMAST) and the 13-item Short MAST (sMAST). These scales have been used most often as screening instruments to assign individuals as having no alcohol-related problems or as alcohol abusive or dependent. The items assess the individual's perception of control over drinking and the presence of alcohol-related personal and interpersonal problems. Early factor analytic evaluations of the MAST suggested four primary factors: recognition of alcohol problems by self and others; legal, work, and social problems; help-seeking, and marital/family difficulties. Despite its widespread use, there have been a number of critiques of the MAST, raising concerns about its psychometric properties and its dimensionality.

Another measure of alcohol-related difficulties, the Drinker Inventory of Consequences (DrInC), was developed in the context of Project MATCH, a large-scale clinical trial evaluating the efficacy of three psychotherapies and the process of client-treatment matching with alcoholics. This 50-item scale was developed to assess 5 *a priori* dimensions of alcohol-related negative consequences: interpersonal, physical, social, impulsive, and intrapersonal. Each scale provides both lifetime and recent (past 3 months) measures of adverse consequences, and scales can be combined to assess total negative consequences. Both lifetime and current versions of the DrInC are also available for collaterals/significant others to complete for male and female clients. A brief 15-item version of the DrInC, the Short Index of Problems (SIP), is also available.

The Alcohol Use Inventory (AUI) is a comprehensive measure that includes subscales dealing with the negative consequences of drinking. The overall AUI consists of 228 items and 24 scales. Among these are measures of negative consequences including loss of control over behavior when drinking, social role maladaption, psychoperceptual withdrawal (e.g., delirium), psychophysical withdrawal (e.g., hangovers), and marital conflict. In addition to these negative physical, psychological, and social consequences, the AUI also assesses the perceived benefits derived from drinking (e.g., drinking to help manage moods, drinking to improve sociability), drinking styles (e.g., compulsive drinking, gregarious/social versus isolated drinking), and how to deal with drinking problems (e.g., prior attempts to stop drinking, readiness for help). This measure has been used to identify unique patterns of drinking style, benefits, and consequences at the individual client level as well as to derive client typologies at a programmatic level.

ALCOHOL-RELATED COGNITIVE–EXPECTATIONAL FACTORS

The third broad domain to be considered for inclusion in a more comprehensive assessment represents the beliefs the individual holds about the perceived benefits that can be derived from alcohol/drinking and the availability of adequate coping strategies to deal with situations that may represent a high risk for relapse. The former beliefs are described as *outcome expectancies*, while the latter are described as *self-efficacy expectancies*.

Outcome Expectancies

A large number of measures of alcohol-related outcome expectancies have been developed. The major differences among these measures include their length, the use of ratings of the strength of the expectancy or the certainty/likelihood that certain outcomes will occur, and the relative focus on positive outcomes relative to negative outcomes. These measures, particularly those focusing on positive outcomes, are often viewed as tapping the dimension of the motivation or reasons for drinking. The original scale to be developed in this area, and the one that has received the most use, is the Alcohol Expectancy Questionnaire (AEQ). There are versions for both adults and adolescents. It assesses six factor-analytically derived subscales: 1) positive global changes in experience, 2) sexual enhancement, 3) social and physical pleasure, 4) social assertiveness, 5) relaxation/tension reduction, and 6) arousal/interpersonal power. Compared to other measures in this group, the AEQ is relatively long (90 items), focuses only on positive expectancies related to drinking, and does not allow rating of the strength of the expectancies or the likelihood of occurrence. This led to the development of briefer measures such as the Alcohol Effects Questionnaire (AEFQ), which is relatively brief (40 items) and focuses on positive as well as negative expectancies (e.g., alcohol-related aggression, cognitive and physical impairment, and carelessness). A further refinement has been made in the Alcohol Expectancy Questionnaire – 3rd Revision (AEQ-3) (i.e., third revision of the Alcohol Expectancy Questionnaire). In addition to maintaining the brevity and focus on negative expectancies found in the AEFQ, the AEQ-3 provides a response format that allows a measure of the strength of endorsement of a given expectancy. The Alcohol Beliefs Scale (ABS) made further advances by incorporating information not only about the strength of endorsement, but also dose-related changes in the anticipated effects of alcohol on judgment, problem solving, depression, aggression, stress, and group interaction (e.g., one to three standard drinks, four to six standard drinks, and "when drunk"), and the perceived usefulness of alcohol in inducing a number of emotions or behaviors. Other measures of outcome expectancies, each with empirical support for their use, include the Drinking Expectancy Questionnaire (DEQ), the Comprehensive Effects of Alcohol Scale (CEOA), and the Effects of Drinking Alcohol (EDA) scale.

Another outcome expectancy measure to mention is the Negative Alcohol Expectancy Questionnaire (NAEQ). It is noteworthy in that it does not include any positive benefits of alcohol but focuses instead on expectations about the negative consequences of alcohol/ drinking. Thus, unlike the previously described expectancy measures that may assess motivation to drink (e.g., an approach motivation), the NAEQ appears to assess a behavioral deterrent to drinking (e.g., an avoidance motivation). In comparing the NAEQ with other measures, it appears generally that the positive expectancies are related to more frequent drinking, a greater number of drinks consumed per drinking day, and poorer drinking-related treatment outcomes. On the other hand, the NAEQ appears related to less drinking and to better outcomes.

No one measure of outcome expectancies is perfect; each has both benefits and limitations. Given the wide variety of expectancy measures from which to choose, the decision of which measure to use needs to be guided by the assessment question being asked, the relative weight being placed on positive versus negative expectancies, the degree to which one knows the strength and perceived probability of certain outcomes occurring, and the perceived usefulness of alcohol in achieving those outcomes.

Self-Efficacy Expectancies

In addition to expectancies about the anticipated effects of alcohol, the individual also holds certain beliefs about the availability and likelihood of using emotional and behavioral coping strategies needed to deal effectively with situations that may threaten his/her goal of abstinence or reduced alcohol consumption. These beliefs are described as *self-efficacy expectancies*. As operationalized in assessment instruments, these expectancies are often measured as a function of how tempted to drink a person is in a given situation and how confident that he/she is not to drink.

Instruments developed to assess drinking-related self-efficacy have been based primarily on the work by Marlatt and colleagues concerning the types of interpersonal and intrapersonal situations that represent high risks for relapse. Two of the most frequently used measures of efficacy, typically used together, are the Inventory of Drinking Situations (IDS) and the Situational Confidence Questionnaire (SCQ). The IDS as originally developed contained 100 items, but an abbreviated 42-item version is now available. In both versions, clients are asked to indicate how frequently they had drunk heavily in the past year in each of the situations/settings described. This represents a form of cue strength, with the assumption that those situations associated with heavier drinking occasions may be associated with higher levels of temptation. The scale assesses eight dimensions that, based on theory and empirical support, represent a high risk of relapse: unpleasant emotions, physical discomfort, pleasant emotions, testing personal control, urges and temptations, conflict with others, social pressure to drink, and pleasant times with others. The SCQ, a 39-item complement to the IDS, assesses the perceived confidence that the individual has about his/her ability to be in each of the situations without drinking heavily. While clinicians can use either of these measures to assess self-efficacy, looking at patterns of frequency of drinking heavily in a given situation in conjunction with ratings of confidence may provide more useful information. For instance, one would assume that those situations with high frequency of drinking and low levels of confidence might be particularly problematic.

Two other measures of drinking-related self-efficacy are the Alcohol Abstinence Self-Efficacy Scale (AASE) and the Drink Refusal Self-Efficacy Questionnaire (DRSEQ). The 40-item AASE also asks individuals to rate the level of temptation they would feel across a number of high-risk situations and their confidence about not drinking in them. The 31-item DRSEQ asks individuals to rate their level of certainty from "I am very sure I would drink" to "I am very sure I would not drink." A major difference between these two measures and the IDS/SCQ is that they focus on the individual's belief that he/she will not drink or will be able to maintain abstinence in high-risk situations, whereas the IDS/SCQ asks about the person's ability to keep from drinking heavily. As such, there are measures of self-efficacy available for both abstinence-oriented and harm reduction programs. It has been suggested that it might be useful to consider measures of alcohol-related outcome expectancies and self-efficacy measures in combination. One might expect differences in drinking behavior and treatment outcomes of individuals with different combinations of these two cognitive-expectational variables (e.g., strong positive outcome expectancies with high levels of temptation and low confidence versus strong negative outcome expectancies with low temptation and high confidence).

Relapse Risk

These self-efficacy measures provide an index of relapse risk. A number of other measures have been developed recently that also appear to be useful in determining the likelihood of relapse. The first is the Reasons for Drinking Questionnaire (RFDQ). The RFDQ is an adaptation for use with alcoholics of a measure originally developed for use in predicting relapse among heroin addicts. It was developed in light of what were felt to be limitations in the method of coding relapse precipitants using Marlatt's relapse taxonomy, which resulted in an overrepresentation of negative emotional precipitants and an underrepresentation of temptation and craving as precipitants. In the adaptation, alcoholic clients were asked to rate how important they felt that each of 16 items, representing 13 potential relapse precipitants from Marlatt's model, was in their most recent relapse episode. Three factor-analytically derived dimensions were found in the alcoholic sample: negative emotions; social pressure and positive emotion; and a mixed factor characterized by physical withdrawal, wanting to get high, testing personal control, and urges to drink. The negative emotions factor was particularly predictive of subsequent drinking outcomes as measured by peak blood alcohol levels on a day of relapse, the duration of the drinking episode, and the likelihood of a subsequent relapse.

The Assessment of Warning-Signs of Relapse (AWARE) is another recently developed measure of relapse risk. It is based on the relapse prevention model developed by Terrance Gorski. A pool of 37 relapse "warning signs" was compiled from Gorski's model of a post-acute withdrawal syndrome. The individual is asked to rate how applicable each of the items is to his/her experience. The scale was subsequently reduced to 28 items on the basis of item and factor analyses. The results suggest the measure to be unidimensional; higher scores on the measure were related to higher rates of subsequent relapse.

SUMMARY

Alcohol dependence is a complex, multifaceted problem with multiple factors contributing to its development, maintenance, and treatment. The assessment process is meant to assess this broad array of factors and to provide information that can be useful in better understanding the client's alcohol use disorder and in informing the type, intensity, setting, and duration of treatment. Since the assessment process typically occurs relatively early in the client's interactions with treatment, it also provides an opportunity to try to further reinforce the individual's commitment to treatment, capitalize on the motivation evidenced in help-seeking, and target treatment to the individual's readiness to change.

SUGGESTED READINGS

Donovan DM: Assessments to aid in the treatment planning process. In: Allen JP, Columbus M (eds.), Assessing Alcohol Problems: A Guide for Clinicians and Researchers. Rockville, MD: National Institute on Alcohol Abuse and Alcoholism Research Monograph, U.S. Department of Health and Human Services, Public Health Service, National Institutes of Health, 1995, pp. 75–122.

Donovan DM: Assessment and interviewing strategies in addictive behaviors. In: McCrady BS, Epstein EE (eds.), Addictions: A Comprehensive Guidebook for Practitioners. New York: Oxford University Press, 1998, pp. 187–215.

BIOCHEMICAL MARKERS FOR ALCOHOL CONSUMPTION

Martin A. Javors
Pamela Bean
Thomas S. King
Raymond F. Anton

Over the past 20 to 30 years, a number of biochemical markers have been proposed and assessed for their value in detecting alcohol consumption. To date, none of these biochemical measurements has resulted in a test with high positive and negative predictive value. Nevertheless, accurate markers for the detection of heavy drinking would provide significant diagnostic value for physicians. Often medical problems such as heart disease and psychiatric illness are a direct result of heavy, long-term drinking. Quick, inexpensive, and available tests for ethanol consumption would help physicians diagnose alcohol-related disease. In the past two decades, a number of prospective markers have been studied and proposed as accurate markers for alcohol consumption. The purpose of this review is to summarize the basis and value of these tests.

It has proven most difficult to detect biologically the consumption of alcohol in patients who deny its use. The half-life of ethanol is so short (3–4 hours) that it is often not detectable in serum or urine for more than a few hours after drinking has ceased. As a result of this difficulty in assessing alcoholic drinking behavior biologically, there has been much interest in the search for markers of consumption that have a longer half-life than ethanol. A number of tests for the consumption of alcohol have been developed and are used clinically (mean corpuscular volume[MCV], γ-glutamyltransferase [GGT], other liver enzymes) or in research studies and by the insurance industry (serum carbohydrate-deficient transferrin [CDT], hemoglobin-associated acetaldehyde[HAA], early detection of alcohol consumption [EDAC] scores, and blood phosphatidylethanol [PtdEtOH]). Several recent reviews have described studies evaluating the utility of various markers for alcohol consumption. A common conclusion is that no single test has yet to provide an objective, accurate, biologically based marker for alcohol consumption with 100% sensitivity and specificity except for the direct measurement of ethanol in the blood or breath. Nevertheless, there is optimism that the combination of current and future markers will eventually provide accurate testing for ethanol consumption.

PROPOSED APPLICATIONS

The recognition and detection of ethanol consumption have a number of medical and forensic uses — for instance: 1) early detection of heavy drinking in a general medical practice, 2) monitoring drinking by recovering alcoholics in treatment, 3) monitoring ethanol consumption in those waiting for liver transplants, 4) detection of heavy drinking among professionals responsible for public safety such as airline pilots, 5) blood alcohol concentration (BAC) measurements by law enforcement officers, 6) detection of ethanol consumption among parolees for driving under the influence (DUI) offenses, and 7) detecting heavy alcohol consumption in pregnant women. Identifying drinking in a general medical practice requires the use of markers for consumption as between-subject variables. That is, the marker level of the patient, usually at a single time point, must be compared against the mean value of a population. Although this type of testing is less accurate to assess drinking than a within-subject variable, it has potential for the early detection of heavy drinkers. The measurement of markers for consumption as a within-subject variable to follow recovering alcoholics during their treatment may be more sensitive. Several recent studies have concluded that following a patient over time with marker measurements provides a sensitive assessment of relapse.

CRITERIA FOR ACCEPTABLE TESTS

Acceptable laboratory tests usually proceed through several stages of development prior to their acceptance by the medical community and their availability in local pathology labs. First, the test must provide diagnostic value for physicians who might use the test for the interpretation of pathological conditions in their patients. Second, the cost of the test must not be so expensive that the patient cannot afford it or the insurance companies will not pay for the total cost of the test. Third, the performance of the test must expose the patient to no more than minimal risk. Fourth, the test should have a combination of high sensitivity and high specificity so that the results provide high diagnostic efficiency. That is, test results should include few false positives and false negatives. Fifth, the test must be precise and accurate in that the measurement specifically and without interference reflects the condition being monitored. Lastly, from the laboratory perspective, the test must be able to be performed quickly and with a minimum of training by a laboratory technician.

EVALUATION OF MARKERS

The developmental process for markers of alcohol consumption generally begins in treatment clinics or hospitals after a potential marker has been identified and a technique for its measurement established. A comparison of the levels of a marker among subjects in heavy drinking versus non-drinking populations is made and assessed. The assessment of the value of a marker includes the calculation of sensitivity and specificity at the level of drinking considered harmful. Sensitivity is the percentage of positive tests among drinkers. Specificity is the percentage of negative tests among non-drinkers or social drinkers. Receiver operator characteristic (ROC) analyses also have been used to evaluate the accuracy of markers. In this analysis, sensitivity and specificity are tested at various marker cutoff levels. Positive and negative predictive values also can be calculated to indicate the percentage of true positives and true negatives. More recently, odds ratios have been employed to evaluate marker effectiveness. For example, to test the value of a marker to reflect an increase or decrease in drinking during abstinence, an odds ratio might be used. The odds ratio could compare the odds of a decrease in CDT level within those with a decrease in drinks per drinking day to the odds of a decrease in CDT level within those with an increase in drinks per drinking day. A high ratio indicates an accurate test.

VALUE OF MARKERS

Accurate and sensitive biochemical markers that reflect level of drinking would be invaluable in several ways. Under-reported drinking is common in clinical practice. Physicians and other caregivers utilize very brief interviews or questionnaires about problems with drinking to assess the patient's difficulties with alcohol. In the early stages of heavy drinking, medical problems associated with chronic alcohol abuse may not be clinically apparent. Lack of forthright responses to questionnaires or lack of significant alcohol-associated medical problems masks heavy drinking. Accurate and sensitive biochemical markers would circumvent this lack of important diagnostic information and would allow physicians to warn patients of potentially severe consequences of prolonged, heavy drinking. Under some conditions, biochemical tests are more objective and more reliable than interviews. They are not influenced by patient or family denial and could be more acceptable to treatment providers. Finally, these tests have been valuable to alcoholics in treatment who are serious about quitting and benefit from positive feedback during abstinence. They also can be used to reinforce motivation to quit drinking or reduce consumption.

CATEGORIES OF MARKERS

For the sake of this review, current and proposed markers are categorized into three groups based on their apparent mechanisms. The first group contains MCV, GGT, and EDAC score and is termed toxic effect markers. The mechanism of ethanol to produce elevations in toxic markers is not clear, but the effect of ethanol elevates marker levels above the normal range. The second group, the indirect markers, contains CDT and 5-hydroxytryptophol (5HTOL). For these markers, the effect of ethanol on enzymes causes the elevation of the marker level. The third group consists of so-called direct markers and includes BAC, blood Ptd-EtOH, EtG, fatty acid ethyl esters (FAEEs), and HAA. The mechanism of formation of the direct markers is via the chemical derivatization of ethanol or its principal metabolite, acetaldehyde.

Toxic Effect Markers

Mean Corpuscular Volume (MCV)

Macrocytosis associated with cirrhosis was reported in 1884. Since that time, the association of excessive alcohol consumption with increased size of red cells has been observed and reported. Results of early studies suggested that as high as 90% of male and female alcoholics who admitted to drinking greater than 80 g/day had increased MCV when compared to patients with non-alcoholic liver disease and healthy control subjects. Subsequent studies verified that macrocytosis occurs in a lower percentage of heavy abusers or alcoholics. It should be noted that groups of alcoholics or heavy drinkers were compared against non-drinking controls in most of these studies. Therefore, the clinical sensitivities and specificities were likely to be optimized. More recent studies place the sensitivity of MCV as a marker for heavy alcohol consumption in the 30% to 50% range. However, specificities are low.

It has been reported that "macrocytosis, which is not related to folate deficiency or liver disease, occurs in the majority of alcoholics, often in the absence of anemia, and appears to be an unexplained effect of ethanol." The mechanism by which alcohol causes elevated MCV remains poorly understood. In fact, it was observed that increased MCV in alcoholics (>80 g/day) is not always associated with anemia or folate deficiency. Consequently, it was concluded that ethanol exerted a direct toxic action on the developing erythroblast to produce macrocytosis.

Substances other than ethanol may interfere with the use of MCV as a marker for alcohol consumption. It has been shown that cigarette smoking increases MCV similar to the effect of drinking. Also, it has been reported that use of anticonvulsants can cause false positive tests and that age also might affect MCV. These interferences limit the use of MCV as a marker independent of other markers.

Increased MCV after heavy exposure to alcohol persists for a number of weeks after abstention and may be related to the turnover rate of red blood cells. There is no study to date in which a correlation between amounts of alcohol consumed and increased MCV was observed.

Measurement of MCV is an inexpensive, standard pathology lab test performed with a Coulter counter. However, the use of this marker probably should be limited to a complementary role with other direct or indirect markers because the demonstrated sensitivity of this test is not sufficient for it to be used alone, and, as noted above, interferences reduce its value.

γ-Glutamyltransferase (GGT)

GGT activity in serum has served as the principal biological marker for alcohol consumption for over two decades. GGT is an integral membrane glycoprotein enzyme that catalyzes the transfer of γ-glutamyl groups between γ-glutamyl peptides and small peptides or amino acids. The enzyme has a molecular weight of approximately 85 kDa and consists of two subunits. The lighter subunit contains the catalytic site. Normally, this enzyme plays an important role in the transport of amino acids across cell membranes, in peptide nitrogen storage, in protein synthesis, and in the regulation of tissue glutathione levels. GGT activity is normally highest in the kidney, but is also found in moderate amounts in the pancreas, liver, and prostate and at lower levels in the spleen, lung, bowel, placenta, and thyroid. Serum GGT levels in apparently healthy volunteers are slightly higher in males than in females.

There are two forms of GGT in the adult liver, an adult form and a fetal form. It appears that ethanol selectively induces the transcription of the fetal form of hepatic GGT, which accounts for the increase in serum GGT after excessive alcohol use. The elevation in serum GGT activity is probably due to a combination of hepatic enzyme induction and toxic effects on hepatic cell membranes, depending on the state of the progression of the disease.

Hepatic microsomal injury may be one of the earliest effects of alcohol toxicity associated with high alcohol intake. Although the measurement of GGT in plasma or serum was first proposed as a marker for liver disease, it also was recognized to have a useful role for the diagnosis of heavy drinking. It was reported in 1972 that serum GGT correlated with alcohol intake, but that it took an average of six drinks per day for weeks to raise the level of GGT above normal in 50% of the subjects. This result suggests that the lower limit of sensitivity requires a relatively high intake of alcohol and indicates that the possibility of false negative results must be considered when GGT is used as a marker for consumption.

Elevated serum GGT activity caused by heavy drinking returns to normal levels during abstinence with a half-life of 2 to 3 weeks. In one study, the minimal amount of drinking required to raise serum GGT levels was approximately 75 g/day over the past 30 days. The sensitivity and specificity of GGT for heavy alcohol consumption vary from study to study, depending on the level and chronology of drinking in the population studied. Overall, the sensitivity of GGT for heavy alcohol consumption is in the range of 50% to 75%, while sensitivity is somewhat lower.

A number of factors can affect GGT levels. It should be noted that drugs such as phenobarbital and chlorpromazine raise serum GGT levels. The results of the recent WHO/ISBRA study indicate that GGT levels vary with age and body mass index. Drinkers under the age of 20 years who drank greater than 80 g/day of alcohol did not have elevated GGT levels. The level of drinking in older subjects correlated with GGT levels. Also, GGT performed better as a marker of heavy consumption in individuals with higher body mass indices. Finally, and most importantly, non-alcoholic liver disease should be considered a source of false positive GGT results.

As a final comment, it should be noted that GGT appears to lack accuracy as an independent marker, but it has been shown to be useful when combined with CDT, which may prove to be its most useful role.

Early Detection of Alcohol Consumption (EDAC) Score

Almost two decades ago, researchers at the NIAAA developed a test to distinguish heavy from social drinking by analyzing the results of a panel of standard laboratory tests using quadratic discriminant analysis to estimate whether a given patient was more likely to be in one group or the other. This method proved to be very accurate, but it never caught on at the clinical level because of the complicated nature of the analysis and the recommendation that two control groups, one healthy and one alcoholic, were recommended at each site where the test would be performed. In 1991, a similar project emerged to develop a practical laboratory screen based on routine blood analytes for detecting excessive drinking in primary clinical settings. Using a variety of statistical techniques to analyze the data based on race, gender, and age, a linear discriminant function was developed. The data were obtained by examination of blood chemistry parameters from close to 1,000 heavy and light drinkers recruited from multiple sites. The linear discriminant function assigns a score (the EDAC score) to each subject; heavy and light drinkers are identified with EDAC scores above and below zero, respectively. The EDAC scores have been used successfully since the mid-1990s to assess heavy alcohol consumption and monitor compliance in individuals attending selected primary care settings in the midwestern United States. The version of the test that uses 13 tests includes the following measurements: Na, Cl, K, bilirubin ratio, total protein, albumin, GGT, AST, MCV, white blood cell count, monocytes, cholesterol, and HDL. The apparent value of the EDAC test in research studies indicates that the combination of tests with varying half-lives and detection limits may eventually provide the needed predictive value that is required for the sensitive and specific detection of heavy drinking. The EDAC score is easy to perform and relatively cost-effective. Although this test appears to have important potential for clinical diagnosis and treatment of alcoholic drinking, the sensitivity and specificity of this test for the identification of heavy drinking in a general medical practice and by recovering alcoholic drinkers are not yet well studied. Also, it requires the cooperation of chemical laboratories to calculate values that clinicians can use, a very difficult requirement in busy laboratories.

Indirect Markers

Carbohydrate-Deficient Transferrin (CDT)

The measurement of serum CDT for the detection of heavy ethanol consumption is perhaps the most widely studied of all. According to a large number of studies over the last 15 years, CDT appears to be more sensitive and specific as a marker for alcohol consumption than any other currently available measure, at least in men. The %CDT version of the test was approved by the Food and Drug Administration (FDA) in 2001 for use as a test for the detection of heavy alcohol consumption.

The physical properties and normal physiological function of transferrin were reviewed recently. Transferrin is a protein with a molecular weight of approximately 80 kDa and a single polypeptide chain of 679 amino acids. There are two homologous domains within the molecule, and each can bind one molecule of iron. The C-terminal half of transferrin, at amino acid numbers 413 and 611, contains two complex, oligosaccharide side chains. Up to eight sialic acid residues can be attached at the end of these two carbohydrate chains, four on each chain. At least 9 isoforms of transferrin can be separated on the basis of the number of sialic acid residues. Under normal conditions and in healthy controls, most transferrin molecules contain four sialic acid residues, two on each carbohydrate chain. The physiological function of transferrin is to bind and deliver iron to cells within various tissues.

The history of the discovery of the effect of ethanol on transferrin was recently reviewed by Helena Stibler, a Swedish scientist who is credited with the discovery of CDT. The initial observation with isoelectric focusing revealed that elevated concentrations of isoforms of transferrin with higher pI values appeared in the serum of alcoholic patients. Further studies showed that the higher pI values of these isoforms were a result of fewer sialic acid residues on their carbohydrate side chains — hence the term carbohydrate-deficient transferrin. The isoforms of transferrin whose levels are elevated in the serum of alcoholics have been shown to be asialo- and disialo-transferrin.

The mechanism by which ethanol or its metabolite acetaldehyde causes fewer sialic acid residues to be attached to the transferrin is not completely understood at this time, but effects on the post-translational transfer of carbohydrate side chains to transferrin appear to be involved.

As of 1991, a large number of clinical studies had been done, which included at least 2,500 subjects. These studies mostly involved distinct groups of subjects such as healthy controls and verified alcoholics, and clinical sensitivities between 81% and 100% and clinical specificities between 97% and 100% were reported for the CDT marker. False positives occurred in only about 1% of the subjects in these studies and were thought to be mostly due to severe hepatic insufficiency, a genetically rare D-variant of transferrin, or carbohydrate-deficient glycoprotein (CDG) syndrome. A more recent study of moderate drinkers (greater than 50 g/day for the past month) indicated a clinical sensitivity of 69% and specificity of 92% for CDT. Another study reported a sensitivity of 79% and a specificity of >90% for males who drank over 60 g/day in the month before admission. The sensitivity was only 44% among 18 female abusers.

In a recent, large study of 1,863 subjects (WHO/ISBRA Collaborative Study), the sensitivity and specificity for CDT were 60% and 92% in males and 29% and 92% in females, respectively. In this study, absolute levels of CDT were measured using the CDTect kit, so upper limits of normal of 20 and 26 units/L were used for males and females, respectively. Cut-off values for reported heavy drinking during the previous month for males and females were >80 g/d and >40 g/d, respectively. These sensitivities and specificities are in line with dozens of previous reports. They suggest that a significant percentage of subjects who drank heavily had false negative tests but few false positive tests. The different cut-off levels for drinking between males and females may have accounted for the difference in sensitivity between the genders. When CDT levels in males and females who were drinking equal amounts of alcohol (60 to 90 g/d) were compared by ROC analysis, there was not a significant statistical difference between genders for CDT's performance, suggesting that CDT may be equally responsive in men and women given equal levels of drinking. Regarding age and CDT levels, subjects under 20 years of age did not express elevated CDT levels at any level of drinking as opposed to older subjects. Interestingly, subjects with the lowest body mass index (<20 kg/m^2) had the highest CDT levels at all levels of drinking.

It is important to note that serum CDT levels in healthy controls are slightly higher in women than in men. Also, serum CDT may not be as useful for moderate forms of alcohol abuse in women as it is in men. However, %CDT (CDT as a percentage of total transferrin) does not appear to differ as much between the genders.

It does not appear that drugs other than alcohol interfere with the CDT test. Perhaps the greatest benefit of the CDT test is that the percentage of false positives is relatively low (high specificity). This is in part due to the low incidence of interference with the test. For example, the authors of a recent study concluded that the CDT assay is a highly specific instrument for use in assessing alcohol consumption in a general medical population with no interference by coexisting hypertension, asthma/bronchitis, diabetes mellitus, adiposis/lipid metabolism disorder, angina pectoris, depression, or disorders of the digestive tract. However, false positives can occur because of genetic D-variants, CDG syndrome, primary biliary cirrhosis, hepatocellular carcinoma, viral liver cirrhosis, and pancreas and kidney transplantation or the drugs used to treat these disorders.

Several different methods have been used for the determination of CDT in serum. Presently, a commercial kit is available (%CDT, BioRad), which uses a micro column separation and ELISA-based detection system. One group of investigators showed that sensitivity and specificity of CDT as a marker of alcohol abuse are significantly influenced by alterations in total serum transferrin. Others have concluded that the relative value (% of total transferrin), when compared with the absolute concentration, of CDT in serum was useful as a marker of alcohol consumption in acute alcoholic hepatitis. This approach has been used in more recent studies and seems to reduce the effect of gender because the CDT level is normalized to total transferrin.

The CDT marker also appears to be the best current marker for monitoring the consumption of alcohol. Consumption of between 50 and 80 grams of alcohol per day for at least a week has been shown to increase serum CDT levels in non-alcoholic test subjects, and the half-life of CDT after commencement of abstinence has been determined to be about 2 weeks. CDT measurements may be useful in the monitoring of the treatment of recovering alcoholics. Data suggest that a rise of about 30% over an abstinent baseline level suggests relapse drinking while a fall of about 30% from an actively drinking level suggests a return toward abstinence.

In population screening studies, the sensitivity for lower amounts or intensities of drinking is considerably lower. Clinical specificity has been reported to be 90% or higher in studies where heavy drinkers are compared with social drinkers, less in the general population. At this time, it appears that the specificity of the CDT test for a certain level of drinking will be its greatest value; that is, the percentage of false positives is low relative to other markers. Also, there appear to be few sources of interference to this test. The use of this test will increase with time, especially if a more automated version becomes available.

5-Hydroxytryptophol (Urinary 5HTOL)/5HIAA

The measurement of 5HTOL in urine as a marker for very recent ethanol consumption has been proposed. 5HTOL is normally a minor metabolite of serotonin. Its formation accounts for only about 2% to 4% of the metabolism of serotonin. The major end product of serotonin metabolism is 5-hydroxyindoleacetic acid (5HIAA). It has been proposed that the consumption of ethanol changes the ratio of 5HTOL/5HIAA in urine for a number of hours after the disappearance of ethanol. Approximately 99% of urinary 5HTOL is conjugated, either as the sulfate or glucuronide salt, apparently because of the lipid/water solubility of 5HTOL.

An acute dose of ethanol causes a significant increase in the production of 5HTOL and a corresponding decrease in 5HIAA production by measurements of the compounds in human urine. This shift in metabolism was probably due in part to an increase in the NADH/NAD^+ ratio (NADH is the reduced form of nicotinamide adenine dinucleotide and NAD^+ the oxidized form) by ethanol or the presence of acetaldehyde, both of which may play a role in the inhibition of aldehyde dehydrogenase, thereby blocking the formation of

5HIAA and forcing the aldehyde of serotonin into the reductive side of the metabolic pathway. Similar results were found in rat brain studies using brain microdialysis.

A study of the time course of ethanol-induced changes in serotonin metabolism reported that the increase of urinary 5HTOL correlated with blood ethanol curve; however, a considerable lag time was observed. Urinary 5HTOL levels did not return to baseline until a number of hours after ethanol levels were undetectable. In this study, an ethanol dose of 0.5 g/kg produced an elevated urinary 5HTOL/5HIAA level. The half-life of the urinary 5HTOL/5HIAA ratio appeared to be about the same as that of ethanol.

Two recent clinical studies support the use of this marker as an indicator of recent ethanol consumption. In a group of 69 subjects who were alcohol abstinent, the values of the 5HTOL/5HIAA ratio varied between 4 and 17 pmol 5HTOL/nmol 5HIAA. It was proposed that a ratio of 20 be used as the upper limit of normal (non- and social drinkers) and that ratios >20 be used to indicate recent heavy consumption. Using these criteria, the statistical probability for a false positive was calculated to be less than 0.001. Another group of investigators performed a study in 15 subjects attempting to abstain from alcohol over a 6-month period. They described correlation between elevated urinary 5HTOL/5HIAA ratios and elevated CDT values and suggested that the two measurements could be used in a complementary way for the detection of relapse in alcohol-dependent patients.

Other drugs that inhibit aldehyde dehydrogenase also may increase the urinary 5HTOL/5HIAA ratio. For example, disulfiram, an aldehyde dehydrogenase inhibitor used for the treatment of alcoholism, has been shown to increase the 5HTOL/5HIAA ratio. However, in one study, several drugs and a variety of clinical conditions had no effect on urinary 5HTOL/5HIAA ratio. Ingestion of bananas, which are serotonin rich, or the presence of serotonin-producing carcinoid tumors caused higher rates of 5HTOL secretion, but the 5HTOL/5HIAA ratio did not differ between these subjects and controls. High concentrations of serotonin also are present in tomato and pineapple.

This marker has not yet been well tested, and values for clinical sensitivity and specificity have not appeared in the literature. Nevertheless, this test has potential as an indicator of very recent alcohol use. Elevated levels of 5HTOL/5HIAA appear to remain for several hours after the disappearance of ethanol from the blood. Therefore, the probable utility of the urinary 5HTOL/5HIAA ratio will be as a prospective marker for relapse or in screening for very recent consumption. As an indicator of very recent ethanol use, this test might complement other tests in the assessment of alcohol consumption. This test also will have a place in forensic medicine to determine the post-mortem formation, as opposed to pre-mortem presence, of ethanol in urine. The measurement of 5HTOL and 5HIAA in urine can be made using HPLC with electrochemical detection.

Direct Markers

Direct markers for ethanol consumption are compounds formed after the consumption of alcohol that are chemical derivatives of ethanol. This class of markers includes ethanol and acetaldehyde derivatives such as ethyl glucuronide, FAEEs, Ptd-EtOH, and whole blood associated acetaldehyde (WBAA). The half-lives of direct markers are longer than that of ethanol. The measurement of ethanol itself in breath or blood is included in this group. Excluding the measurement of ethanol, the development of testing of direct markers as indicators of ethanol consumption is a relatively recent event. In humans, approximately 90% to 95% of ethanol is oxidized via hepatic and non-hepatic pathways. The non-oxidative pathways comprise 5% to 10% of the metabolism of ethanol. Sensitive analytical techniques have allowed for the development of testing for direct markers of ethanol consumption.

Blood/Breath Alcohol Levels (BAC)

The direct measurement of ethanol in the blood or other bodily fluids, such as saliva, urine, or sweat, is a specific means by which to detect consumption. Ethanol taken orally is absorbed very quickly from the stomach and the intestine and distributes in total body water. Approximately 80% of ingested ethanol is metabolized in the liver to acetaldehyde, and then blood ethanol and acetaldehyde levels drop quite rapidly after the discontinuance of alcohol ingestion. The half-life of ethanol and acetaldehyde is about 3 to 4 hours. The total elimination rate of ethanol includes the rates of metabolism and excretion as well as the concentration of ethanol in blood when abstinence begins. The maximal elimination rate is approximately 15 mg%/hr in the post-absorption phase of the blood alcohol curve. Therefore, the complete elimination of ethanol at a blood level of 100 mg%, which is the legal intoxication level in many states, would take about 6 hours. These measurements are limited when used for screening in the general population or during treatment, but useful for forensic purposes.

Obvious situations in which direct measurement of blood ethanol concentration is helpful are: 1) in the hospital emergency room to help in the treatment of a patient, 2) for forensic purposes, e.g., a driver might be suspected of being legally intoxicated, 3) in recovering patients, and 4) for use in devices that prevent drivers under the influence from operating a motor vehicle. For these purposes, devices have been developed to measure ethanol concentration in the breath. This method works well in most populations, with the possible exception of the elderly. Significant variability in peak blood alcohol concentrations in subjects who have consumed equal amounts of ethanol has been observed. This variability may be due to different metabolic rates and/or tolerance among alcohol consumers and must be taken into account when interpreting ethanol levels.

Ethanol can also be measured in urine, saliva, and sweat, but these measurements are less frequently used. Ethanol is present in the urine longer than in the blood, but the relationship between urine and blood levels is not always proportional. Blood ethanol levels can be determined by very sensitive laboratory tests that are readily available.

Blood Phosphatidylethanol (Ptd-EtOH)

Ptd-EtOH is an abnormal phospholipid that is formed in the blood only when phospholipids, phospholipase D (PL-D), and ethanol are present. Normally, the catalytic action of PL-D on phospholipids produces phosphatidic acid. However, in the presence of ethanol, the substitution of ethanol onto the phosphate group of the phospholipid is strongly favored over the -OH moiety from water. As a result, Ptd-EtOH is formed instead of phosphatidic acid. This phenomenon is the biochemical basis for the formation of this potentially useful marker.

Recently, a method has been developed for the quantification of Ptd-EtOH in blood by HPLC and evaporative light scattering or electrospray mass spectrometric detection.

One group of investigators followed 15 inpatients in an alcoholic detoxification clinic for 7 days after admission by measuring Ptd-EtOH during that time. They found measurable levels of Ptd-EtOH in red blood cells, but not in leucocytes, serum, or plasma. These levels were reduced by 7 days of abstinence with a half-life of 4.0 ± 0.7 days and gave a good fit for a one-compartment elimination model. This half-life is shorter than those of GGT and CDT, making this marker an attractive adjunct marker for combination. CDT and Ptd-EtOH levels did not correlate in this study, suggesting that these two markers might be used in combination. Others have tested a variety of drugs and concluded that they did not interfere with the test. Regarding the sensitivity of the test, it was determined that a single dose of 50 g of ethanol would not produce detectable levels, but that 50 g/day for a few days would. Very few studies have been conducted to study this marker, and more comprehensive, systematic studies are needed to further confirm the value of this measurement.

Ethyl Glucuronide

Following ingestion, ethanol is primarily oxidatively metabolized. However, approximately 0.5% of ingested ethanol is conjugated with glucuronic acid. The non-volatile, water-soluble metabolite ethyl glucuronate can be isolated and quantified in urine and serum samples. Ethyl glucuronide also has been measured in hair samples from individuals who had recently ingested ethanol. Ethyl glucuronide is not detected in serum or urine samples of individuals who have not been exposed to ethanol recently. Formation of ethyl glucuronide is dependent on the presence of circulating ethanol and peaks approximately 3 hours after the peak in ethanol concentrations. Accordingly, ethyl glucuronide has been touted as a potential marker for alcohol use.

Serum or urine ethyl glucuronide is isolated by liquid-liquid extraction and recently by solid-phase extraction techniques. The metabolite is typically quantified by gas chromatography-mass spectroscopy (GC-MS) as well as by LC/MS-MS. In both analytical methods, deuterium-labeled ethyl glucuronide is used as the internal standard. Limits of determination and limits of detection may be as low as 0.1 mg/L and 0.03 mg/L, respectively, using GC-MS. Similar limits of determination and detection were observed with LC/MS-MS. Ethyl glucuronide may be present in urine samples for at least 80 hours in hospitalized patients undergoing alcohol withdrawal.

In one of a series of similar publications over the past decade, Wurst and colleagues reported on a group of 33 alcoholics with a mean blood alcohol concentration of 183 mg/dL at the time of their hospitalization. They compared levels of ethyl glucuronide in these individuals with levels in non-alcoholic to no-alcoholic-intake controls using GC-MS with deuterium-labeled ethyl glucuronide (d5-EtG). Ethyl glucuronide concentrations in the alcoholic group ranged from 3.6 to 710 mg/L for up to 80 hours following their last intake of ethanol. Ethyl glucuronide was not present in urine samples from controls. These results support the use of ethyl glucuronide as a marker for ethanol exposure. However, they also noted that there was no direct correlation between urine ethyl glucuronide levels and blood alcohol concentrations. This might suggest limited usefulness for this marker as more than a qualitative index for recent alcohol exposure. Nevertheless, they suggest that ethyl glucuronide represents a useful marker for recent alcohol consumption as well as relapse among alcohol abusers.

Drug metabolites often can be measured in hair samples. This also is true of ethyl glucuronide. One group of investigators reported measuring ethyl glucuronide in postmortem hair samples as well as in skin swabs/scrapings from individuals with known use of alcohol immediately prior to death. For comparison, similar samples were collected from social drinkers and from non-ethanol-exposed children. A liquid-liquid extraction was followed by analysis using GC-MS in selected ion monitoring mode. Methyl glucuronide was used as the internal standard. The limit of detection and limit of quantification were 2.2 and 5 ng/mg, respectively. For skin swabs, the limit of detection and limit of quantification were 8.0 and 25 ng/mg, respectively. Recoveries average 81% ± 3%. Measurable levels of ethyl glucuronide were present in some but not all of the groups of alcohol abusers and social drinkers. Ethyl glucuronide was not present in samples from non-alcohol-exposed (children) controls. Another study reported measuring ethyl glucuronide in concentrations up to 4,025 pg/mg in postmortem hair samples of alcoholics and levels ranging from 119 to 388 pg/mg in patients undergoing alcohol withdrawal. Again, ethyl glucuronide was not present in hair samples from individuals who had not ingested alcohol.

Recently, a group of investigators described an immunochemical assay (ELISA using polyclonal antibodies) for determination of serum or urine levels of ethyl glucuronide. Test specificity (percent of true negatives) was 91.6% for serum samples and 76.8% for urine samples, while test sensitivity (percent of true positives) was 90.5% from serum samples and 75.7% for urine samples. Lower limits of detection were 0.31 mg/L for serum samples and 1.33 mg/L for urine samples.

Fatty Acid Ethyl Esters (FAEEs)

Ethanol is metabolized via both oxidative and non-oxidative pathways. The former results in the formation of acetaldehyde. Through the non-oxidative pathway, esterification of ethanol and fatty acids produces FAEEs. Measurable concentrations of FAEEs are normally present only in the circulation of alcohol users and in organs such as the liver and brain damaged by alcohol abuse. The formation of FAEEs may account, at least in part, for the central nervous system and other organ toxicity associated with chronic alcohol abuse.

Apart from their potentially cytotoxic impact, levels of circulating FAEEs may be used as markers for acute as well as chronic alcohol use. Study subjects given alcoholic drinks at a controlled rate over a 90-minute period exhibited closely parallel increases in serum FAEE levels and blood ethanol concentrations. Serum FAEE levels were measurable 24 hours after alcohol intake. Even among test subjects with very low blood alcohol levels (<0.10 g/L), serum FAEEs could be detected, suggesting that FAEE analysis represents a sensitive measure for ethanol exposure. Since the estimated half-life of FAEEs in adipose tissue is significantly greater than that of alcohol itself (16 ± 1.6 hours vs. 4 hours, respectively), the presence of measurable concentrations of FAEEs in this tissue represents a valuable marker for previous alcohol use. Analysis of FAEE concentrations in adipose tissue, easily obtained at necropsy, also may be useful in determining antemortem alcohol intake.

The fatty acid composition of FAEEs is tissue-specific, with different fatty acids present in FAEEs from blood, liver, pancreas, and other tissues. The levels of a particular fatty acid also vary according to the frequency of alcohol abuse. For example, levels of ethyl oleate (E18:1) are higher in chronic alcoholics versus binge alcohol abusers, thus providing a marker that could be used to differentiate patterns of alcohol abuse. Measurement of ethyl arachidonate (E20:4) greater than 200 pmol/g in liver and/or adipose tissue is considered evidence of antemortem ethanol ingestion.

FAEEs most commonly detected in blood and tissue samples include ethyl palmitate (E16:0), ethyl palmitoleate (16:1), ethyl stearate (E18:0), ethyl oleate (E18:1), ethyl linoleate (E18:2), and ethyl arachidonate (E20:4). FAEEs are typically separated by a liquid-liquid extraction and subsequent thin-layer chromatography or by a solid-phase extraction method. Recoveries of individual FAEEs varied from 72% to 87% using solid-phase extraction. Sample storage and preparation are important considerations in the determination of FAEEs. Serum and tissue samples may be stored frozen but should not be exposed to light since FAEEs are light sensitive. Individual FAEEs are quantified using GC-MS with chemical ionization. Electron impact ionization produces identical FAEE fragments, whereas chemical ionization yields a diagnostic ion for each FAEE. Using tissue specimens obtained at autopsy, one group of investigators reported test sensitivity to identify individuals with detectable blood alcohol versus those without detectable blood alcohol as 93% with a specificity of 100%. Among individuals with blood alcohol levels greater than 1.5 g/L, serum FAEE concentrations correlate very closely with blood ethanol concentrations. Peak FAEE levels in these individuals ranged from 1 to 3 μmol/L. Furthermore, serum FAEE remained detectable (0.03–0.24 μmol/L) at least up to 24 hours after ethanol intake when blood ethanol was itself no longer detectable. It was noted, however, that estimation of peak serum FAEE levels cannot be extrapolated from serum FAEE levels 24 hours after ethanol ingestion.

FAEEs also have been measured in hair samples using liquid-liquid extraction coupled with headspace solid-phase microextraction extraction and GC-MS to detect selected FAEEs (ethyl myristate, E14:0; ethyl palmitate, E16:0; ethyl oleate, E18:1; ethyl stearate, E18:0). Corresponding deuterated d_5-FAEEs are typically employed as internal standards. One group of investigators reported detection limits from 0.01 ng/mg for ethyl 18:0 to 0.04 ng/mg for ethyl oleate (E8:1). Intra-assay variation among the measured FAEEs ranged from 3.5% to 15.5%. The predominant FAEE was ethyl oleate (18:1) in all samples of hair from individuals ingesting alcohol. Negative results, or trace amounts of ethyl palmitate (E16:0), were noted among nondrinkers. FAEE levels were higher in alcoholics (1–29 ng/mg) than in social drinkers (<0.8 ng/mg). Detection of FAEEs in hair samples is not affected by the use of hair care products including shampoo, dye, and bleaching, although use of alcohol-based hair lotions may generate false positive results. Analysis of hair samples for the presence of FAEEs may represent a useful marker for current or past alcohol use.

Measurement of accumulated FAEEs in meconium also has recently been described as a marker for heavy maternal drinking in the second trimester of pregnancy. Meconium FAEE concentrations were analyzed using solid-phase extraction and GC-MS with chemical ionization. The lower limit of detection was 50 ng/g of meconium. Though not always present in every sample, oleic and linoleic acid ethyl esters were present in highest concentrations when present in samples. FAEEs in meconium samples provide a potentially valuable marker for fetal alcohol exposure, additional to maternal interview.

Clearly, FAEEs represent sensitive and specific markers for recent as well as chronic alcohol ingestion. Quantification of FAEEs in blood, liver, and other organs as well as hair samples provides readily obtainable means by which to assess alcohol ingestion. Unfortunately, the number of clinical laboratories currently capable of measuring FAEEs is limited, thus reducing the practical use of FAEEs in the clinical evaluation of alcohol abuse patterns.

Hemoglobin-Associated Acetaldehyde (HAA)

Acetaldehyde is the major catabolic product of ethanol metabolism. After alcohol ingestion, acetaldehyde circulates in plasma or penetrates erythrocytes to remain inside these cells as free, unstable, short-lived compounds. Acetaldehyde preferentially partitions into the red cell, presumably as a CO_2 analogue, and, like CO_2, has a high binding affinity for hemoglobin. At the same time, acetaldehyde also binds to a number of plasma proteins, including albumin and hemoglobin, to form stable protein-acetaldehyde adducts. The combination of free and protein-bound acetaldehyde is called whole blood acetaldehyde. Healthy volunteers ingesting moderate amounts of alcohol show free (plasma and erythrocyte) acetaldehyde concentrations that peak 30 minutes after the last drink. Both plasma and red blood cell free-acetaldehyde return to levels not significantly different from baseline by 3.5 hours. However, the protein-bound acetaldehyde, 90% of which is in the form of hemoglobin-associated acetaldehyde, remains elevated for approximately a month.

Measures of acetaldehyde-protein adducts provide a potential means by which drinking behavior might be quantified in a manner analogous to the use of glycosylated hemoglobin assays in another chronic disease, diabetes mellitus. Measurement of increased acetaldehyde-adduct formation by HPLC has been reported since the late 1980s to distinguish between drinkers and non-drinkers. The procedure used at that time required careful, daily preparation of reagents and skilled technicians to run the test. Commercial laboratories were unable to obtain the quality of results expected of a well-standardized and validated test. Nonetheless, using this pioneering procedure as a research tool, *in vitro* experiments and animal studies demonstrated that elevations in WBAA are a function of both the quantity and frequency of alcohol consumption.

The WBAA test was introduced in the U.S. in 1990, after the design of an improved HPLC assay with the advantages of effective automation and a user-friendly preparation of stable reagents to assure proper quality control. The improved procedure, adapted for routine use, provides valuable insights to detect alcohol abuse because, unlike GGT, WBAA elevations are believed to be evident prior to liver damage.

Combination of Tests

Some authorities have conjectured that the combination of test results for the identification of consumption would produce higher sensitivities but lower specificities. For instance, it has been reported that the combination of CDT and GGT produced higher sensitivity without lowering specificity for heavy drinking (>60 g/day). The tests were combined so that if either test was positive, the combination of tests was considered positive, but both tests had to be negative or normal for the combined marker test to be negative. Another group of investigators used this same strategy and found that the performance of the combined test was significantly better than that of either %CDT alone or GGT alone, as evaluated by calculating sensitivity and likelihood ratio at a specificity of 0.85 and by comparing areas under ROC curves statistically. Also, the combination of GGT and CDT has been reported to produce higher correlations with reported drinking than for either marker alone.

Factors that Affect Marker Levels and Diagnostic Accuracy

A number of factors have been shown to influence the levels of potentially useful diagnostic markers for alcoholic drinking levels. The effect of these factors must be characterized before a marker can find its place among the more established tests. Levels may vary based on age, gender, therapeutic agents, body mass index, as well as non-alcoholic and alcoholic pathologies. The development of sensitization or tolerance to ethanol-induced elevation of markers may be important. For example, there have been suggestions in the literature that elevation of GGT and CDT may become sensitized during heavy ethanol consumption. That is, GGT and CDT levels may rise more quickly during relapses in alcoholics that have abstained for some period of time, then "slip" into drinking again.

Clinical Applications

Clinical Utility of Alcohol Abuse Biomarkers

In an era of cost constraints, newly emerging diagnostic procedures must demonstrate an advantage in terms of clinical outcome. Do the test results affect the way in which the physician manages the patient and improve the overall mortality, morbidity, and cost of care? In clinical practice, a common question is, "If the patient has a positive test, how likely is he/she to have the condition?" or "If the patient has a negative test, how likely is he/she not to have the condition?" Regardless of the biochemical marker used, a single data point must be accurate in delivering this response, especially if the test is being used to determine alcohol abuse. To answer these questions, we must examine the clinical utility of these diagnostic tests in several areas as described below.

Confirmation of Suspicion of Alcohol Abuse

It is widely known today that the initial screening tests perceived by insurers as the most helpful in identifying potential abusive drinking are GGT, elevated HDL-C, and AST. Indeed, elevations of AST and HDL-C are associated with high positive rates of CDT, whereas elevations of GGT are associated with high positive rates of HAA. Thus, in the presence of an unproven suspicion of alcohol abuse as evidenced by elevations in a number of screening tests or other suspicious factors, CDT and HAA show optimal performance as confirmatory tools for harmful drinking.

Screening for Alcohol Abuse in the General Population

One of the largest known studies on alcohol abuse or dependence among family care practices confirmed that conventional laboratory tests are of little use for detecting alcohol abuse or dependence in a primary care setting without first having a suspicion of alcohol-related problems. The study concludes that the %CDT test performed poorly and cannot be used as a screening instrument in a general practice population with a 9% past-year prevalence of alcohol abuse or dependence. The EDAC test was recently evaluated as a screening tool to assess heavy drinking in 1,680 insurance applicants. Ninety-three percent of applicants showed a negative EDAC test. The 7% (n = 134) who screened positive for the EDAC test were then sequentially tested (reflex testing) with CDT and HAA. Sixteen percent (22/134) showed a positive confirmatory test. Among these 16% of subjects, 41% (9/22) showed no elevations in liver enzymes or HDL-C results. These results suggest that the EDAC screen may provide an efficient alternative-screening tool for the identification of heavy alcohol consumption as it identifies applicants with both normal and abnormal liver enzymes and HDL-C.

Routine Health Examination

A recent, large-scale study suggests that CDT can provide useful information to primary care clinicians when studying patients with pre-existing illnesses. Indeed, it was found that 57% of persons with diabetes and hypertension use alcohol but that less than 20% were asked about alcohol use by their physician. The findings suggest that a CDT test and an alcohol use history should be obtained as part of the initial assessment in general practitioners' offices. Recent studies also have reported a significant correlation between plasma HDL concentrations and biomarkers of harmful alcohol drinking. In men in particular, CDT has shown an extremely strong correlation with elevated HDL-C levels; men with HDL-C >70 mg/dL and >80 mg/dL had CDT positive rates more than 10-fold and 14-fold higher, respectively, than men with HDL-C levels <70 mg/dL. Based on these studies, HDL-C may represent a useful routine marker for recent excessive alcohol intake, and high HDL-C levels should potentially alert clinicians to investigate a patient's recent pattern of alcohol consumption.

Monitoring Abstinence and Relapses

A change in CDT over time can be used as an outcome measure in alcoholism treatment research because CDT changes with drinking status. Abstinent patients have an average 30% decrease in CDT, while patients who relapse to heavy drinking have an average 30% increase in CDT when relapse is defined as 2 drinking days over the past 2 weeks. Also, a recent study concluded that a change in both CDT and GGT could be used simultaneously to improve detection of relapse drinking. This type of comparison may be used during longitudinal testing in a person in recovery. In addition to the CDT test, the performance of the EDAC and HAA tests was recently analyzed in a group of patients after discharge from residential treatment. In the relapse group, the EDAC had a sensitivity of 52%, which was greater than the sensitivity of the CDT test (19%) and the HAA assay (16%). This study concludes that combining two or three biomarkers of alcohol abuse improves the detection of relapse episodes in these patients.

Forensic Applications

A recent study concludes that the analysis of FAEEs in hair is a useful diagnostic tool to prove heavy drinking behavior in fatalities. In a similar study, the comparison of FAEE with GGT, GPT, and MCV produced a relatively high sensitivity of FAEEs for the detection of alcohol abuse. On the basis of a cut-off value of 1.0 ng/mg, 15 of the 19 cases (80%) were positive and 2 additional cases were just below this limit. When a cut-off of 1.0 ng/mg is used, strong alcoholics can be distinguished from teetotalers and moderate social drinkers with relatively high accuracy. Thus, FAEEs in hair can be an efficient tool to support the clinical diagnosis of alcohol abuse, particularly in combination with, or as a supplement to, the classic markers of alcohol abuse. Also, CDT has been reported to be stable in post-mortem serum for many hours after death and may be useful in detecting chronic alcohol exposure prior to death.

Public Safety (Pilots, DUI Offenders)

A study carried out in a large workplace in the transport sector offered employees the opportunity to undergo an alcohol screen and check their alcohol habits during their routine health examination. Findings suggest that the Alcohol Use Disorders Identification Test (AUDIT) and CDT are complementary instruments for alcohol screening in a routine workplace health examination, and each has value for identifying a different segment of the risky drinking population.

Differential Diagnosis

CDT also is a good tool for differential diagnosis when the clinician wants to identify alcohol abuse among other medical conditions. For instance, there is ample evidence that alcohol misuse can lead to irreversible physical injuries and neuro-psychiatric disorders. Approximately 20% of sequentially received specimens for peripheral neuropathy testing were positive for CDT in the absence of autoantibodies, suggesting an alcohol-related etiology. In fact, elevated serum concentrations of CDT can identify alcohol misuse in patients with idiopathic peripheral neuropathies and non-inflammatory myopathy. Similarly, in 102 patients with biopsy-verified liver diseases, CDT values were normal in all of the 87 non-alcohol-abusing patients, irrespective of type or degree of liver disease. Alcoholic patients (87%) with current abuse showed elevated CDT values, while in abstaining alcoholics with remaining liver disease the values were normal. No correlations were found between CDT level and volume density of liver fibrosis or steatosis. The only significant correlation was between CDT concentration and the level of present daily alcohol consumption in the alcoholic patients. These results indicate that CDT can be used as a marker of present but not previous alcohol abuse, even in patients with various liver diseases. In a more recent study, it was discovered that an elevated CDT value might not accurately represent alcohol consumption in patients with advanced liver disease. In fact, CDT may be a marker for the degree of liver impairment in alcoholic and non-alcoholic liver disease.

SUMMARY

The use of markers to identify heavy consumption of alcohol for a variety of purposes is an important and expanding part of medical practice. Indirect markers such as GGT and CDT have been extensively studied and are well established as indicators of heavy consumption. However, these two markers alone or even in combination do not have the diagnostic sensitivity and accuracy to serve as standalone tests. More recently, analytical advancements have allowed scientists the ability to measure the very low levels of alcohol or acetaldehyde conjugates in blood. These "direct" markers are in the early stage of their development, but they may provide additional laboratory tests for the assessment of problematic alcohol consumption.

SUGGESTED READINGS

Aertgeerts B, Buntinx F, Ansoms S, Fevery J: Screening properties of questionnaires and laboratory tests for the detection of alcohol abuse or dependence in a general practice population. Br Genl Pract 51(464): 206–217, 2001.

Anton RF, Dominick C, Bigelow M, Westby C, in collaboration with the CDTect research group: Comparison of Bio-Rad %CDT TIA and CDTect as laboratory markers of heavy alcohol use and their relationships with gamma-glutamyltransferase. Clin Chem 47(10):1769–1775, 2001.

Anton RF, Lieber C, Tabakoff B: Carbohydrate-deficient transferrin and gamma-glutamyltransferase for the detection and monitoring of alcohol use: results from a multisite study. Alcohol Clin Exp Res 26(8): 1215–1222, 2002.

Doyle KM, Cluette-Brown JE, Dube DM, Bernhardt TG, Morse CR, Laposata M: Fatty acid ethyl esters in the blood as markers for ethanol intake. JAMA 276(14):1152–1156, 1996.

Javors M, Johnson B: Current status of carbohydrate deficient transferrin, total serum sialic acid, sialic acid index of apolipoprotein J, and serum β-hexosaminidase as markers for alcohol consumption. Addiction (in press).

Meerkerk GJ, Njoo KH, Bongers IM, Trienekens P, van Oers JA: The specificity of the CDT assay in general practice: the influence of common chronic diseases and medication on the serum CDT concentration. Alcohol Clin Exp Res 22(4):908–913, 1998.

Varga A, Hansson P, Lundqvist C, Alling C: Phosphatidylethanol in blood as a marker of ethanol consumption in healthy volunteers: comparison with other markers. Alcohol Clin Exp Res 22(8):1832–1837, 1998.

Wurst FM, Kempter C, Metzger J, Seidl S, Alt A: Ethyl glucuronide: a marker of recent alcohol consumption with clinical and forensic implications. Alcohol 20(2):111–116, 2000.

ASSESSING MEDICAL CONSEQUENCES OF ALCOHOLISM

Shimi K. Kang
David Gastfriend

Alcohol has pervasive consequences for the human body. The medical consequences of alcohol represent some of the most important public health problems confronting society. They are among the most common causes of hospital visits, and the fourth leading cause of death among adults aged 25–65 years in urban areas. Substance abuse in general and related health problems add $114 billion each year to the cost of health care in the United States. Additional costs include lost employment opportunities and crime that occur because of alcohol.

Alcohol's direct effect on the body's vital organs is profound. In addition, vast physiologic and morphologic changes occur from chronic alcohol exposure. In combination, these effects leave the alcohol abuser with an abnormal response to alcohol, drugs, other toxins, and even basic nutrition. Almost all body tissues are vulnerable to deleterious effects of alcohol. For this reason, this chapter is organized along the classic medical review of systems. Remarkably, almost all of the medical consequences of alcoholism are fully reversible with abstinence and nutritional replacement. For the purposes of this chapter, the few disorders that are unfortunately permanent despite alcohol cessation and treatment will be specifically noted.

CENTRAL NERVOUS SYSTEM

The central nervous system is one of the body systems most frequently and most seriously affected by alcohol. The deleterious effects of alcohol are caused by direct toxic effects on neuronal membranes, by neuronal damage from withdrawal after chronic intoxication, or by nutritional deficiency.

Wernicke's Encephalopathy and Alcohol Amnestic Disorder (Korsakoff's Dementia)

Wernicke's encephalopathy refers to an acute or subacute disease manifested by nystagmus, sixth nerve and conjugate gaze palsies, gait ataxia, and mental disturbances such as confusion, apathy, and drowsiness. The condition somewhat mistakenly termed Korsakoff's dementia refers to these symptoms combined with an intense anterograde amnesia that is more severe than the general level of cognitive impairment—thus, it is not a true dementia. The current nosology for this condition is *alcohol amnestic disorder*. These disorders begin when heavy drinking causes intestinal malabsorption and thiamine (vitamin B_1) deficiency. The etiology is not well understood, but proposed mechanisms include altered cerebral energy metabolism, decreased nerve-impulse transmission at synapses, or impaired DNA synthesis. Patients may be genetically predisposed to the syndrome, and treatment involves administration of thiamine 100 mg/d for at least three months. Untreated, it carries a mortality of 15%, and only one third of those with complete short-term memory impairment will demonstrate clinically relevant recovery even with full treatment. Brain imaging and autopsy studies typically show microhemorrhages in the mammillary bodies, in the dorsomedial nucleus of the thalamus, and in the periventricular gray matter of the brain. Electroencephalographic patterns may show diffuse slowing in the initial phase of the illness in about half of patients.

Dementia

Dementia can occur because of both the direct effects of alcohol and specific vitamin deficiencies. It is possible that 15%–30% of nursing home patients have alcohol-induced dementia. Brain imaging studies typically show deterioration of the corpus callosum, cerebral atrophy, and white matter hyperintensities. Ventricular enlargement and sulcal widening also are characteristic. Although abstinence and nutritional repletion can significantly improve cognition for some patients, some aspects of alcohol dementia are irreversible despite vigorous treatment.

Marchiafava-Bignami syndrome involves degeneration of the corpus callosum and has been reported in wine drinkers of Italian heritage. Symptoms include confusion, dysphasia, seizures, and, at the extreme end of the spectrum of corpus callosum degeneration, dementia.

Delirium

Delirium can result, and may be secondary to alcohol withdrawal or to such consequences of chronic alcohol dependence as stroke, hemorrhage, subdural hematoma, or a hepatic or toxic leukoencephalopathy.

Stroke

Hemorrhagic, embolic, and thrombotic stroke may be more common in alcoholics owing to underlying hypertension, hyperlipidemia with atherosclerotic disease, and/or coagulopathies. Coagulopathy may also be responsible for an increased incidence of subdural hematomas in those who suffer head trauma.

Alcoholic Coma

Coma is common in those with a blood alcohol level (BAL) of 500 mg/dl, and is lethal in half of these patients. However, severe chronic drinkers with BALs $\geq$ 500 mg/dl may be relatively unaffected owing to acquired tolerance. If low BALs are associated with profound stupor and coma, complicating illness or the ingestion of another sedative drug should be suspected.

Seizures

Seizures are the most common serious neurologic problem in alcoholics. They are usually isolated and generalized and occur during the first two days of alcohol withdrawal. Electroencephalographic and computed tomography studies are typically normal, and in the absence of further alcohol ingestion, seizures usually do not recur. Special electrolyte monitoring including the correction of magnesium deficiency should be performed, as this may increase the seizure threshold.

Cerebellar Disorders

Alcohol-induced cerebellar degeneration results in a rapidly progressive permanent incoordination and is seen in less than 1% of people with alcohol dependence. More commonly, ataxia of gait and the extremities occurs, with leg ataxia being more prevalent than arm ataxia. The characteristic stance is a wide-based gait with the trunk tilted slightly forward and arms held slightly away from the sides. Ataxia usually follows a history of poor nutrition and long-standing heavy alcohol use.

Cerebellar syndrome is clinically and pathologically similar to Wernicke 's encephalopathy but connotes the isolated cerebellar manifestations without ocular and mental signs. Dysarthria and postural tremor are commonly observed, with either an abrupt or insidious onset, and then may remain unchanged for many years.

Central Pontine Myelinolysis

Central pontine myelinolysis is a devastating condition that usually occurs in nutritionally debilitated alcoholics in the setting of rapid correction of hyponatremia. The resulting pseudobulbar manifestations may include emotional lability, pathologic crying, speech difficulties, facial paralysis, quadriplegia, confusion, coma, and death.

Alcoholic Amblyopia

Central scotomas and decreased visual acuity for near and distant objects develop over days to weeks in alcoholic amblyopia. These changes are always bilateral and symmetrical, and funduscopic exam may show mild hyperemia, blurring of disk margins, and mild papillitis. A retrobulbar neuropathy known as tobacco-alcohol amblyopia may also produce double vision and decreased acuity.

Peripheral Neuropathy

Chronic alcohol intake leading to the destruction of peripheral nerves is seen in 5%–15% of chronic alcohol abusers. Damage first occurs to the smaller nerves in the feet and hands, with the legs being generally affected before the arms; hence the term "stocking-glove" distribution. Common symptoms include weakness, burning paresthesias, and pain. Characteristic signs include lower extremity atrophy, muscle tenderness, decreased Achilles and patellar reflexes, and impaired superficial sensation over the shins and feet. A "burning feet" syndrome also may occur, and manifests as a distressing sensation of heat, usually on the soles of the feet, made worse with contact or stimulation.

At later stages of severe alcohol dependence, motor neuropathy with loss more common in the distal rather than the proximal muscles can occur. Foot or wrist drop may be seen first, followed by shoulder and hip girdle weakness, and rarely complete limb paralysis. End stage alcoholism may be associated with autonomic neuropathy, leading to orthostatic hypotension and gastric emptying abnormalities.

Effects on Motor Activity

All types of motor performance can be affected by alcohol, whether it be the simple maintenance of standing posture, control of speech, or highly complex motor skills. All motor tasks are more slowly and inaccurately executed with alcohol use. Even mild intoxication is associated with significant adverse effects on hand-eye coordination. Alcohol intoxication causes decreased peak saccadic velocity, which results in fragmentation of smooth eye pursuit movements.

Effects on Intelligence

Intellectual capabilities including memory, learning, and judgment are impaired by alcohol intoxication. The amount and concentration of alcohol are important determinants of mental function. Low alcohol concentrations produce an increase in low-amplitude fast activity on the electroencephalograph, and higher alcohol levels cause slowing and synchronization, which can manifest as depression of consciousness. Most people presenting for alcohol detoxification show signs of intellectual impairment. Brain imaging studies demonstrate that 40%–70% show signs of enlarged ventricles possibly secondary to decreased brain tissue. It is likely that both ventricular size and IQ testing recover with abstinence. Although controversial and unclear, the etiology of cognitive impairment could be a combination of trauma, vitamin deficiencies, neuronal membrane deformation, neurotransmitter disruptions, and other direct neurotoxic effects of alcohol.

Memory Deficits

Memory deficits can occur in all alcohol consumers along the spectrum of mild impairment to alcohol amnestic disorder and dementia. The term "blackout" has a specific meaning: a transient period of amnesia during intoxication and often without evidence of other neuropsychologic impairment, usually in the context of rapid elevation of blood alcohol content. Blackouts are possibly due to effects on short-term memory function and may be an early predictor of alcohol dependence disorder.

Pathologic Intoxication

Pathologic intoxication is a rare, extreme, excitatory effect caused by alcohol in a small proportion of the population. It is characterized by a bizarre outburst of indiscriminate fury, combativeness, and destructive behavior in persons without a history of alcoholism or mental or neurologic disease.

GASTROINTESTINAL SYSTEM

Effects on the Upper Gastrointestinal Tract

Glossitis and stomatitis are likely due to poor nutrition. Peptic esophagitis with complicating strictures may result from injury of the esophageal mucosa by ethanol. Late stage alcoholism with portal hypertension can lead to potentially fatal bleeding from Mallory-Weiss tears and esophageal varices.

Effects on the Liver

Alcohol is metabolized primarily in the liver following gastrointestinal absorption. Adverse liver changes can occur with the consumption of as little as 20 g/d of alcohol for women and 40 g/d for men.

The toxicity of alcohol on the liver is thought to be secondary to the use of alcohol by liver cells as a "preferred fuel." Even a small dose of alcohol disturbs gluconeogenesis (sugar production) and shunts carbohydrate moieties into fat production. The sequence of liver damage begins with acute fatty metamorphosis (with repeated blood alcohol levels of 80 mg/dl), followed by alcoholic hepatitis, then irreversible perivenular fibrosis, and ultimately cirrhosis. End stage liver disease results in liver cell failure and portal hypertension with complicating splenomegaly, jaundice, coagulopathies, hormonal changes, esophageal varices, or spontaneous bacterial peritonitis from ascites.

Heavy alcohol use certainly exacerbates infectious hepatitis and interferes with the success of treatment. The combination of alcoholism and hepatitis C causes enhanced liver toxicity, with damage seen in excess of that expected from the simple additive effects of each.

A condition of potentially fatal liver damage occurs with the co-administration of as little as 2.5 g/d of acetaminophen (Tylenol) in the context of greater than six standard drinks of alcohol per day.

Effects on the Stomach

Alcohol favors colonization of the bacillus *Helicobacter pylori*, which produces ammonia and, in turn, contributes to gastritis and the further colonization of bacteria associated with the development of ulcers—more so with beer and wine. Thus, although causative in hemorrhagic gastritis, alcohol does not directly cause ulcer disease. Alcohol also may work synergistically with *H. pylori* to delay healing and worsen already present ulcers. Alcohol is responsible for an increased incidence of gastroesophageal reflux disease and problems with peristalsis secondary to autonomic neuropathy. High alcohol concentrations result in delayed gastric emptying of the solid portions of a meal but enhanced gastric emptying of the liquid portions.

Effects on the Small Intestine

The small intestine is exposed to high concentrations of ethanol during drinking episodes, which leads to changes in its cellular structure, metabolism, and circulation. Alcohol predisposes to hemorrhagic erosions of intestinal villi and duodenitis. These, in combination with an increase in motility, cause defective absorption of important bodily nutrients, which can have a variety of medical consequences.

Effects on the Colon

Hemorrhoids may result secondary to portal hypertension due to liver damage. Alcohol also causes decreased non-propulsive colonic activity and increased propulsive motility, potentially exacerbating hemorrhoids.

Effects on the Pancreas

Alcohol can cause pancreatic enzyme leakage due to the fragility of the cellular storage structures. This can lead to inflammation that would result in the blockage of pancreatic ducts, with further stimulation of digestive enzymes. The combination of these processes leads to both acute and chronic pancreatitis. With recurrent episodes, endocrine and exocrine insufficiency may result in diabetes, malabsorption, and fat-soluble vitamin deficiencies.

CARDIOVASCULAR SYSTEM

Cardiac Changes

Of all those with alcoholism, 25% will eventually develop some form of cardiovascular disease. The pathogenesis is mostly due to the toxicity of alcohol on striated muscle, which may produce cardiac muscle inflammation, cardiomyopathy, dysrhythmias, and left ventricular abnormalities.

Secondary damage from alcohol-induced hypertension and elevation in blood lipids and cholesterol can also contribute significantly to cardiovascular morbidity. For example, coronary artery disease is about six times greater in alcoholics (four or more drinks per day) and causes 20% more mortality. During alcohol withdrawal, all cardiac problems and electrocardiographic abnormalities are exacerbated, and new signs and symptoms also may arise.

The cardiac response to ethanol reflects the physiology of the subject, rate and quantity of alcohol ingested, and previous use. In those with left ventricular dysfunction, the depressant effects of alcohol predominate, causing a decrease in cardiac output. Alcohol also causes changes in regional blood flow and tends to increase skin, splanchnic, and myocardial blood flow and reduce blood flow to brain, muscle, limbs, and pancreas. This altered blood flow may be associated with subsequent organ injury.

Alcoholic Cardiomyopathy

Alcohol dependence can lead to two categories of cardiac dysfunction: thiamine dependent (alcoholic beriberi) or thiamine independent (alcoholic cardiomyopathy). Alcoholic cardiomyopathy is of unknown pathophysiology. Chronic alcoholics (usually greater than 10 years of heavy drinking) are found to have myocardial hypertrophy and varying degrees of myocardial and perivascular fibrosis at autopsy. The most common early complaint is breathlessness, and in the early stages symptoms appear to be out of proportion to signs of heart failure. Cough, often occurring at night, and flu-like illness are often identified. Other common symptoms include easy fatigability (reflecting a low and fixed cardiac output), palpitations associated with cardiac dysrhythmias, anorexia, edematous swelling, and abdominal discomfort caused by hepatic and intestinal congestion. As the disease progresses, physical findings of cardiac cachexia ensue, although initially weight loss is obscured by fluid retention. Blood pressure is often normal or low, and several murmurs may be audible, including gallop rhythm with loud S3 and S4 with accentuated pulmonic closure, diminished S1, and soft apical systolic murmur. Echocardiography will demonstrate features of dilated cardiomyopathy, and electrocardiographic findings are not specific. Alcoholic cardiomyopathy is generally irreversible, although some symptomatic relief can certainly occur with abstinence.

Beriberi

Beriberi is a rare cause of heart disease in alcoholics and is recognized as a thiamine-dependent cardiomyopathy. Cardiomegaly, hyperdynamic circulation, circulatory congestion, and thiamine responsiveness characterize beriberi.

Holiday Heart Syndrome

This is a condition of acute cardiac rhythm and/or conduction disturbance (particularly supraventricular tachycardias) after heavy alcohol consumption in otherwise healthy people. Atrial fibrillation is the most common rhythm disorder and usually converts to normal sinus rhythm within 24 hours. The syndrome may recur, but its clinical course is benign, and specific antiarrhythmic therapy is not usually needed. The mechanism of this syndrome is not certain, but proposed mechanisms include increased secretion of epinephrine and norepinephrine, a rise in the level of free fatty acids, or as an indirect result of acetaldehyde, the primary metabolite of alcohol. The most common symptom is palpitations, but occasionally patients experience near syncopal symptoms, dyspnea on exertion, and angina.

Hypertension

Mild elevations in blood pressure can be the result of alcoholism, especially if there is pressure fluctuating over time. As little as 1 g/kg body weight per day of ethanol over 5 days can result in a significant pressure increase—even more so in those with previous hypertension. Since hypertension is the leading risk factor for stroke, alcohol tends to increase the incidence of hemorrhagic stroke, embolic stroke secondary to cardiac thrombus, and cerebral ischemic infarction. Hypertension is frequently seen in alcohol withdrawal, even in those without a previous history, and can lead to significant complications. The type of beverage used, race, and age may influence the impact of alcohol consumption on blood pressure. For example, beer, wine, saki, and whiskey are particularly associated with increased blood pressure. Also, those over 50 years old are more sensitive to the effects of alcohol on blood pressure.

Effects on Cholesterol Levels

Hyperlipidemia develops because lipogenesis is promoted by the altered redux state secondary to ethanol oxidation. This altered redux state is characterized by a preference for ethanol rather than lipid as fuel for the liver, causing fat accumulation in the liver, which is a stimulus for lipid secretion into the bloodstream. As alcoholism proceeds to severe hepatic damage, the impairment of the liver's secretory capacity may actually produce the opposite effect, leading to relative malnutrition and cachexia. Alcohol also has an acute myocardial depressant effect that decreases lipid metabolism and increases formation of abnormal metabolic by-products such as fatty acid ethyl esters.

HEMATOLOGIC SYSTEM

Alcohol can have a profound effect on the body's hematologic system, resulting in a variety of anemias, leukopenias, and coagulopathies. Overall, a picture of pancytopenia can occur because of bone marrow toxicity and/or splenic sequestration from portal hypertension-induced splenomegaly. Additionally, macrocytic anemia results from folic acid and B_{12} deficiency, abnormal red blood cell release from the bone marrow, and membrane defects. Microcytic anemia may result from iron deficiency and ongoing upper gastrointestinal blood loss. Normocytic anemia may result from a state of chronic disease, bone marrow suppression, or both. A decreased hematocrit may result solely from expanded plasma volume. White cell deficiency and particularly lymphopenia could predispose the alcohol abuser to infections. Thrombocytopenia from bone marrow suppression and splenic platelet sequestration, in combination with decreased hepatic production of clotting factors, all contribute to gastrointestinal bleeding, easy bruising, and other coagulopathies.

Alcoholic liver disease may alter red blood cell membrane lipids that can manifest as macrocytes, target cells, burr cells, and schistocytes—all leading to hemolytic anemia and acanthocytosis.

Malnourished alcoholics often have ringed sideroblasts, possibly as a result of inhibition of heme synthesis, and can develop sideroblastic anemia. Also, depressed serum and red blood cell phosphate levels may lead to spherocytosis, decreased red blood cell membrane fluidity, decreased adenosine triphosphate production, and acute hemolysis.

IMMUNE SYSTEM

Alcohol is associated with decreased immune functioning, resulting in an increased risk of infection and cancer.

Infection

The alcohol abuser may be prone to infection from malnutrition, splenic dysfunction, leukopenia, granulocyte dysfunction (decreased adherence to capillary walls and less mobilization to inflammatory sites), and an impaired gag reflex. Aspiration pneumonia, empyema, HIV, sexually transmitted diseases, brain abscess, meningitis, spontaneous bacterial peritonitis, and tuberculosis are frequent in heavy drinkers with an increased rate of mortality and longer, more costly hospital stays.

Cancer

Alcoholics have higher rates of cancer of the aerodigestive system (lip, oral cavity, tongue, pharynx, larynx, esophagus, stomach, and colon), breast, liver, bile duct, and lung. This is true even when confounding factors of diet, smoking, and lifestyle are excluded. Ingestion of as little as one or two drinks per day is associated with a moderately increased risk of breast cancer. Alcohol's role in cancer is primarily that of a co-carcinogen; that is, it enhances the carcinogenic activity of other carcinogens such as tobacco. Other possible mechanisms of cancer induction include local irritation of the lung or digestive tract lining, or impaired immune system function that would otherwise identify and destroy cancer cells. For example, lower T cells and thymus-derived lymph factors may all be contributing factors for increased cancer rates in alcoholics.

MUSCULOSKELETAL SYSTEM

Muscle

Muscle inflammation can result from alcohol binges, and muscle wasting, especially in the shoulders and hips, can develop from chronic heavy alcohol consumption. Inflammation can produce compartment syndromes or rhabdomyolysis, a condition characterized by acute muscle pain, rapid muscle tissue destruction, and potential kidney failure that is specifically associated with tissue necrosis from pressure sores during states of unconsciousness. Alcoholic myopathy (which is classified as acute, chronic, or subclinical) is either due to the direct impact of ethanol on skeletal muscle or secondary to metabolic derangements because skeletal muscle does not oxidize ethanol. Acute myopathy manifests as patchy, often distal muscle tenderness, sometimes associated with weakness, neuropathy, and very high levels of creatinine kinase. Chronic myopathy from long-standing alcohol abuse presents as a symmetric proximal muscle weakness frequently with associated neuropathy and a moderate rise in creatine kinase but without tenderness. Subclinical myopathy has characteristics of both the acute and chronic forms.

Bones

Decreased bone density and strength (osteoporosis) occurs in alcoholics, possibly related to changes in parathyroid hormone and cortisol. In the bone marrow, increased osteoclast activity and decreased osteoblast activity result in further osteopenia. Osteonecrosis, such as that of the femoral head, may also occur with heavy alcohol consumption. All of these, in addition to trauma, lead to increased incidence of bone fractures.

PULMONARY

Alcohol intoxication can lead to respiratory depression with complicating aspiration and chemical and/or infectious pneumonitis. Tachypnea can occur secondary to infection, respiratory alkalosis from liver disease, or alcohol withdrawal.

RENAL

Altered kidney function in a chronic alcohol user can often be attributed to liver disease. This, in addition to the renal effects of alcohol intoxication, causes impaired regulation of uric acid, fluids, and electrolytes. Cirrhosis can result in the generally fatal complication of renal ischemia in hepatorenal syndrome. Dilutional hyponatremia, hypokalemia, hypophosphatemia, and hypomagnesemia can develop because of sodium retention with chronic liver disease. Hypomagnesemia as a result of diuretic use, hypokalemia, and hyperparathyroidism is common and leads to hypocalcemia that responds only to magnesium replacement. Hyperuricemia can result in renal failure, but it more commonly presents as the swollen, red, and exquisitely tender great toe of gout. Alcohol abuse leads to acid-base disturbances, and metabolic acidosis may result from lactic acidosis (sepsis, injury, pancreatitis, post-ictal) or ketoacidosis. Respiratory acidosis develops in cases of intoxication with respiratory depression. Metabolic alkalosis may result with prolonged vomiting or profuse diarrhea. Respiratory alkalosis may be seen in alcohol withdrawal or in cirrhosis due to endogenous toxins. Dehydration, often contributing to prerenal failure, is common in heavy drinkers with presenting symptoms of vomiting, diarrhea, and diuresis.

METABOLISM

Glucose

Alcohol leads to carbohydrate-regulation abnormalities due to impaired liver and pancreatic response. Decreased insulin sensitivity during alcohol withdrawal and impaired insulin response during acute alcohol consumption can result in states of either very high or very low blood glucose. A life-threatening condition known as alcoholic lactic acidosis or ketoacidosis characterized by nausea, vomiting, abdominal pain, and abnormal blood glucose can occur, resulting in decreased electrolytes, such as sodium, potassium, magnesium, calcium, and phosphorus.

Protein

Alcohol leads to cerebral atrophy by decreasing brain protein synthesis. Although effects on liver protein synthesis have not been found, alcohol does interfere with protein secretion by the liver, and this may be the basis for the "ballooning" effect of hepatocytes seen in cell necrosis in alcoholic liver injury.

HORMONES AND SEXUAL FUNCTION

Parathyroid hormone, insulin, adrenocorticotropic hormone, prolactin, cortisol, and growth hormone levels may all be altered by alcohol consumption. Men may experience resulting decreased testosterone production, decreased sperm count and motility, sexual dysfunction, and infertility. They also may have testicular atrophy and gynecomastia with end stage liver disease due to the abnormal production of estrogen. Women may experience early or delayed menopause and menstrual irregularities such as dysmenorrhea or metrorrhagia because of malnutrition, coagulopathies, or both. Amounts as little as one standard drink per week are associated with decreased fertility in women.

NUTRITION

Alcohol is a source of "empty calories"—making alcoholism one of the major causes of nutritional deficiency in the United States. Contributing factors include direct toxicity to tissues, interference with nutritional absorption and metabolism, decreased nutrient intake, and nutrient loss from the body. Thiamine (vitamin B_1) deficiency leads to Wernicke-Korsakoff syndrome, beriberi heart disease, and polyneuropathy. Vitamin B_6 deficiency causes neurologic, hematologic, and dermatologic disorders.

Folic acid and vitamin B_{12} depletion leads to megaloblastic anemia and associated neurologic deficits. Zinc deficiency is associated with rough, dry skin, mental lethargy, disordered taste, and poor appetite. Vitamin A, B_2, C, D, E, and K, magnesium, calcium, folate, phosphate, and iron also have been found to be deficient in alcoholics. Improved nutrition and abstinence are necessary to correct these deficiencies; however, active replacement with thiamine, folic acid, and multivitamins for at least three months is often indicated because malabsorption may prevent adequate correction even with resumption of good nutritional intake. Severe cases should receive acute intramuscular thiamine, because malabsorption is often a complication.

SLEEP

Alcohol can be stimulating and results in initial and middle insomnia, periodic limb movements, and daytime fatigue although, paradoxically, many alcoholics require a drink to quell withdrawal-related sympathetic arousal in order to fall asleep. Even moderate alcohol at dinner, in non-alcoholic middle-aged men, has been shown to diminish rapid eye movement stage sleep. After cessation of chronic alcohol consumption, rapid eye movement rebound results in vivid dreams that may cause the individual to awaken; thus, the rapid eye movement stage cycle is not completed, and there is ongoing sleep deprivation.

Obstructive sleep apnea can be caused or worsened by alcohol owing to its depressant effects on respiration and relaxation of the upper airway.

PREGNANCY

Heavy consumption during pregnancy, generally considered to be over 2 oz of absolute alcohol per day, is associated with birth defects in 32%–50% of cases. Increased rates of miscarriage are associated with consuming 1–2 standard drinks per week during the first or second trimester. Fetal alcohol syndrome is caused by chronic alcohol consumption during pregnancy. It is characterized by decreased prenatal and postnatal growth (below the 10th percentile), craniofacial abnormalities, and impaired central nervous system development. Central nervous system involvement includes developmental delay, intellectual impairment, brain malformation, head circumference below the third percentile, and other signs of neurologic abnormalities. Craniofacial dysmorphology includes microphthalmia and/ or short palpebral fissures, elongated midface, poorly developed philtrum, thin upper lip, and flattening of the maxillary area. Alcohol-related birth defects or fetal alcohol effects are terms used to describe hyperactivity, learning disabilities, and other behavioral problems secondary to alcohol use in pregnancy that do not meet the full criteria for fetal alcohol syndrome.

OTHER

Other areas affected by alcohol include oral changes such as gum disease, tooth decay, and parotid gland enlargement. Skin conditions such as eczema and psoriasis are seen, and dystrophic changes of the skin of the lower legs and feet are common including stasis edema and pigmentation, glossiness, and thinness of skin. Trauma from motor vehicle accidents, physical abuse and/or sexual abuse can be frequently seen in heavy drinkers. Perioperative complications such as withdrawal, infection, bleeding, pneumonia, delayed wound healing, and dysrhythmias are also seen with alcohol dependence.

PHYSICAL EXAMINATION

A comprehensive physical examination should always be performed, noting areas of reported symptoms and those of particular importance for alcohol dependence. Early on, there is usually little evidence of alcohol abuse, and patients may have few signs other than elevated blood pressure. At later stages, significant signs appear, the most ominous being in the neurologic system and the liver. Both obvious and subtle changes should be noted, according to body systems. A list of important abnormalities is presented in Table 8.1.

MENTAL STATUS EXAMINATION

Common findings are signs of intoxication, withdrawal, retrograde or anterograde amnesia, encephalopathy, delirium, dementia, or major psychiatric consequences and/or co-morbidity. Patients with

Table 8.1.   Common Physical Examination Abnormalities in Alcohol Abuse and Dependence

Vital signs

Tachycardia, abnormal respiratory rate, hypertension, postural hypotension, temperature elevation, malnutrition (height & weight for body mass index)

Skin

Jaundice, perspiration, pallor, bruises, track marks, spider nevi, palmar erythema, hyperpigmentation of lower legs, poor skin turgor

Head, eyes, ears, nose, throat

Head—microcephaly, meningeal signs, lymphadenopathy, head trauma;
Oral Cavity—malignant lesions, glossitis, stomatitis, parotid enlargement, dental hygiene, gum disease;
Nasal Cavity—signs of bleeding;
Eyes—visual fields, extraocular muscles (ophthalmoplegia, lateral gaze palsy), nystagmus, dilated or constricted pupils, scleral icterus, fundi—blurred disc, papillitis, hyperemia

Pulmonary

Infection—tuberculosis, aspiration, infectious/chemical pneumonia, empyema

Breasts

Lumps, masses, gynecomastia

Cardiovascular

Enlarged heart, displaced apical pulse, thrills, heart sounds, arrhythmia, murmurs, hypertension, peripheral edema

Gastrointestinal

General Abdomen—obesity, caput medusae, ascites, tenderness; Epigastric – gastritis, peptic ulcer disease
Right Upper Quadrant—hepatitis, cholecystitis
Left Upper Quadrant—splenomegaly, pancreatitis
Hepatic—enlargement, edge firmness, tenderness
Rectum—hemorrhoids

(Continued)

Table 8.1.   Continued

Musculoskeletal

> *Muscle*—atrophy, tenderness, weakness
> *Bone*—signs of fracture, spinal tenderness,
> signs of gout

Central nervous system

> Cranial nerves, tremor, peripheral neuropathy,
> myopathy, motor weakness, limb & gait
> ataxia (wide-based, slow, uncertain, short-
> stepped gait), asterixis, cerebellar signs,
> positive Romberg's sign, deep tendon reflex
> changes

Reproductive

> Sexually transmitted diseases, loss of sexual
> hair, testicular atrophy, early menopause

long-standing alcoholism can sometimes present disheveled and unkempt, but appearance can just as easily be well kept. Those with Korsakoff syndrome will be alert and oriented but lack the ability to provide an appropriate recent history and manifest anterograde and retrograde amnesia and confabulation. Affect can range from normal to apathetic to acute delirium in those with alcohol withdrawal. No characteristic speech pattern or perceptual disturbances exist unless the patient presents in acute intoxication or withdrawal. Mood may vary from agitated to constricted to depressed. Thought form and content may vary from impoverished to expansive and frankly psychotic.

LABORATORY ABNORMALITIES

The most common blood test abnormalities due to alcoholism include elevated liver function tests, elevated creatine phosphokinase, elevated uric acid, hypercholesterolemia and other lipid abnormalities, and changes in hematologic components (hemoglobin, mean corpuscular volume, white blood cells, platelets, partial thromboplastin time/International Normalized Ratio). Although liver function abnormalities are often found in the initial screening of alcohol users, only about one in five people actually present with clinically significant hepatic damage. Gamma-glutamyl transferase is the most sensitive and earliest indicator of alcohol consumption, and it increases in response to direct induction by ethanol. Alanine aminotransferase and aspartate aminotransferase do not usually change unless liver cells have actually been altered. Liver function tests may return to normal within 4–12 weeks of abstaining and may increase rapidly with resumption of drinking. Carbohydrate-deficient transferrin, a blood protein responsible for transfer of iron, will show decreased levels after one week of about six drinks per day. Other lab abnormalities may include positive infection testing for HIV, tuberculosis, hepatitis, and other sexually transmitted diseases and markers such as blood methanol levels, levels of unusual alcohols such as dolichols, beta-hexosaminidase, and unusual forms of red blood cell constituents.

CONCLUSIONS

Medical consequences of alcohol abuse and dependence are vast and range from the covert to the obvious. Meticulous effort by the physician in history-taking, physical exam, and laboratory testing often pays off, both (1) in the discovery of health problems in need of care and (2) as an incentive for the patient to redouble efforts at self-protection. Assessment of medical consequences, if performed diligently and sensitively, can be highly motivating for alcohol-dependent patients. Integration of the medical data with intervention and rehabilitation counseling is empowering, and is, therefore, of vital and lasting benefit.

ACKNOWLEDGMENT

The authors wish to extend their appreciation to Mia Zarharna, B.Sc., for her assistance in bibliographic research and editorial preparation of this chapter.

SUGGESTED READINGS

Agarwal DP, Seitz HK: Alcohol in Health and Disease. New York: Marcel Dekker Inc., 2001.

Enoch M-A: Problem drinking and alcoholism: diagnosis and treatment. Am Fam Phys 65:441–450, 2002.

Evert DL, Oscar-Berman M: Alcohol-related cognitive impairments: an overview of how alcoholism may affect the workings of the brain. Alcohol Health Res World 19(2):89–96, 1995.

Graham AW, Schultz TK (eds.): American Society of Addiction Medicine (ASAM), Principles of Addiction Medicine, Third Edition. Chevy Chase, MD: ASAM Inc., 1998.

Hennekens CH: Alcohol and risk of coronary events. In: Zakhari S, Wassef M (eds.), Alcohol and the Cardiovascular System. NIAAA Research Monograph No. 31. NIH Pub. No. 96–4133. Washington, D.C.: U.S. Government Printing Office, 1996, pp. 15–24.

ASSESSING THE BRAIN SEQUELAE OF ALCOHOLISM USING NEUROIMAGING

Mark S. George
Hugh Myrick
Xingbao Li
Raymond Anton

Many of the profound sequelae of chronic heavy alcohol use were discovered years ago through pathological studies at autopsy. However, the recent development of new tools for structural and functional brain imaging has extended this earlier knowledge. One can now noninvasively assess, with neuroimaging, the brain sequelae of alcohol use. So far, imaging studies have demonstrated that chronic alcohol consumption causes cortical loss, some of which is reversible with abstinence. Additionally, alcohol acts as a global central nervous system (CNS) depressant, with chronic use resulting in reduced activity, from which it may take a month or more to recover. Finally, these imaging tools are also beginning to shed light on which brain regions are active when an alcoholic has the urge to drink. Neuroimaging studies have helped improve understanding of the brain effects of alcohol and will likely continue to advance understanding in this area.

ASSESSING THE EFFECTS OF ALCOHOL ON BRAIN STRUCTURE

Brain Atrophy

It is very clear that chronic alcohol use causes brain damage, and that the entire brain volume shrinks. Neuroimaging techniques such as computerized tomography (CT) and magnetic resonance imaging (MRI) have documented ventricular volume enlargement as well as deficits in gray and white matter volumes in alcoholics as compared to non-alcoholic subjects. This cellular loss is greater in older alcoholics than younger alcoholics, even after the duration and amount of alcohol consumed are taken into consideration. The loss in both gray and white matter is different from what has been found in other neurodegenerative disorders such as Alzheimer's disease, in which the cell loss is gray matter alone. In addition, the gray and white matter loss in alcoholics is most pronounced in the frontal lobes. Interestingly, some, but not all, of the brain volume loss associated with alcoholism has been found to reverse within a few weeks of abstinence.

Gender Differences

While many studies have evaluated brain structure in alcoholic men, alcoholic women have received less research attention. Women may be more vulnerable to the brain effects of alcohol; while they develop alcoholism later in life, they often manifest adverse consequences of alcoholism sooner than do male alcoholics, a phenomenon often referred to as "telescoping." For example, two early studies using CT found that male and female alcoholics had a similar effect on the ventricle:brain ratio despite the fact that the women had less daily alcohol consumption. This led to the hypothesis that women may be more vulnerable to the toxic effects of alcohol. However, a follow-up MRI study failed to replicate these findings. Thankfully, more recent MRI studies have significantly added to this literature. One group of investigators evaluated 43 alcohol-dependent men and 36 alcohol-dependent women as well as 39 healthy control subjects. They found that the alcoholic women had greater white and gray volume loss as well as increased sulcal and ventricular volumes compared to control females. Furthermore, the difference in brain volume loss, particularly in the gray matter, was greater in the female than male alcoholics. However, another research team performed volumetric MRI measurements on age-matched and length of sobriety–matched alcoholic men and women as well as age-matched healthy controls. While the alcoholic women showed no differences in brain volume indices in comparison to healthy control women, alcoholic men showed volume deficits compared to non-alcoholic men. These findings are consistent with a separate positron emission tomography (PET) study in which alcoholic men had deficits in energy utilization whereas these deficits were not found in alcoholic women. Thus, while some studies have supported the idea that women are more vulnerable to the detrimental brain effects of alcohol than are men, more research is needed to conclusively settle the issue. The role of diet and other comorbid conditions need further exploration as well.

Group Effects Versus Individual Assessment

While the studies discussed above all find that alcoholics have smaller brains than non-alcoholics, for several reasons structural imaging such as CT or MRI is not routinely used on an individual basis to assess alcohol effects. First, there are many other disease processes that can cause brain atrophy, such as Alzheimer's disease. Thus, although one can clinically observe atrophy on the MRI scan of an alcoholic, this finding is non-specific for the diagnosis of alcoholism. Secondly, the degree of atrophy across individuals varies greatly, perhaps due to factors such as gender, brain reserve, nutrition, head trauma, and other factors. This adds to the non-specificity of structural scanning as an assessment tool. Finally, most alcoholics do not have structural brain scans predating their heavy alcohol use. When those are available, they are often from older scanners with poor image resolution. Thus, although structural atrophy has been found in most longitudinal and cross-sectional brain imaging studies in alcoholics, these scans are not particularly useful within a given individual for diagnosis or monitoring.

ASSESSING THE EFFECTS OF ALCOHOL ON BRAIN FUNCTION

In addition to examining brain structure, neuroimaging technology has also been utilized to examine brain function in alcoholism. These studies have evaluated brain activity after cessation of alcohol use, as well as after sustained abstinence. In addition, neuroimaging has been used to advance our understanding of the brain regions involved in producing or maintaining alcohol craving states.

Brain Function Immediately after Stopping Alcohol Use

Unfortunately there are relatively few neuroimaging studies in close temporal proximity to alcohol withdrawal. One group of authors in 1992 used PET scans in recently abstinent alcoholics (6–32 days) and healthy controls and found that alcoholics had lower overall brain metabolic rates. In a follow-up study in 1994, ten alcoholic men were serially scanned using the glucose-PET method at 8, 16, and 30 days after their last use of alcohol. These scans were then compared over time as well as with scans from 10 age-matched nonalcoholic healthy controls. On the initial scan 8 days after alcohol cessation, alcoholics showed lower brain metabolism in numerous brain regions compared to the control group. Over the period of abstinence, brain metabolism improved significantly. A different research team found a significant reduction in global cerebral blood flow (CBF) in 12 subjects in the first two days of withdrawal with the ^{133}Xe inhalation method. However, they reported relatively high temporal and low parietal flows coupled with aggravated symptoms of alcohol withdrawal. Another group of investigators studied cerebral perfusion in 15 alcoholics with single photon emission computerized tomography (SPECT) during day 1 or 2 of acute alcohol withdrawal and again 3 weeks later. During acute alcohol withdrawal, relative perfusion was elevated in the bilateral inferior temporal regions and reduced in the bilateral superior temporal regions.

To evaluate the role of the pattern of alcohol use on regional brain activity, our group at The Charleston Alcohol Research Center at MUSC studied fourteen adults with brain perfusion SPECT on days 7–9 following their last drink and 2–3 days since their last detoxification medication. Seven healthy adults were scanned as control subjects. The alcoholics, compared with controls, had widely reduced relative activity in cortical secondary association areas and relatively increased activity in the medial temporal lobes. To evaluate differential brain effects based on multiple alcohol withdrawals (alcohol withdrawal–sensitization or kindling), five alcoholic patients with > 1 previous alcohol detoxifications were compared with five patients in their first detoxification. Contrary to our initial hypothesis, those individuals with multiple detoxifications had significantly *lower* relative activity in bilateral anterior temporal poles, amygdala, and in visual cortex compared to individuals with only one prior alcohol detoxification. The finding of limbic hypo-metabolism seen in the post-withdrawal period in the multiple detoxification group was felt to represent a "shutdown" following limbic hyperactivity during the acute withdrawal. Thus, while functional neuroimaging studies examining the basal "resting" state of the brain following alcohol cessation have demonstrated that chronic alcohol use globally reduces neuronal activity for several weeks, the limbic area seems to exhibit increased activity during this period. However, the number of prior detoxifications may modulate the responsivity of the limbic system, since individuals with multiple previous detoxifications seem to experience more craving and relapse than those without such a history. Clearly more imaging studies are needed, paying particular attention to alcoholism disease subtypes (first detoxification versus multiple detoxifications, chronic daily drinking versus bingeing), and changes over time as a function of withdrawal. Functional imaging scans reveal group effects but are not routinely used for individual assessment, for many of the same reasons discussed above about structural imaging.

Using Brain Imaging to Understand the Brain Circuits Involved in Alcohol Craving

Recently, imaging technologies (PET, SPECT, and functional magnetic resonance imaging (fMRI)) have been used to flush out the brain circuits involved in craving substances of abuse. The vast majority of these studies have been done in cocaine craving. Less work has been published in the alcohol area but similar findings are emerging.

One group of investigators in 1995 using SPECT imaging reported increased blood flow in the right caudate nucleus during craving induction in alcoholics. Later, another group, utilizing PET imaging, used a challenge of m-chlorophenylpiperazine to induce craving in alcohol subjects and controls. While no subjective craving was elicited, activations were found in the cerebellum, posterior cingulate, and thalamus in the alcohol group. Our group at MUSC recently pioneered the use of fMRI to evaluate alcohol cue-specific brain activation. Our study found that alcoholics, as a group, had activation in the anterior thalamus and left dorsolateral prefrontal cortex when they were viewing alcohol-specific images after a sip of alcohol. A matched group of social drinkers did not have any alcohol cue-specific brain activation. We recently extended this finding with a new cohort in a more sophisticated scanner with real time measurements of craving. Activity in the prefrontal cortex strongly correlated with subjective craving ratings. Recent studies have used visual or olfactory cues within the fMRI scanner to elicit craving for alcohol and have reported cue-specific activation in the superior temporal lobe, cerebellum, and putamen. Taken together, these studies demonstrate that a variety of alcohol-specific cues can induce brain activation in alcoholics within the MRI environment. They also imply that there is an appetitive and motivational circuit in the brain that is activated during stimulation by sensory alcohol cues and linked to craving for alcohol. This circuit is similar to the one activated when cocaine users see cocaine paraphernalia, or even when chocolate addicts view or smell chocolate.

Although these imaging studies offer dramatic proof of the neural circuitry underlying alcohol addiction, several of the most important research questions remain unaddressed. For example, is activity in this circuit different in alcoholics as a function of their daily alcohol use and exposure (e.g., conditioning and learning), or is this circuit somehow different in individuals who are likely to go on to develop alcoholism (e.g., is this a vulnerability circuit)? In ongoing work, our group at MUSC is testing whether different potential alcohol medication treatments block this cue-induced activation within the fMRI scanner. Our group and others are thus pioneering the use of fMRI as a prescreening tool prior to using medications in expensive and lengthy clinical trials.

In summary, functional brain imaging can demonstrate the short-term effects of chronic alcohol use. It appears from some studies that these brain changes differ as a function of chronic alcohol use patterns. Exciting new work is also demonstrating that a craving circuit for alcohol is different in individuals with alcohol dependence compared to control drinkers. It is unclear whether these craving circuit changes are true sequelae of alcohol use, or rather indicate a vulnerability or predisposition. Finally, although these tools work well for groups of alcoholics, they have little value at present for individual diagnosis, assessment, or monitoring.

LIMITATIONS IN INTERPRETING NEUROIMAGING DATA

Is it Alcohol, or Something Else?

While neuroimaging techniques have found changes in both brain structure and function in alcoholics, there are several limitations in assuming that alcohol itself may be the causative agent in producing these sequelae. For example, chronic alcoholism is often associated with poor nutritional intake that could lead to a reduction in brain volume. For instance, alcohol use can lead to a deficiency in thiamine, and consequently Korsakoff's syndrome, that is associated with mamillary body damage. Alcohol use may be associated with other end-organ damage that could influence brain volume. This is particularly true in the case of alcohol-related liver disease that could lead to encephalopathy. Additionally, there are many co-morbid psychiatric disorders, such as depression and drug dependence, that often accompany alcoholism. These co-occurring disorders may have an impact on brain volumes. Finally, alcoholics are thought to experience minor head trauma that could likely result in reduced brain volume.

IMPORTANCE OF CHANGES OVER TIME

The effect of the amount of lifetime alcohol consumption and the pattern of alcohol use are also important factors to consider in interpreting imaging data. The amount of alcohol consumed over an individual's lifetime would seem to affect brain volumes owing to the cumulative effect of neurotoxicity. However, evidence for a cumulative effect has not been found. The time interval between last drink and imaging could lead to brain volume differences. Longitudinal studies have found that there may be some reversal of volume loss with abstinence. This increase in brain volume is not due solely to rehydration. In contrast, further volume loss has been documented with continued alcohol use over a 5-year longitudinal study. Therefore, the timing of imaging studies from the individual's last drink is important for valid interpretation.

CONCLUSIONS

The development of new neuroimaging tools has revolutionized the ability to image and understand the brain sequelae of chronic alcohol use. We now understand that chronic daily alcohol use causes brain atrophy, which is partially reversible with abstinence. Moreover, alcohol causes global as well as regional reductions in overall function, which can take over a month of abstinence to reverse. Finally, alcoholics have different brain activity in a motivational circuit when they are exposed to alcohol-related cues than do social drinkers. It is unclear whether this is a consequence of, or the cause of, repeated alcohol use.

These important advances in understanding alcohol sequelae at the group level have as yet not been translated to the care and management of individual patients. However, it is abundantly clear that new neuroimaging tools will be discovered in the future, and that as our science develops, using imaging to understand alcohol effects will only increase as a field. It has the potential of one day being able to monitor individual patients, and perhaps even to predict who is at risk for developing alcoholism. More research is needed.

ACKNOWLEDGMENTS

The authors acknowledge grant support from the Charleston Alcohol Research Center (ARC) (NIAA 2 P50 AA10761). Dr. Myrick also is funded through NIAAA K23 AA00314 and the VA Research and Development Service, Ralph H. Johnson Department of Veterans Affairs Medical Center. Drs. George and Li would like to acknowledge additional grant support from the Stanley Foundation, the National Alliance for Research on Schizophrenia and Depression (NARSAD), the Borderline Personality Disorders Foundation (BPDRF), NINDS grant RO1-AG40956, and the Defense Advanced Research Projects Agency (DARPA). Dr. George has also received grant support from Cyberonics (VNS) and Neotonus (Neuronetics) (TMS) for clinical trials.

SUGGESTED READINGS

George MS, Anton RF, Bloomer C, et al: Activation of prefrontal cortex and anterior thalamus in alcoholic subjects on exposure to alcohol-specific cues. Arch Gen Psychiatry 58:345–352, 2001.

George MS, Teneback CC, Malcolm RJ, et al: Multiple previous alcohol detoxifications are associated with decreased amygdala and paralimbic function in the post-withdrawal period. Alcohol Clin Exp Res 23(6): 1077-1084, 1999.

George MS, Teneback C, Bloomer CW, et al: Using neuroimaging to understand alcohol's brain effects. CNS SPECT Int J Neuropsychiat Med 4(1):88–92, 1999.

Hommer D: Functional imaging of craving. Alcohol Res Health 23(3): 187–196, 1999.

Treatment Modalities

PSYCHOTHERAPY IN ALCOHOLISM TREATMENT

Carlo C. DiClemente
Lisa Jordan
Angela Marinilli
Melissa Nidecker

Research evidence supports the efficacy of some forms of psychotherapy and psychosocial interventions in the treatment of alcohol abuse and dependence. The evidence supports a shift from more generic or psychodynamic psychotherapy approaches to treatments that concentrate on drinking behavior and problems directly linked to drinking. Although most research studies attempt to examine defined and manualized treatments, practitioners increasingly have become more eclectic in their treatments. Behavioral approaches have been combined with cognitive ones, focused on attitudes and expectancies, to create a cognitive-behavioral therapy (CBT). Twelve-step–trained counselors use many cognitive and behavioral strategies in their groups. Attendance at Alcoholics Anonymous (AA) meetings and the AA Big Book Study often are an integral part of detoxification, outpatient, inpatient, and residential programs. In addition, motivational approaches based on the notion of patients' differential readiness to change have been incorporated into many different interventions. Research on these combined approaches as well as on how psychosocial treatments interact with various pharmacological agents to assist the drinker in avoiding alcohol is just beginning to examine the contributions of individual treatment components and the effectiveness of using them in combination.

This chapter describes the most frequently used and researched psychotherapies for treatment of alcohol abuse and dependence. We will describe each treatment and highlight research on the efficacy of each of these approaches, pointing out countraindications for use. Research comparing these approaches has not supported the unique treatment efficacy or superiority of any one the therapies reviewed. However, findings in Project MATCH, a large randomized clinical trial comparing different psychosocial treatments, suggest that treatments with a history of efficacy, offered by well-trained, skilled therapists who believe in their approach and execute that approach in a faithful and competent manner, can assist alcohol-dependent and abusing clients in making significant reductions in the intensity and frequency of drinking as well as promote abstinence. We will begin with an overview of the MATCH trial and its findings since they play a significant role in the reviews of cognitive and cognitive-behavioral, twelve-step, and motivational enhancement treatment approaches.

PROJECT MATCH

Project MATCH compared three alcoholism treatment methods and consisted of two parallel but independent studies: one study was conducted with patients who had received only outpatient treatment, and the other study included patients who had participated in either an inpatient or a day hospital treatment program and were currently receiving aftercare. The study was designed to test the efficacy of matching clients to one of three conceptually different treatments based on various client characteristics. Treatments included CBT, in which patients learned coping skills to reduce alcohol use; twelve-step facilitation (TSF), based on the principles of AA; and Motivational Enhancement Therapy (MET) designed to increase patient readiness to change. All treatments were delivered individually over twelve weeks with both CBT and TSF having weekly sessions and MET having only four sessions over the twelve weeks. Each of these treatments produced significant and long-lasting reductions in alcohol consumption, with 30% to 40% of the sample abstinent during the final three months of the follow-up period. Although the treatments were distinct, no single treatment was found to be substantially more effective than another. There were a few matching effects and other findings that will be described in the sections on the individual psychotherapies.

Overview of Cognitive-Behavioral Treatments

Cognitive-behavioral interventions are currently among the most widely used treatments for a broad spectrum of psychiatric disorders and have been researched for use in the treatment of alcohol disorders for over a quarter of a century. These interventions emphasize the importance of thoughts, feelings, and expectancies as well as the more traditional behavioral approaches using counter-conditioning and contingency management in addressing the problem of alcohol misuse. In contrast to strict behavioral models that focus almost exclusively on the environmental cues and reinforcers (Chapter 11), cognitive-behavioral models examine expectancies about alcohol effects, self-efficacy, and other attributions thought to mediate the behavioral process from perception of alcohol-related stimuli to eventual alcohol use.

Practitioners' use of cognitive-behavioral approaches in alcoholism treatment differs widely in terms of length of intervention (brief vs. long-term), modality (individual vs. group; inpatient vs. outpatient), and focus (specific vs. general behaviors). However, each variation of CBT has two important components in common. First, all variations of CBT focus on the client's ability to cope with life stressors, including confronting and dealing with alcohol-related stimuli. Deficits in coping skills are thought to maintain excessive drinking by causing individuals, who are attempting to abstain, to resume drinking when under stress. Second, CBT includes cognitive restructuring and coping skills training designed to combat cognitive and behavioral coping deficits that contribute to one's use of drinking as a central coping mechanism. This training includes educating clients on irrational thinking and automatic thoughts, teaching skills to identify risky situations in which coping skills are needed, modeling, role-playing, and behavioral rehearsal. The rationale behind teaching these techniques is to assist the individual in identifying situations in which he or she is likely to use alcohol, as well as to facilitate a sense of mastery in situations that may trigger drinking behavior.

In addition to focusing on drinking behavior itself, CBT approaches also target other problem areas in a person's life. It is believed that these problem areas are directly and indirectly related to alcohol consumption and, therefore, need to be considered in treatment. For example, if depressive thoughts are an antecedent to drinking behavior for an individual, CBT will focus on situations that elicit depressive thoughts, as well as the cognitive and behavioral processes that surround one's drinking during a depressed mood. If these processes can be altered, alcohol-related stimuli or alcohol cues will become less of a trigger for drinking behavior. Similarly, if social or employment skills are deficient, a more comprehensive version of this type of treatment can be used. One group of investigators used an eight-week CBT intervention specifically geared toward coping with depression (CBT-D) and produced greater reductions in post-treatment depressive symptoms when compared with depressed drinkers who received a relaxation control therapy.

There are other popular variations of CBT including Relapse Prevention and Rational Emotive Behavior Therapy. Relapse Prevention (RP) has been found to have its greatest effects in treating alcoholism as compared with treating other addictive behaviors. RP posits that certain factors and situations (e.g., negative or positive emotional states, interpersonal conflict, social pressure) lead to relapse, and it focuses on developing skills that are beneficial in the prevention of relapse episodes. The cognitive and behavioral strategies used in the RP model focus on specific, immediate determinants of relapse (e.g., high-risk situations, coping skills, self-efficacy, expectancies) as well as global strategies that focus on more covert antecedents of relapse (e.g., lifestyle imbalances, cognitive distortions, urges and cravings). Studies generally support RP's effectiveness in reducing the frequency and intensity of relapse episodes, but its effectiveness has not been found to be superior to other types of alcoholism treatments.

Rational Emotive Behavior Therapy (REBT) also uses cognitive and behavioral principles to treat individuals with alcohol problems. REBT views alcoholism as being determined by an interaction between a person's social learning history and genetic, familial, and cultural factors. Treatment focuses on helping the client make a conscious decision to change drinking behavior and develop effective cognitive strategies to change self-defeating thoughts and to develop higher frustration tolerances for maintaining abstinence, since these variables are thought to be precursors for alcohol use. The literature supporting REBT's effectiveness for treating alcoholism is scant. One recently conducted meta-analysis of REBT outcome literature identified only six studies since 1970 that focus on REBT as a treatment for alcoholism. Each of these studies was flawed methodologically in some way (e.g., lack of random assignment, no control conditions), leading the authors to surmise that no conclusions can be drawn about REBT's unique effectiveness at the present time.

MATCHING CLIENTS TO CBT

Several interesting indications and contraindications for the use of CBT approaches have emerged recently. Project MATCH demonstrated the efficacy of CBT in certain populations. For instance, using a subsample of 397 outpatients diagnosed with social phobia in addition to alcoholism, socially phobic female alcoholics (but not males) showed delayed relapse to drinking when treated with CBT in comparison to TSF. In addition, women, who received either CBT or TSF, reported higher increases in levels of social support while in CBT treatment than those women who received MET. A similar study supported the efficacy of CBT for drinkers with panic disorder with or without agoraphobia.

Data from Project MATCH also demonstrated small but significant differences among treatments for outpatients on measures of alcohol consumption and negative consequences related to alcohol during the twelve weeks of treatment. Both CBT and TSF patients demonstrated more abstinence during treatment than those receiving MET.

Overall, it appears that CBT techniques may be somewhat more beneficial than some other treatments in reducing alcohol-related events in patients with some forms of psychopathology, particularly anxiety-related disorders. However, for the general population seeking alcohol treatment, the benefit of using CBT over other effective treatments is not strongly substantiated. Evidently, matching client characteristics to hypothesized mechanisms of CBT makes little difference in drinking outcomes. However, CBT remains among the most widely used and researched interventions for alcohol use, attesting to its acceptability and perceived efficacy.

Overview of Twelve-Step Facilitation Therapy

Twelve-Step Facilitation Therapy (TSF) is a treatment approach that is based on the AA model of treatment for alcoholism. TSF was developed for use in the MATCH clinical trial, with expert consultation from the Hazelden Foundation, the pioneers of the "Minnesota Model" treatment programs. Similar to other "Minnesota Model" programs, the underlying assumption of TSF is that alcoholism is a spiritual, as well as a medical, disease. TSF treatment is administered by a professional counselor over a set period and is designed to assist the client to achieve abstinence and enhance commitment to attend AA. The TSF counselor focuses on the twelve steps of AA, with a primary emphasis on steps 1 through 5. Consistent with the first three steps of AA, TSF focuses on acceptance of the disease, recognition of loss of control over alcohol, and acceptance of the goal of abstinence. In addition, clients recognize the hope provided by faith and belief in a Higher Power that can help them overcome the problems associated with alcoholism. Clients are encouraged to recognize the AA path as their best chance for success. Aside from the emphasis on acceptance and surrender, clients learn about the ways in which their thinking has been affected by alcohol, including the problem of denial.

As implemented in Project MATCH, TSF is a twelve-session intervention in which the therapy sessions are highly structured and include some cognitive behavioral strategies, such as symptom inquiry, review and reinforcement of AA participation, setting and modifying goals for attendance, and other "recovery tasks." Each session has a theme, and clients are provided with written materials, including AA literature, meditation books, and other materials with which the therapist is familiar. In TSF, the primary role of the therapist is as an educator and facilitator of the client's change process.

Although TSF was designed as a twelve-session intervention, the number and timing of sessions are flexible and have been modified in subsequent trials. Significant others may be involved in the sessions, or not, at the discretion of therapist and client. TSF may also be used in conjunction with other treatment modalities.

RESEARCH ON TSF

Research findings regarding TSF must be interpreted in light of the long history of research on AA and the impossibility of designing truly randomized studies of self-help groups. Numerous studies have found an association between AA participation and positive treatment outcome. According to the 1998 AA membership survey, 47% of active members had remained sober for over five years, while another 26% maintained sobriety for at least one year but less than five. From these findings, it is evident that those who "work the program" are likely to benefit, but little is known about those who are unable or unwilling to make use of AA. The search for characteristics of clients who attend and benefit from AA has examined sociodemographic characteristics, diagnosis, treatment history, quality of social support, childhood background, and a host of other factors. Few consistent findings have emerged. Some studies have shown that individuals with comorbid psychopathology report lower levels of AA attendance and are less likely to benefit from AA-oriented treatment. Similarly, a recent meta-analytic study indicated that AA participation is generally more strongly related to drinking outcomes in outpatient, rather than inpatient, samples. In light of these findings, research on TSF, which prepares clients for post-treatment AA involvement, is particularly relevant.

In the Project MATCH trials, TSF was shown to be an effective treatment resulting in significant reductions in both drinks per drinking day and percent of days abstinent at follow-up. Compared with clients in the CBT and MET treatments, outpatient TSF clients were significantly more likely to remain completely abstinent (24%) during the first year after treatment than those in the other two groups (14% and 15%). In addition, participants who received MATCH as an aftercare treatment and met criteria for greater alcohol dependence had better post-treatment drinking outcomes when they participated in TSF.

Other research based on the Project MATCH trials examined pretreatment social network characteristics and support for drinking as predictors of TSF engagement and outcomes. In general, outpatient clients with large daily networks (i.e., individuals in their social networks with whom they had daily contact) and more abstainers or recovering alcoholics in their networks showed better post-treatment drinking outcomes. However, for clients with high concentrations of substance abusers in their social networks, the TSF intervention was found to be particularly effective compared with similar MET clients during the early weeks of treatment and at the three-year post-treatment interview. These findings suggest that adding abstainers and recovering alcoholics to social networks improves both the short- and long-term outcomes for clients who are in the early stages of recovery. Involvement in AA or other self-help groups provides a readily available means of making these important network changes. Ethnicity may also interact with TSF effectiveness and attendance, with Hispanic clients reporting lower rates of AA attendance both prior to and following outpatient TSF treatment.

Although Hispanic clients reported being equally committed to AA-related practices and beliefs (e.g., working the steps, celebrating sobriety anniversaries, obtaining a sponsor) and were just as likely to benefit from AA attendance in terms of sobriety measures, they were less likely to respond to clinicians' encouragements to attend meetings.

In summary, the literature on TSF and post-treatment AA involvement suggests that it is an effective intervention for many clients, particularly for those whose social networks promote continued drinking. In addition to providing a means of altering "people, places, and things," it is likely that post-treatment AA involvement is conducive to increasing clients' self-efficacy and motivation, as well as promoting active coping mechanisms and providing specific guidance on lifestyle and cognitive changes. TSF is an intervention that is based on a long history of self-help for substance abuse problems and may be particularly useful for outpatient clients who need support for maintaining sobriety.

Overview of Motivational Enhancement Therapies

Lack of motivation to change among substance abusers is a common challenge faced by therapists and counselors treating individuals struggling with addiction. Motivation for change directly impacts attendance and participation in therapy as well as adherence to treatment guidelines. Unlike confrontational approaches to substance abuse treatment that emphasize labeling, argumentation, and prescribed treatment goals, motivational therapies adopt a client-centered, directive approach designed to build and maintain motivation for changing substance abuse patterns by exploring and resolving ambivalence about change. Research suggests that motivational interventions for alcohol abuse and dependence are more effective than no treatment controls and are equally as effective as more extensive psychotherapies.

Motivational interventions are generally brief, ranging from one to four sessions that vary in duration from 30 to 60 minutes each. Motivational therapies employ distinct principles and techniques that reflect a collaborative, client-centered, and empathic style. When using motivational approaches for problem and dependent drinkers, the task of the therapist is to create an environment that enhances the client's own motivation for, and commitment to, change. The therapist seeks to encourage intrinsic motivation for change by calling upon the client's inner resources and tapping sources of support within existing helping relationships.

From the perspective of motivational therapies, one's motivation to change is not considered a static personality problem (e.g., denial), but a state of readiness to change. A model for understanding the context and process of behavior change, called the Transtheoretical Model of Change (TTM), is frequently used in conjunction with motivational therapies for substance abusers. This model describes how people move through a series of stages in the process of behavior change, from precontemplation (where people see no reason to change) to action and maintenance (where people are actively modifying their behavior and sustaining change).

Therapists using motivational approaches with problem and dependent drinkers embrace several key techniques as they explore with their clients ambivalence about changing. These techniques include reflective listening, eliciting self-motivational statements, examining advantages and disadvantages of drinking or changing drinking, providing feedback regarding personal risk or impairment related to drinking, and minimizing resistance to change. While motivational approaches are not confrontational, they are directive. Therefore, although argumentation and labeling are avoided, the therapist directs the client toward motivation for change and offers advice and feedback when appropriate.

An example of a manualized motivational intervention for alcohol abuse and dependence is the Motivational Enhancement Therapy (MET) implemented in Project MATCH. As mentioned above, during the twelve weeks of treatment, patients in CBT and TSF consumed alcohol less frequently and reported fewer alcohol-related consequences compared with patients in MET. However, the one-year post-treatment results demonstrated significant and sustained reductions in drinking outcomes in all three of the treatment groups, with no substantial differences in post-treatment drinking behavior by type of treatment. In fact, the strongest treatment-matching effect indicated that outpatients with elevated degrees of state/trait anger had better drinking outcomes when given MET compared with the CBT and TSF treatments. Post-treatment outcomes indicate that the briefer motivational therapy performed on a par with more intensive psychotherapies for outpatient and aftercare patients and is more beneficial to those outpatients struggling with elevated levels of anger and hostility. These patients may respond to the client-centered, empathic spirit of motivational approaches that are designed to reduce resistance to treatment.

A number of studies also support the efficacy of motivational therapies in reducing problem drinking. One randomized, controlled trial compared MET with nondirective reflective listening (NDRL; person-centered therapy on issues of interest to the client) and a feedback condition with no further counseling (NFC) with 122 mildly to moderately alcohol-dependent patients. Six-month follow-up results indicated that only 43% of patients treated with MET reported heavy drinking (ten or more drinks on at least six occasions) compared with approximately 63% of patients receiving NDRL and 65% of those given feedback only. Another study compared two types of feedback sessions for problem drinkers: directive-confrontational (argumentative, handled client resistance by emphasizing evidence of alcohol problems, using the label "alcoholism" when appropriate) and client-centered feedback (empathic style using reflective listening, de-emphasized diagnostic labels). Results showed that in general, confrontation by the therapist (e.g., challenging, sarcasm, disagreeing, head-on disputes) was met with resistance from patients in the form of arguing, interrupting, and negative responses. In contrast, therapist behavior such as listening and restructuring was significantly related to positive, self-motivational responses from patients. One-year drinking outcomes showed that confrontation predicted drinking behavior with greater confrontation, producing more drinking.

Motivational techniques also have been used at the beginning of treatment to increase motivation to change drinking behavior. One research team randomly assigned 51 patients entering a standard, cognitive-behavioral six-week day hospital program for alcohol dependence to one of two pre-treatment conditions. The intervention was a two-session motivational intervention consisting of one 60-minute session and a 5- to 10-minute meeting conducted one week later. Patients were encouraged to discuss their concerns about drinking, positive and negative consequences of alcohol use, and how continued use or abstinence would affect their lives. The control group received an educational intervention that included information about myths and facts related to alcohol as well as long- and short-term effects of alcohol use. Patients in the motivational condition showed greater problem recognition compared with those in the control condition. Following the intervention, the motivational group showed lower levels of ambivalence regarding change and increased problem recognition and reported more steps to change drinking behavior than did the control group.

In conclusion, motivational therapies for alcohol abuse and dependence focus on building intrinsic motivation to change using a client-centered, directive, and empathic style designed to explore and resolve ambivalence about change. While such therapies are typically brief, they appear to be as effective as more extensive psychotherapies. In addition, motivational interventions may provide additional benefit to highly resistant and/or hostile patients. Additional research is needed to evaluate the potential use of motivational approaches as a "pre-treatment" adjunctive therapy for alcohol abuse and dependence.

CONCLUSIONS AND RECOMMENDATIONS

This review indicates that there are several psychotherapies, representing different philosophies and techniques, that can be used effectively in the treatment of alcohol abuse and dependence. Cognitive-Behavioral, Twelve-Step, and Motivational therapies are those that have received the most research support and are currently the most popular of the psychotherapies. There are other approaches including behavioral, network, social system, and pharmacotherapy approaches to intervention that are included in other chapters of this handbook and that can be used instead of, or in conjunction with, the psychotherapies described in this chapter. However, we offer the following conclusions and recommendations for using psychotherapy in the treatment of alcohol abuse and dependence:

1. Cognitive-Behavioral, Twelve-Step, and Motivational approaches should be offered by therapists who are properly trained in these treatments and who have the skills and belief systems that would support the different therapies. Individual therapists have been found to produce more efficacious or less efficacious outcomes using these treatments.
2. For individuals whose drinking may pose serious and immediate medical consequences, more extensive treatments such as the twelve-session TSF or CBT seem to be more effective in promoting abstinence during the early phase of outpatient therapy when compared with a less intensive motivational treatment.
3. Cognitive-behavioral approaches seem to address co-existing psychiatric problems such as anxiety and depression more productively than do the other types of therapies.
4. Motivational enhancement interventions seem particularly useful for alcohol abusers and for those individuals who are more angry or hostile when they come into treatment.

5. Twelve-Step therapy with its emphasis on the use of AA support group attendance seems to be most useful for those drinkers who have a social network that is saturated with alcohol-using and abusing members.
6. Psychotherapies are delivered in both individual and group formats. The TSF and CBT treatments are often delivered in groups and may be more amenable to a group format. MET more often is delivered in an individual format. However, there are new initiatives to use motivational approaches in a group setting.
7. Several studies are under way to examine the interaction of psychotherapy with pharmacotherapy interventions. The results will be instructive in how to combine various forms of psychosocial or psychotherapy approaches with different types of medication used in the treatment of alcohol problems.
8. Our understanding of the mechanisms and the process of change that underlie the efficacy of psychotherapies is still incomplete. It is likely that there will continue to be advances in the nature and scope of the psychotherapy approaches that can be recommended for the treatment of alcohol problems.

SUGGESTED READINGS

Babor T, DelBoca F (eds.): Project MATCH: The Book. Cambridge, UK: Cambridge University Press, 2003.

DiClemente CC: Addiction and change: How addictions develop and addicted people change. New York: Guilford Press, 2003.

DiClemente CC, Velasquez M: Motivational interviewing and the stages of change. In: Miller WR, Rollnick S (eds.), Motivational Interviewing: Preparing People for Change. Second Edition. New York: Guilford Press, 2002, pp. 201–216.

Irvin JE, Bowers CA, Dunn ME, Wang MC: Efficacy of relapse prevention: A meta-analytic review. J Consult Clin Psychol 67:563–570, 1999.

Monti PM, Kadden RM, Rohsenow DJ, et al: Treating Alcohol Dependence. Second Edition. New York: Guilford Press, 2002.

Morgenstern J, Longabaugh R: Cognitive-behavioral treatment for alcohol dependence: A review of evidence for its hypothesized mechanisms of action. Addiction 95:1475–1490, 2000.

Nowinski J, Baker S, Carroll K: Twelve Step Facilitation Therapy Manual: A Clinical Research Guide for Therapists Treating Individuals with Alcohol Abuse and Dependence. U.S. Department of Health and Human Services, Publication No. 94–3722, 1999.

BEHAVIORAL INTERVENTIONS FOR PROBLEM DRINKING: COMMUNITY REINFORCEMENT AND CONTINGENCY MANAGEMENT

Stephen T. Higgins
Kenneth Silverman
Sarah H. Heil

In this chapter, we provide an overview of the community reinforcement approach (CRA) and contingency-management (CM) procedures for treating problem drinking (i.e., alcohol abuse and dependence). Both interventions are efficacious for the treatment of problem drinking as well as other forms of problematic drug use. Interestingly, CRA and CM were first introduced to the area of substance abuse in the early 1970s as interventions for problem drinking. Despite strikingly positive results from several controlled studies supporting their efficacy in reducing problem drinking, little more was done with these treatments in the alcohol field for several decades. During that hiatus, research continued, also with impressive results on efficacy, on the use of CM and (more recently) CRA for the treatment of problematic use of illicit drugs.. Use of these treatments outside of research settings remains limited, which is the case for most empirically based substance abuse treatments. Part of the discontinuity between treatments that have been shown to be efficacious in controlled studies and those used in community clinics has to do with differences in treatment philosophy. Financial constraints are also an important factor. Community clinics often operate on limited budgets that interfere with their ability to adopt and train staff in research-based interventions. In any event, there has been a re-emergence of research interest in CRA and CM for problem drinking, perhaps because their success in the treatment of problems connected with illicit drug use. This chapter introduces readers to CRA and CM by describing the conceptual framework on which they are based and the general features of the interventions, as well as briefly summarizing results from controlled studies on efficacy.

CONCEPTUAL FRAMEWORK

CRA and CM are based on the concepts and principles of conditioning and social learning theory. Within that framework, use of alcohol and other drug is considered to be learned behavior that is maintained by the unconditioned reinforcing effects of abused drugs in combination with the social and various forms of conditioned reinforcement derived from a drug-abusing lifestyle.

Drugs that humans abuse act on basic reinforcement or reward centers of the central nervous system, which are designed to support learning related to the survival of the individual and the species (e.g., procurement of food and water, sexual reproduction, etc.). By acting on these brain centers, abused drugs directly increase the probability that drug self-administration will be repeated in the future. This is not a phenomenon that is unique to humans. Most drugs that are abused by humans are readily and voluntarily consumed by a variety of other species, which suggests that pharmacological reinforcement is, biologically, a normal event. That is, no particular physical, psychological, or social abnormality or deviance is necessary for humans or other organisms to voluntarily consume most abused drugs.

Within this conceptual framework, all healthy humans are considered to possess the necessary neurobiological systems to experience drug-produced reinforcement and hence to develop drug use, abuse, and dependence. Indeed, drug use is considered a normal, learned behavior that falls along a continuum ranging from little use and few problems to excessive use and many untoward effects. The same basic principles of learning are assumed to operate across this continuum, which raises the question of individual differences in vulnerability to problem drinking and other problematic drug use. If we are all biologically vulnerable, why is it that some humans develop the problems whereas others do not? Obviously, the scientific community does not yet fully understand individual differences in vulnerability to drug use, abuse, and dependence, but progress has been made. An essential point to make regarding individual differences is that such variability is a basic characteristic of all biological phenomena, often taking the form of an inverted U-shaped curve. Vulnerability to problematic drug use is no exception. Research shows that biological (e.g., familial or early-onset) alcoholism, acquired individual characteristics (e.g., educational attainment), and environmental context (availability of drugs in one's immediate environment) can significantly affect the probability of developing problematic drug use. No one of these variables is deemed to be necessary for problematic drug use to emerge. Instead, they are variables that affect the probability or risk for emergence of problematic use.

Humans are social animals, and social and related environmental circumstances exert a profound influence on all aspects of human drug use. They influence whether and when one comes into contact with drug use, which drugs one is likely to use, the social circumstances surrounding such use, rituals and norms regarding frequency and quantity of drug use, etc. Social/cultural circumstances also greatly influence the availability of other social and material reinforcers (e.g., vocation, hobbies, family life) that can serve as alternatives to, or substitutes for, the reinforcement derived from drug use. CRA and CM are designed to reorganize the environments of problem drug users so as to systematically weaken the influence of pharmacological and social reinforcement obtained through drug use and strengthen alternatives and substitutes. Primary emphasis is on decreasing drug use by increasing the availability and frequency of alternative reinforcing activities, especially those that are incompatible with a drug-abusing lifestyle. Drug use also can be decreased by systematically arranging for reinforcing events to be lost or aversive events to be delivered as consequences of drug use. The following sections provide more detail on how these general concepts and strategies are implemented in CRA and CM interventions.

COMMUNITY REINFORCEMENT APPROACH

The overarching goal of CRA is to rearrange and improve the quality of the reinforcers obtained by patients through their social, recreational, vocational, and family activities. The goal is for these sources of reinforcement to be available and to be of high quality when the patient is sober, and unavailable, or less available, when drinking occurs. Plans for how to rearrange these alternative sources of reinforcement are individualized to conform to each patient's unique situation.

CRA has several key components: (1) Immediate barriers to treatment engagement, such as pending legal matters, homelessness, or other crises, are addressed in the first or second session, usually through coordination with relevant community agencies. In regard to pressing legal matters, for example, therapists may help the patient get representation through the local public defender's office. (2) Patients are taught how to functionally analyze their drinking in order to learn the antecedents that regularly trigger drinking as well as the consequences derived from drinking that help to maintain it (e.g., the camaraderie of drinking buddies). Therapist and client solve the problem of how to rearrange the environment so that contact with antecedents of problem drinking is minimized. They also work on skill training to promote effective management of certain types of problems or mood states that often precede problem drinking. Also important is planning for healthier ways to obtain some of the desirable consequences that the client previously obtained through drinking. (3) Those who are unemployed or employed in jobs that are risky for drinking are given vocational counseling. (4) Marital and family therapy is often provided. Couples or other family members receive training in positive communication skills to facilitate negotiation of contracts that reciprocally reinforce changes in one another's behavior, including abstinence from problem drinking on the part of the client. For those without family, attempts are sometimes made to identify someone in the community who is willing to serve as a surrogate family member. (5) Social and recreational counseling is implemented. Clients are counseled to interact with friends and relatives who have low tolerance for drinking and to avoid interactions with drinkers. Participation in Alcoholics Anonymous and other self-help groups can be very useful for clients who are willing to participate. Therapists spend a considerable amount of time helping clients identify and plan healthful recreational activities that can function as substitutes for drinking. (6) Unless it is medically contraindicated, disulfiram therapy monitored by a significant other or clinic staff member who will ensure medication compliance is a prescribed recommendation for all problem drinkers.

The seminal CRA study was conducted with 16 severe alcoholics who were admitted for treatment of alcoholism to a rural state hospital located in southern Illinois. These men were divided into eight matched pairs. Paired members were randomly assigned to receive CRA plus standard hospital care or standard care only. Standard hospital care consisted of 25 1-hour didactic sessions involving lectures on Alcoholics Anonymous, alcoholism, and related medical problems. After discharge from the hospital, CRA patients received a tapered schedule of counseling sessions, beginning on a once- or twice-weekly basis during the first month and then on a once-monthly basis across the next several months.

During the 6-month follow-up period after hospital discharge, reported time spent drinking was 14% for participants in CRA versus 79% for those in standard treatment. Those treated with CRA also had significantly better outcomes in the percentage of time patients were unemployed and institutionalized.

Subsequent research with CRA focused on improving the treatment as well as extending it to new populations, including homeless, alcohol-dependent individuals. Space constraints permit us to highlight only a few of those developments.

Disulfiram therapy was not part of the original CRA treatment. It was added as a step to improve CRA and again tested against standard care, first in an inpatient setting and later in an outpatient clinic. CRA with disulfiram was more efficacious than standard care that also included advice to take disulfiram (i.e., the physician provides a prescription for the medication but takes no steps to ensure medication compliance). In assessments conducted for 6 months after hospital discharge, outcomes achieved with CRA were superior to those achieved with standard care in terms of percent of time spent drinking, time unemployed, time away from family, and time spent institutionalized. The CRA group reported spending the majority of time abstinent during a 2-year follow-up period; comparable data were not reported for the standard treatment group.

Another study by the same group of investigators focused on isolating the contribution made by monitored disulfiram therapy to outcomes obtained with CRA. Male and female alcohol-dependent outpatients received usual care plus disulfiram therapy without compliance support, usual care plus disulfiram therapy with significant others to support compliance, or CRA in combination with disulfiram therapy and support from significant others. CRA in combination with disulfiram and compliance procedures produced the greatest reductions in drinking; disulfiram in combination with compliance procedures but without CRA produced intermediate results; and the usual care plus disulfiram therapy without compliance support produced the poorest outcome. Interestingly, married patients did equally well with either the full CRA treatment or disulfiram plus compliance procedures alone. Only unmarried subjects appeared to need CRA treatment plus monitored disulfiram to achieve abstinence. It therefore appears that spouses can play a significant role in maintaining disulfiram compliance.

CRA also has been adapted to assist the significant others of treatment-resistant problem drinkers by encouraging the drinkers to enter treatment. The CRA intervention includes education about alcohol problems, information and discussion of the positive consequences of abstinence from alcohol, assistance in involving the designated client in healthy activities, increasing the involvement of the significant other in social and recreational activities, and training the significant others in how to respond to drinking episodes (including dangerous situations) and how to recommend treatment entry to the designated client. Several studies on this topic suggest greater efficacy of the CRA approach compared with more traditional approaches involving confrontation. The majority of designated clients whose families received the CRA intervention entered treatment and decreased their problem drinking, whereas none or few of those in the comparison conditions did so.

In sum, the empirical evidence supporting the efficacy of CRA in treating problem drinking is strong, even when the clinical situation is complicated by homelessness. The evidence is also good regarding the efficacy of CRA in helping families facilitate treatment entry among individuals who are not motivated to receive treatment. CRA appears to have much unrealized potential for the treatment of problem drinking among other special populations, such as those with serious mental illness or complications related to other illness (e.g., HIV or other infectious disease). Although this topic was not covered earlier, there also have been successful extensions of CRA to outpatient treatment of those with cocaine and opiate dependence.

CONTINGENCY-MANAGEMENT INTERVENTIONS

CM interventions involve the explicit and direct application of the conditioning principles of reinforcement and punishment to increase useful or desired behaviors or to decrease problematic ones. Under these procedures, clients receive tangible consequences contingent on displaying clinically important target behaviors. CM interventions require the designation of three critical elements: an objective, observable target mode of behavior that must be increased or decreased; a tangible consequence that can be delivered promptly and reliably by a treatment provider contingent on display of the target response; and specification of a contingency or the rules according to which the consequence will be delivered by the treatment provider.

CM interventions have been used most frequently to reinforce or increase desirable behaviors. In those cases, the consequences that appear appealing or attractive to clients are provided contingent on display of the target behavior. When that contingency increases the frequency of the target behavior, the operant process of reinforcement is exemplified and the goal of the procedures is accomplished. Alternatively, contingencies can be arranged so that punishing events occur if clients use alcohol or fail to display important treatment behaviors. CM interventions have been used extensively in the treatment of drug abuse. They have been used less often to treat clients with alcohol problems, although important work has been done in this area to promote alcohol abstinence or medication compliance, or to increase other behaviors deemed important to the treatment process, such as regular attendance at counseling sessions.

Directly Promoting Abstinence

Some of the earliest evidence that CM interventions could be used to reduce drinking and promote abstinence from alcohol came from research with alcoholic adults who were given the opportunity to drink under controlled laboratory conditions. The research showed that drinking could be decreased by CM interventions in which subjects earned money or access to an enriched environment in exchange for abstinence from drinking, or by imposition of a financial penalty or a brief period of social isolation contingent on drinking.

The seminal trial that examined the efficacy of CM in the treatment of problem drinking was conducted with chronic offenders arrested for public drunkenness. Twenty recent arrestees were randomized to a CM or a control group. Through the support of several cooperating social service agencies, those in the CM group earned housing, employment, medical care, and meals by reducing their drinking. Sobriety was assessed through direct staff observation of gross intoxication and randomly administered expired breath-alcohol-level assessments (BALs). Those with BALs of less than 0.01% continued to receive services, whereas those with BALs of 0.01% or more, or gross intoxication, had services terminated for 5 days. Subjects in the control group received the same goods and services as those in the CM group independent of BALs or intoxication. Subjects in the CM and control groups were arrested an average of 1.7 ± 1.2 times and 1.4 ± 1.1 times during a 2-month baseline period. During the 2-month intervention period, arrests decreased by more than 80% in the CM group, although they remained relatively unchanged in the control group.

After a relatively long period without research on CM in the treatment of alcohol abuse/dependence, a clinical trial was reported in which 42 alcohol-dependent clients who entered an intensive outpatient substance abuse clinic were randomized to standard treatment plus CM or standard treatment only. Clients in both groups met with a research assistant daily during intensive treatment and weekly during aftercare to provide a breath sample. In the CM group, clients earned the chance to draw from a bowl and win a prize for each negative BAL they submitted and for each of three preset activities they completed each week. Prizes ranged in value from $1 to $100. Of the clients assigned to the CM condition, 84% remained in treatment for the 8-week treatment period, compared with only 22% of those assigned to the standard treatment-only condition. By the end of the treatment period, 69% of the clients in the contingent group had not yet experienced a relapse to alcohol use, compared with 39% of those in the standard treatment condition.

Increasing Medication Compliance

CM interventions also can be used to increase medication compliance. Although disulfiram can be an effective pharmacotherapy for some problem drinkers, many refuse to take it on a regular basis. To address this limitation, CM interventions have been used to increase and sustain disulfiram ingestion. Efforts to promote disulfiram ingestion with CM were made first in individuals with dual dependency on heroin and alcohol who received methadone. Methadone is an opioid agonist and is an effective treatment for heroin dependence. Taken daily and in adequate doses, methadone can prevent withdrawal signs and symptoms associated with abrupt termination of heroin use, and can reduce heroin use. As an opioid medication, methadone itself is attractive to patients and can serve as a reinforcer. One group of investigators used methadone to reinforce and promote disulfiram ingestion. Under a novel CM intervention, alcoholic methadone-maintenance patients were required to ingest disulfiram as a condition for obtaining their daily methadone dose. The research showed that this intervention could increase disulfiram ingestion and decrease drinking in this population.

Increasing Counseling Attendance

CM interventions also have been used to increase participation in treatment. One research team conducted a series of experimental studies that examined the efficacy of mandated treatment in jailed criminal opulations. In one study, 19 alcoholics who had served alcohol-related sentences in the penitentiary were randomized either to a group whose attendance in outpatient alcoholism treatment was a parole requirement or a control group whose attendance after the first appointment was urged but not required. Subjects in the compulsory group were instructed that failure to attend a scheduled clinic visit was a violation of parole for which they would be returned to prison to serve out their time (typically several years). Treatment-compulsory subjects had considerably higher rates of treatment attendance and improved long-term outcomes than the treatment-voluntary subjects.

In sum, although relatively little research has been conducted on the use of CM interventions to treat problem drinking, the available research has shown the efficacy and versatility of these interventions. The research has shown that CM interventions can be used to increase a range of important clinical behaviors, from abstinence to medication compliance and treatment attendance. Abstinence is clearly the most important behavior to address, although it does pose a special challenge to CM interventions because of the difficulty involved in objectively monitoring alcohol intake. Urinalysis provides an objective marker of illicit drug use in most users during the several days preceding the test; however, the practical objective measure of alcohol use in the general community is BAL. Unfortunately, BALs provide evidence of use only during the few hours preceding the test. This absence of a biological marker with appropriate detection duration makes it difficult to reinforce or punish alcohol use. Nevertheless, one investigator's work suggests that relying on a combination of observations by others in the subject's natural environment and randomly scheduled BALs can surmount this difficulty.

The studies illustrate a critical point about the types of consequences that can and should be used in CM interventions. The investigators used reinforcers or punishers that were tailored to the various treatment populations and situations. In ideal cases, the commodities or services used were already being dispensed to the patients on a noncontingent basis as a part of routine clinical care. For example, one author used access to housing, employment, medical care, and meals, which were already being provided by local social service agencies. He simply arranged a contingency in which participants could get access to those services only if they remained abstinent. Others have used access to methadone treatment, a service that was also being delivered otherwise on a noncontingent basis, to promote disulfiram ingestion. Furthermore, in the best CM interventions, the consequences that were employed had substantial value to clients. What could be more valuable than the food, shelter, and medical care that the former author offered his participants if they remained abstinent from alcohol? Few consequences could have been more influential than the jail time that participants in an earlier study would have faced for failing to attend treatment. Practitioners who think creatively about identifying and control access to such valuable consequences could experience considerable success in treating patients with CM interventions.

SUMMARY AND CONCLUSIONS

In this chapter, we reviewed how, within a conditioning and learning theory framework, drug (including alcohol) use is considered a normal, learned behavior that falls along a continuum ranging from light use with no problems to heavy use with many untoward effects. Treatment strategies based on this conceptual framework aim to weaken the reinforcement obtained from drug use and related activities and increase and strengthen the material and social reinforcement obtained from other sources, especially from participation in activities deemed to be incompatible with a drug-abusing lifestyle. CRA and CM procedures are based on this general strategy and are effective in treating problem drinking and other substance use. CRA and CM offer a range of empirically based and effective strategies that have the potential to enrich the therapy options available to practicing clinicians.

ACKNOWLEDGMENTS

Preparation of this chapter was supported by research grants RO1 DA09378, RO1 DA08076 and RO1 AA12154 from the National Institute on Drug Abuse and the National Institute on Alcohol Abuse and Alcoholism.

SUGGESTED READINGS

Budney AJ, Higgins ST: The Community Reinforcement plus Vouchers Approach: Manual 2: National Institute on Drug Abuse Therapy Manuals for Drug Addiction. Rockville, MD: National Institute on Drug Abuse, NIH publication # 98–4308, 1998.

Higgins ST, Petry NM: Contingency management: incentives for sobriety. Alcohol Res Health 23:122–127, 1999.

Higgins ST, Silverman K: Motivating Behavior Changes Among Illicit Drug Abusers: Research on Contingency Management Interventions. Washington, D.C.: American Psychological Association, 1999.

Meyers RJ, Miller WR: A Community Reinforcement Approach to Addiction Treatment. Cambridge, UK: Cambridge University Press, 2001.

Petry NM, Martin B, Cooney JL, Kranzler HR: Give them prizes, and they will come: contingency management for treatment of alcohol dependence. J Consult Clin Psychol 68:250–257, 2000.

MEDICATIONS FOR THE TREATMENT OF ALCOHOLISM

Nassima Ait-Daoud
Bankole A. Johnson

Alcoholism treatment has progressed since the early 1990s as a result of better understanding of the biological basis for addiction. Earlier studies targeted the enzymatic processes associated with ethanol metabolism that provoke an adverse chemical reaction to deter further alcohol consumption if reinstatement of drinking follows abstinence. Preclinical studies have advanced scientific knowledge of the neurotransmitters that are involved in the expression of alcohol drinking and other behaviors associated with its abuse liability. These studies have implicated several target neurotransmitter systems, particularly those interacting with the dopamine (DA), serotonin (5-HT), opioid, gamma-aminobutyric acid (GABA), N-methyl-d-aspartate (NMDA), alpha-amino-3-hydroxy-5-methylisoxazole-4-propionic acid (AMPA), and kainate glutamate receptors. There is new knowledge showing that some alcoholics may possess a biological predisposition to the disease. These biologically vulnerable individuals, compared with those whose alcoholism is more psychosocially determined, could, therefore, be expected to experience a differentially greater treatment benefit from specific adjunctive medication targeted toward correcting or ameliorating the underlying abnormalities. Medication combinations may provide an added therapeutic treatment effect, thereby enabling development of more effective treatment strategies. This review focuses on the development of medications that are designed to reduce the desire to drink, promote abstinence, or both.

DISULFIRAM

Disulfiram alters the breakdown of alcohol in the body by inhibiting acetaldehyde dehydrogenase, thereby causing a chemical (acetaldehyde) to build up in the blood. If alcohol is consumed, acetaldehyde levels are increased and unpleasant symptoms such as nausea, vomiting, palpitation, dyspnea, lowered blood pressure, and (occasionally) collapse can occur. Association of these unpleasant symptoms with drinking discourages further alcohol consumption.

Disulfiram has been used for treating alcoholism since the 1940s. Newer studies, however, have cast doubt on its effectiveness and safety. The most rigorous trial was a multisite, double-blind, controlled study of veterans conducted by Fuller and coworkers in 1986. In that study, disulfiram neither improved abstinence nor prolonged the time to first drink after a period of abstinence. Although disulfiram use was associated with some reduction in drinking frequency, compliance rates with the treatment regimen were low. Indeed, the only types of alcoholic individuals who might benefit from disulfiram treatment are those with high compliance and supportive spouses—just the type of alcoholic patients who are likely to maintain abstinence without any pharmaceutical aid. Although disulfiram implants can enhance compliance, their efficacy is doubtful.

Finally, disulfiram use can be associated with life-threatening illnesses such as hepatitis, and this drawback has limited its use even among highly motivated alcohol-dependent individuals.

OPIOIDS

Alcohol has important effects that are mediated primarily in the endogenous opioid system via endorphins. Endorphins, traditionally known to modulate nociceptive responses, also mediate the appreciation of euphoria. In animals, ethanol intake stimulates the release of endogenous opioids, and alcohol-preferring animals, compared with wild strains, show enhanced endorphin release when ethanol is consumed.

Preclinical studies show that the opioid antagonist, naltrexone, reduces ethanol intake. In 1994, naltrexone (50 mg orally) was approved by the Food and Drug Administration as an adjunct to psychosocial support for treating alcoholism. Naltrexone treatment appears equally effective, and may be more so, when coupled with supportive compared with coping skills relapse prevention therapy. Nevertheless, 5 months after naltrexone discontinuation, relapse rates were no different between those who received naltrexone and those who were given placebo.

Although the majority of clinical trials have supported naltrexone's efficacy in treating alcoholism, there have been some exceptions. Multicenter trials (especially in the United Kingdom and the United States) with naltrexone have generally met with less success than single-site investigations. This may be because naltrexone's treatment effect appears to be in the small-to-medium range. Naltrexone's therapeutic effects appear to diminish with time and may not be evident 3 months after treatment cessation. Further, naltrexone compliance rates of less than 80% (especially if there is a lack of engagement in psychosocial treatment) tend to yield no greater therapeutic benefits than placebo. Indeed, adverse event rates can account for up to 14% of study withdrawals among those who received naltrexone. Naltrexone doses above 300 mg/day have been associated with life-threatening hepatotoxicity and are not recommended. The ramifications for a potential interaction between nonsteroidal anti-inflammatory agents and naltrexone to elevate liver enzymes and bilirubin level are still being investigated. Slow naltrexone titration, building up from 25 mg to 50 mg over 3 to 5 days, increased subject compliance and tolerability. Unfortunately, no dose-ranging studies have as yet been published; thus, it is unknown whether higher naltrexone levels may be associated with greater efficacy. Future development of depot naltrexone preparations, if efficacious, would obviously be of clinical importance as a new method of medication delivery.

Nalmefene, a mu-opioid antagonist reported to be less hepatotoxic than naltrexone, has yet to be clearly demonstrated as being superior to placebo. Although there is a published report of nalmefene-associated improved drinking outcomes from a randomized, double-blind, clinical trial, the use of one-tailed statistical tests to compare the nalmefene vs. placebo groups has made it difficult to assess the full magnitude of the treatment response. Additionally, the results of a large, 12-week multicenter U.S. trial did not demonstrate significantly different drinking outcomes between nalmefene (20 mg/day or 80 mg/day) and placebo as an adjunct to cognitive behavioral coping skills therapy.

In sum, naltrexone's (50 mg/day orally) effectiveness in treating alcoholism has been demonstrated in the majority of clinical trials undertaken. Naltrexone's effectiveness depends on high medication compliance levels. Thus, skilled implementation of naltrexone administration is required to obtain the best therapeutic results. Potentially, this may limit naltrexone's use in community-based clinics that deliver generic treatment for alcoholism. The development of depot preparation forms of naltrexone may ease compliance issues. Determining which type of alcoholic individual may respond to naltrexone treatment is an important area of current research. This knowledge would enable naltrexone treatment to be directed to those alcoholics who are most likely to achieve a therapeutic benefit. Results from the U.S. multicenter COMBINE study, conducted by the National Institute on Alcohol Abuse and Alcoholism, are awaited eagerly.

N-METHYL-D-ASPARTATE (NMDA)

NMDA Antagonists

Animal studies show that the abstinence-promoting neurochemical effects of acamprosate may be related primarily to its central nervous system interactions with the excitatory amino acid (EAA), glutamate. Acamprosate (1) attenuates ethanol consumption in rodents without affecting water intake, albeit in a two-lever choice paradigm; (2) suppresses conditioned cue responding for ethanol in dependent animals, even after prolonged abstinence (mechanistically analogous to negative craving in humans); (3) reduces the neuronal hyperexcitability associated with alcohol withdrawal that can manifest as increased glutamate and decreased central dopamine levels, particularly in the nucleus accumbens; (4) inhibits brain *c-fos* expression, an immediate early gene associated with alcohol withdrawal; and (5) antagonizes voltage-gated calcium channels, thereby preventing alcohol withdrawal-induced supersensitivity. Of the mechanistic processes described in humans, the most prominent as an explanation for acamprosate's therapeutic potential for treatment of alcoholism may be its ability to modulate the intensity of postalcohol cessation craving (i.e., negative craving), particularly on exposure to situations at "high risk" for provoking alcohol use.

Although there are few human laboratory studies of acamprosate, a recent double-blind, placebo-controlled magnetic resonance study showed that humans who received acamprosate had reduced brain activity in areas with dense NMDA innervation. These results are consistent with the findings of decreased central glutaminergic activity obtained from *in vivo* microdialysis studies of acamprosate-treated, alcohol-dependent rats. Hence, both preclinical studies and a human imaging study provide support for the therapeutic potential of acamprosate in the treatment of alcoholism.

Evidence for the efficacy of acamprosate in the treatment of alcoholism is largely drawn from the results of testing more than 3000 alcoholic subjects in several European multicenter trials. These studies have shown that acamprosate doses between 1.3 g/day and 2 g/

day are associated with about half the relapse rates seen with placebo. Earlier studies did, however, contain important methodological problems that have caused difficulty in comparisons with U.S. trials testing other medications. These problems include the use of insensitive self-reported drinking measures, nonstandardization of psychosocial treatments, and inconsistent diagnostic criteria for alcoholism. Later European studies (conducted in the 1990s) overcame these problems and again demonstrated efficacy of acamprosate in enabling alcoholic subjects to maintain abstinence. Treatment effects appear to be similar to those of naltrexone. Acamprosate is well tolerated, with the most common adverse event being mild diarrhea. Acamprosate is an approved medication for treating alcoholism in several European countries. Unfortunately, however, the recent U.S. multicenter trial of acamprosate did not demonstrate acamprosate's superiority over placebo as a treatment for alcoholism, and it will not be licensed, at the present time, for this indication by the Food and Drug Administration unless further confirmatory studies are undertaken. The future results of the National Institute of Alcohol Abuse and Alcoholism's (NIAAA's) COMBINE study, may, if positive, aid the approval of acamprosate for treating patients with alcoholism in the United States.

In sum, acamprosate is a promising medication for treating patients with alcoholism and is widely used in Europe for this indication. Failure of the U.S. multicenter trial to demonstrate acamprosate's efficacy in treating alcoholism has resulted in the Food and Drug Administration's refusal to license it in this country for this indication.

ALPHA-AMINO-3-HYDROXY-5-METHYLISOXAZOLE-4-PROPIONIC ACID (AMPA)

AMPA Antagonists

Midbrain and cortical dopamine pathways mediate alcohol's rewarding effects (including craving) associated with its abuse liability. Alcohol intake increases gamma-aminobutyric acid (GABA) receptor activity. GABA inhibits midbrain dopamine neurons and facilitates their neurotransmission. AMPA and kainate glutamate antagonists oppose GABA activity, thereby decreasing dopamine neurotransmission. This effect is exaggerated in chronic alcoholic individuals, who have enhanced glutamate binding sites in the brain.

Topiramate is a sulfamate fructopyranose derivative that facilitates GABA (through a non-benzodiazepine $GABA_A$ receptor site) and antagonizes AMPA and kainate glutamate receptors (all contributing to decreasing central dopamine). It should, therefore, be of therapeutic benefit in treating alcoholism. Based on this concept, we showed in a double-blind, randomized clinical trial (N = 150) that topiramate (up to 300 mg/day), compared with placebo, decreases drinking, reduces craving, and promotes abstinence among alcohol-dependent individuals. Self-reported drinking reductions were confirmed by decreases in plasma gamma-glutamyl transferase (GGT), the biochemical marker of heavy alcohol consumption. Treatment effect sizes were in the medium range. Tolerability of topiramate was enhanced by a dose-escalation regimen—taking 8 weeks to

Table 12.1.   Topiramate Dose-Escalation Schedule

Week	AM Dose	PM Dose	Total Daily Dose
1	0 mg	(1) 25-mg tablet	25 mg
2	0 mg	(2) 25-mg tablets	50 mg
3	(1) 25-mg tablet	(2) 25-mg tablets	75 mg
4	(2) 25-mg tablets	(2) 25-mg tablets	100 mg
5	(2) 25-mg tablets	(1) 100-mg tablet	150 mg
6	(1) 100-mg tablet	(1) 100-mg tablet	200 mg
7	(1) 100-mg tablet	(1) 100-mg + (2) 25-mg tablets	250 mg
8	(1) 100-mg + (2) 25-mg tablets	(1) 100-mg + (2) 25-mg tablets	300 mg
9	(1) 100-mg + (2) 25-mg tablets	(1) 100-mg + (2) 25-mg tablets	300 mg
10	(1) 100-mg + (2) 25-mg tablets	(1) 100-mg + (2) 25-mg tablets	300 mg
11	(1) 100-mg + (2) 25-mg tablets	(1) 100-mg + (2) 25-mg tablets	300 mg
12	(1) 100-mg + (2) 25-mg tablets	(1) 100-mg + (2) 25-mg tablets	300 mg

This dose-escalation schedule is similar to that provided in the Physicians' Desk Reference.
Numbers in parentheses indicate the number of tablets administered.

achieve the 300 mg/day maximum dose (Table 12–1). The most common adverse events were dizziness, paresthesia, and psychomotor slowing. All participants in this trial received a brief behavioral treatment to enhance medication compliance. Brief behavioral compliance-enhancement treatment (BBCET) emphasizes that medication compliance is crucial in changing the drinking behavior of alcohol-dependent individuals. Minimal interventions are effective and beneficial treatments for alcohol dependence. BBCET also has a practical advantage in that nurses or general practitioners in a primary-care setting can deliver it while they are dispensing and monitoring the medication. BBCET was modeled on the clinical management condition in the collaborative depression trial conducted by the U.S. National Institute of Mental Health, which was used as an adjunct to the medication condition. For this study, BBCET was conducted by trained nurse practitioners who used a standardized manual (see Appendix pages 282–301 for the manual).

Uniquely, this topiramate trial was based on a neuroscientific hypothesis before animal testing was done. Obviously, some serendipity must have been associated with this clinical discovery because much is still unknown about the neuropharmacology of alcohol-seeking behavior. Animal studies are needed to expand our knowledge of topiramate and its direct effects on drinking alcohol. Additionally, despite these promising results, topiramate's efficacy in treating alcoholism remains to be further established by confirmatory clinical trials. Nevertheless, the potential usefulness of

AMPA/kainate antagonists in treating alcoholism may herald an exciting new vista for developing novel medications.

SEROTONIN (5-HT)

Various serotonergic agents have been studied since the 1980s as potential treatments for alcoholism. Increased knowledge about the various 5-HT receptor subtypes has encouraged the testing of relatively specific agents.

Selective Serotonin-Reuptake Inhibitors (SSRIs)

Preclinical studies show that depletion of 5-HT in the brain is associated with decreased ethanol preference. SSRIs also have been shown to reduce ethanol drinking in both operant and conditioned-drinking animal models. These effects of SSRIs have been attributed to a reduction of alcohol reward (by chronic suppression of central dopamine) or a decrease in general consummatory behavior.

Despite these encouraging preclinical results, the clinical data have been inconsistent on SSRIs as single agents for the treatment of alcoholics without major depressive disorder. Early studies suggested that SSRIs reduce alcohol consumption in problem drinkers. Nevertheless, other investigators, in separate, well-executed, double-blind clinical trials, have failed to show the superiority of SSRIs over placebo among a heterogeneous group of treatment-seeking alcoholics. Interestingly, predicated on the findings of human laboratory studies that alcoholics with an early onset of disease may have reduced levels of 5-hydroxyindole-acetic acid (5-HIAA), one of the research teams re-examined their data. Paradoxically, they found that the SSRI, fluoxetine, compared with placebo, did not improve the drinking outcomes of early-onset alcoholics. In contrast, these investigators found that SSRIs appear to benefit late-onset alcoholics. Early-onset alcoholics differ from their late-onset counterparts by having a more significant family history and a greater propensity toward impulse-dyscontrol and antisocial behaviors. It is, therefore, tempting to speculate that the relationship between abnormality of 5-HT function and the onset of alcoholism is not a simple deficiency state but may be due to differential expression of genotypic differences in the serotonin system. This topic is revisited (see later) in the subsection on 5-HT$_3$ receptor antagonists.

SSRIs may be useful in the treatment of alcoholics with either comorbid depression or late-onset alcoholism; however, further studies are needed to confirm these results, given that in most studies tricyclic antidepressants provided to similar populations tend to reduce the dysphoric symptoms with little effect on drinking behavior.

In conclusion, SSRIs do not appear to be effective treatment for a heterogeneous alcoholic group. SSRIs may, however, be useful as treatment for late-onset alcoholism or for alcoholism complicated by comorbid major depression.

5-HT$_1$ Partial Antagonists

Animal studies have suggested that the 5-HT$_{1A}$ partial antagonist, buspirone, may be an agent for reducing ethanol consumption. Buspirone decreased volitional alcohol consumption by 30% to 60% in macaque monkeys; however, although buspirone (0.0025–0.63 mg/kg) suppressed drinking in alcohol-preferring rats that displayed moderate consumption, buspirone (>2.5 mg/kg) increased alcohol consumption without affecting water consumption. Although buspirone is a partial 5-HT_{1A} antagonist, the net effect of its repeated administration is to enhance 5-HT function via postsynaptic facilitation (which is more sensitive than the autoreceptor) and to down-regulate autoreceptor function. These studies provided some basis for testing buspirone in the treatment of alcoholism.

Several clinical studies that tested the effectiveness of buspirone in the treatment of alcoholics without comorbid anxiety have mostly yielded negative results. Nevertheless, there is some evidence that alcoholics with comorbid anxiety may benefit from buspirone treatment.

Hence, buspirone does not appear to be effective treatment for a heterogeneous alcoholic group. Buspirone may, however, be useful as treatment for alcoholism complicated by comorbid anxiety disorder.

5-HT$_2$ Antagonists

In a series of animal studies, the 5-HT_2 receptor antagonist, ritanserin, has been shown to attenuate ethanol consumption. Rats selectively bred for alcohol preference also exhibit reduced drinking behavior after treatment with the 5-HT_2 antagonists, amperozide and FG 5974. 5-HT_2 receptor antagonists may reduce ethanol intake by becoming substitutes for its pharmacobehavioral effects via enhancement of burst firing in dopaminergic mesocorticolimbic neurons, or through chronic administration-induced reciprocal feedback inhibition of central dopaminergic activity. Although the preclinical evidence for potential efficacy of these 5-HT_2 receptor antagonists may be relatively stronger for amperozide and FG 5974, only ritanserin has been tested clinically.

Ritanserin's effectiveness as a treatment for alcohol dependence has been tested in a rigorous multicenter clinical trial. In that study ($N = 423$), ritanserin (2.5 mg/day or 5 mg/day) was not superior to placebo as adjunctive medication to cognitive behavioral therapy for treating alcoholism. Hence, at these doses, ritanserin does not appear to be an effective treatment for alcoholism. A later study that compared ritanserin (10 mg/day) vs. placebo in alcoholics also did not show efficacy for the medication. It is plausible that higher ritanserin doses may be more efficacious. Testing higher ritanserin dosages is, however, limited by the fact that 5-HT_2 receptor antagonists dose-dependently prolong the QTc interval on the electrocardiogram, thereby increasing the potential for cardiac arrhythmias and sudden death.

In conclusion, ritanserin at pharmacologically relevant clinical doses does not appear to be an effective treatment for alcoholism. There are at present no clinical data on the use of other 5-HT_2 antagonists as treatment for alcoholism.

5-HT$_3$ Antagonists

Animal studies demonstrate that the 5-HT_3 receptor modulates some of the biochemical and behavioral effects of alcohol. Like other drugs of abuse, alcohol increases midbrain dopamine release, an effect associated with its abuse liability (i.e., rewarding) potential. 5-HT_3 receptor antagonists have been shown to block dopamine activity in several animal paradigms and to suppress ethanol preference and drinking (almost without exception) across a wide range of paradigms and in many animal species.

In the human laboratory, we extended these animal findings by being the first to demonstrate that ondansetron reduces some of alcohol's positive subjective effects, including the desire to drink. Others also have shown that ondansetron reduces alcohol preference in humans. One research team, in a preliminary 6-week clinical trial, found that ondansetron (0.5 mg/day but not 4 mg/day) was efficacious in treating moderate alcohol abusers, especially when a small cohort of severely dependent individuals was excluded from the analysis. In a larger double-blind, randomized clinical trial (N = 321), we showed that ondansetron (1, 4, and 16 μg/kg b.i.d.) is superior to placebo as an adjunct to cognitive behavioral therapy in decreasing drinking, reducing craving, and promoting abstinence among early-onset alcoholics. Ondansetron was not an effective treatment for late-onset alcoholics. Self-reported drinking reductions were corroborated by decreases in a biochemical marker of heavy alcohol consumption, serum carbohydrate-deficient transferrin (CDT). Of the ondansetron doses, the 4 μg/kg b.i.d. dose was the best although it was not significantly (i.e., statistically) better than the other doses. A recently completed clinical trial also has confirmed that ondansetron (4 μg/kg b.i.d.) is significantly superior as a treatment for early-onset compared with late-onset alcoholics. Body weight dosing for ondansetron can be achieved by appropriate titration of the readily available pediatric elixir.

Predicated on the finding that SSRIs improve the drinking outcomes of late-onset alcoholics and on our discovery that ondansetron is efficacious in treating early-onset alcoholics, we hypothesize that these differential treatment effects may be due to differing distribution frequencies of alleles at the 5-HT transporter. Ongoing studies are specifically testing ondansetron's efficacy in treating alcoholics who vary genetically at the 5-HT transporter over and above the effect of onset age.

In sum, ondansetron is a promising medication for treating individuals with early-onset alcoholism. Molecular genetic differences between subtypes of alcoholics may explain the variation in treatment response to specific types of serotonergic agents. Determining the critical molecular differences associated with response to a particular serotonergic agent would allow specific treatments to be targeted to those who would benefit most.

DOPAMINE

Dopamine Antagonists

Augmentation of DA-innervated mesocorticolimbic pathways has been implicated as playing a mediating role in the expression of alcohol-seeking behavior. DA-receptor antagonists are, therefore, obvious candidate medications for the treatment of patients with alcoholism.

In animals, a variety of DA2/DA3 antagonists such as haloperidol, tiapride, and SCH 23390 have been shown to attenuate low-dose ethanol-induced hyperactivity (i.e., because higher doses of ethanol are associated with sedation). Interestingly, however, only tiapride and SCH 23390 did not adversely affect the righting reflex in the rats. These results suggest that tiapride and SCH 23390 would be preferential to haloperidol as treatment agents for alcoholism.

In humans, tiapride (100 mg t.d.s.) was demonstrated in a randomized, placebo-controlled clinical trial of 54 alcoholics to be superior to placebo at increasing abstinence, self-esteem, and life satisfaction. Drinking levels also were significantly lower in the tiapride group than in the placebo group. Importantly, tiapride is quite sedating and, like other neuroleptics, can cause extrapyramidal symptoms. Tiapride also lowers the seizure threshold and may, therefore, be associated with the provocation of delirium tremens in recently abstinent alcoholics.

Thus, although DA2/DA3 antagonists possess potential as treatment agents for alcoholism, their side-effect profiles may limit their widespread use.

Dopamine Agonists

Low-dose DA2/DA3 agonists such as bromocriptine and 7-OH DPAT can reduce ethanol consumption in animals. Although seemingly paradoxical to the theory that abused drugs augment central dopamine function and their treatment conversely requires dopamine antagonism, dopamine agonists at a low dose may preferentially affect the autoreceptor with the chronic effect of reduced dopamine turnover.

In humans, although an earlier report suggested that bromocriptine may reduce alcohol craving, subsequent studies have found no effect on alcohol-drinking or related behaviors. Also, the high potential for nausea with these compounds limits any potential utility. Given this latter reservation and the negative findings, dopamine agonists do not hold much promise as effective treatments for alcoholism.

NEW VISTAS

Delta- and Other Mu-Opioid Antagonists

Research suggests that other opioid antagonists, such as those at the delta receptor (e.g., ICI 174864, naltriben, naltrindole), suppress ethanol drinking across species, including alcohol-preferring rats. More research is, however, needed in both animals and humans to better characterize this response.

Calcium Channel Antagonists

Preclinical studies have provided evidence for the involvement of dihydropyridine-class calcium channel antagonists in mechanistic processes associated with ethanol intake. Dihydropyridine-class calcium channel antagonists (e.g., isradipine, nimodipine) suppress ethanol intake in both nonselectively and selectively bred alcohol-preferring animals; block ethanol discrimination; and inhibit the development of tolerance. Disappointingly, a small laboratory study found that isradipine did not reduce alcohol's abuse liability. Also, dihydropyridine-sensitive calcium channels do not appear to be altered in humans, even after long-term alcohol exposure. Although these studies apparently diminish the promise of these agents for treating alcoholism, it would be premature to rule out this possibility entirely until larger scale and definitive human laboratory and clinical studies have been conducted.

Puerarin

Recently, isoflavinoids extracted from the Chinese root plant, *Pueraria lobata*, have shown some evidence in animal paradigms of being able to suppress ethanol consumption in alcohol-preferring (P) and Fawn Hooded rats. Multiple monoaminergic systems have been hypothesized to be associated with these effects of puerarin, but no definitive conclusions have been reached. No human studies have been conducted.

Neuropeptide Y (NPY)

Due to their co-localization with dopamine-innervated mesocorticolimbic neurons, neuropeptides may modulate ethanol response. Alcohol-preferring (P) compared with alcohol–non-preferring (NP) rats possess less neuropeptide Y (NPY) in the amygdala and hippocampus, and low-dose intracerebroventricular administration of NPY in Wistar rats is associated with anxiolysis. Event-related potential studies show that NPY has alcohol-like effects such as increased latency of the cortical N1 component and decreased P3 amplitude in the amygdala. Taken together, these effects suggest that NPY could be an endogenous substitute for alcohol and may be useful as an anti-withdrawal agent. This hypothesis awaits clinical testing.

COMBINATION TREATMENTS

Multiple neurochemical pathways may be deranged as either "state" or "trait" effects on drinking behavior. Thus, combining effective medications that work at different neurotransmitters may produce a synergistic or (at least) an added or superior response. Although this hypothesis is instinctively alluring, knowledge is in its infancy about how the various neurotransmitters interact in the living brain of dependent individuals and how this may vary under different stages of the alcoholism disease. Hence, the practical option at present is to combine medications with some demonstrated effectiveness in the clinical setting and to evaluate treatment response.

Several medication combinations are currently being tested in clinical trials. Of these, a few are of special interest. Presently, NIAAA is sponsoring the multicenter COMBINE study, which is testing the combination and individual effects of naltrexone and acamprosate. Interestingly, a published trial done in Europe has provided initial evidence for an added effect in combining naltrexone and acamprosate. Additionally, we have provided preliminary evidence that the combination of ondansetron and naltrexone is likely to be superior to either alone in the treatment of early-onset alcoholism. A confirmatory large-scale clinical trial is ongoing. Finally, studies are ongoing to test the combination of naltrexone with SSRIs.

EXTRAPOLATING FROM ANIMALS TO HUMANS: SOME CAVEATS

Animal studies have greatly expanded our knowledge about the neurochemical basis of alcoholism. Animal studies have been particularly useful for studying alcohol-seeking processes under controlled conditions; the impact of species and strain differences (as a prelude to the development of molecular genetic concepts) in drinking behavior; the development of neurochemical concepts that may allow parallel comparisons with the human experience of initiation, acquisition, maintenance, recovery, or drinking reinstatement; and toxicology. There are, however, some important difficulties in extrapolating directly from animals to humans, and there are, as yet, no direct parallels. Therefore, rigorous testing of putative therapeutic medications in randomized clinical trials remains the gold standard for determining efficacy.

CLINICAL TRIALS RESEARCH: PATHS FOR DEVELOPMENT

Pharmacotherapy trials have become more sophisticated since the early 1990s. Parameters for determining efficacy are under intense development, and the use of biochemical markers to corroborate self-report is increasing. Standardization of psychosocial treatments (now conceptualized as a "dose of psychotherapy") in clinical studies has occasioned greater confidence in comparing efficacy across clinical trials. Improved statistical models should enable clearer interpretation of clinical improvement.

Important challenges remain. Subtyping alcoholics to determine who would benefit the most from a particular medication lies at the heart of optimizing treatment efficacy. Further, differences in subtype may reflect underlying biomolecular variations that could be characterized to allow *a priori* determination of treatment choice. Dose-ranging studies, despite their expense, should be the standard paradigm to ascertain the optimal balance between effectiveness and adverse events. Finally, scientific advances should be used to generate hypotheses that can be tested in clinical trials.

CONCLUSIONS

This decade has seen an explosion in our knowledge about the behavioral and biological underpinnings of alcoholism. Built on this foundation, important advances have been made in the development of therapeutic medications for the treatment of alcoholism. Naltrexone has been approved for treating alcoholics in the United States. Acamprosate is widely used in Europe. Promising medications such as ondansetron and topiramate may usher in a new era of biological targets for treatment agents. Combination therapies with ondansetron, naltrexone, and acamprosate should facilitate development of even more efficacious treatments for alcoholism.

ACKNOWLEDGMENTS

We thank the National Institute on Alcohol Abuse and Alcoholism for its support of Assistant Professor Nassima Ait-Daoud (grant K23 AA 00329–01) and Professor Bankole A. Johnson (grants AA 10522–08 and 12964-01).

We deeply appreciate the skilled technical assistance of the staff at the South Texas Addiction Research and Technology (START) Center, Department of Psychiatry, The University of Texas Health Science Center at San Antonio. We also are grateful to Robert H. Cormier, Jr., for his assistance with manuscript preparation.

SUGGESTED READINGS

Cornelius JR, Salloum IM, Ehler JG, Jarrett PJ, Cornelius MD, Perel JM, et al: Fluoxetine in depressed alcoholics: a double-blind, placebo-controlled trial. Arch Gen Psychiatry 54:700–705, 1997.

Johnson BA, Ait-Daoud N, Bowden CL, DiClemente CC, Roache JD, Lawson K, et al: Oral topiramate for treatment of alcohol dependence: a randomised controlled trial. Lancet 361:1677–1685, 2003.

Johnson BA, Ait-Daoud N, Prihoda TJ: Combining ondansetron and naltrexone effectively treats biologically predisposed alcoholics: from hypotheses to preliminary clinical evidence. Alcohol Clin Exp Res 24: 737–742, 2000.

Johnson BA, Ait-Daoud N: Neuropharmacological treatments for alcoholism: scientific basis and clinical findings. Psychopharmacology 149: 327–344, 2000.

Kiefer F, Jahn H, Tarnaske T, Helwig H, Briken P, Holzbach R, et al: Comparing and combining naltrexone and acamprosate in relapse prevention of alcoholism: a double-blind, placebo-controlled study. Arch Gen Psychiatry 60:92–99, 2003.

Kranzler HR, Pierucci-Lagha A, Feinn R, Hernandez-Avila C: Effects of ondansetron in early- versus late-onset alcoholics: a prospective, open-label study. Alcohol Clin Exp Res 27:1150–1155, 2003.

Pettinati HM, Volpicelli JR, Kranzler HR, Luck G, Rukstalis MR, Cnaan A: Sertraline treatment for alcohol dependence: interactive effects of medication and alcoholic subtype. Alcohol Clin Exp Res 24:1041–1049, 2000.

Sellers EM, Toneatto T, Romach MK, Somer GR, Sobell LC, Sobell MB: Clinical efficacy of the 5-HT3 antagonist ondansetron in alcohol abuse and dependence. Alcohol Clin Exp Res 18:879–885, 1994.

MODELS FOR INTEGRATING PSYCHOTHERAPEUTIC AND PHARMACOLOGICAL INTERVENTIONS IN THE TREATMENT OF ALCOHOL DEPENDENCE

Helen M. Pettinati
Roger D. Weiss
Julie Madaras

Combining psychosocial and pharmacological interventions to treat alcohol dependence is a relatively recent and novel approach in addiction medicine. Combining biological with psychological treatments is especially favored by those who maintain that alcohol dependence is comparable with other recurrent medical disorders. In other areas of medicine, chronic and recurrent disorders are typically treated from an integrated pharmacological and psychological perspective. Pharmacotherapy can positively alter brain chemistry, whereas psychosocial strategies can enhance motivation for wellness, teach lifelong coping skills, increase a patient's self-esteem, and improve interpersonal relationships. In addition, pharmacological and psychological approaches can interplay in such a way that each strengthens and increases the effectiveness of the other treatment.

Research support for treatment models in addiction that integrate pharmacotherapy and psychosocial interventions has been demonstrated for methadone maintenance treatment and for the use of behavioral couples therapy to enhance compliance with disulfiram in alcohol-dependent patients. However, integration of pharmacotherapy and psychotherapy is used less often in the treatment of substance-dependent patients than in other areas of psychiatry and medicine, where this practice has some empirical support. For example, in comparison with either psychosocial therapy or pharmacotherapy alone, combination therapy has increased treatment retention and improved outcomes in depressed psychiatric outpatients. Thus, pharmacotherapy and psychosocial intervention together may improve a patient's quality of life in a way that is not possible with either treatment alone.

In the United States, alcohol dependence has historically been viewed as a moral, spiritual, and/or psychosocial illness, both in origin and presentation. It has not traditionally been seen as a biological illness, despite psychiatry's constant efforts to transcend the ancient mind-body dichotomy. Nonetheless, failure to see the biological side of addiction has resulted in limited usage of pharmacotherapy in the treatment of alcohol dependence. That is, in the treatment of alcohol dependence, pharmacotherapy has had a narrow role, primarily for detoxification or treating coexisting disorders. Consequently, alcohol treatment today predominantly consists of psychosocial rather than pharmacological or integrated interventions. Nonetheless, important gains have been made since the early 1990s toward understanding a potential role for medications in managing alcohol dependence. Furthermore, models for treating alcohol dependence that integrate psychotherapeutic and pharmacological interventions are currently being developed and tested systematically.

PSYCHOSOCIAL TREATMENTS FOR ALCOHOL DEPENDENCE

The treatment of alcohol dependence has traditionally included individual and/or group psychotherapeutic interventions and support groups such as Alcoholics Anonymous (AA). Research has continually demonstrated good response rates to various psychosocial interventions, and there is now good evidence that relatively brief interventions can be as effective as more intensive treatments in some patient populations and treatment settings. Results from Project MATCH (Matching Alcoholism Treatments to Client Heterogeneity), a National Institute on Alcohol Abuse and Alcoholism (NIAAA)-supported, national multisite treatment study of 1726 alcohol-dependent patients, underscored the effectiveness of three different types of psychosocial treatments for alcohol dependence. Findings from this study demonstrated that patients receiving either 12 sessions of twelve-step facilitation (TSF) or cognitive behavioral therapy (CBT) or 4 sessions of motivational enhancement therapy (MET) were able to show successful outcomes in reduced drinking as well as in other areas of psychological and social functioning.

PHARMACOLOGICAL TREATMENTS FOR ALCOHOL DEPENDENCE

Pharmacotherapy has, historically, been used infrequently in the treatment of alcohol dependence, except for detoxification or treatment of coexisting disorders. However, recent theories of alcohol dependence have focused on dysfunction of several complex neurochemical systems, including opioid, dopaminergic, and serotonergic systems. These theories presuppose that biological treatments may be useful in the acute treatment and long-term management of alcohol dependence. To this end, pharmacotherapy has increasingly become an area of intense study in addiction medicine since the early 1990s and has become a more attractive option for treating alcohol dependence.

In the United States, two medications are currently approved by the Food and Drug Administration for the treatment of alcohol dependence: disulfiram (Antabuse) in 1948 and naltrexone (ReVia) in 1994. Both medications have been scientifically shown to be effective in reducing excessive alcohol drinking in patients who are adherent to taking the respective medications as prescribed. Disulfiram works by altering the metabolism of alcohol via inhibition of the enzyme aldehyde dehydrogenase, thereby producing a buildup of the metabolite acetaldehyde. This is associated with unpleasant symptoms such as flushing, nausea, and headache, which are sufficiently strong to cause patients who drink alcohol to immediately stop drinking after taking disulfiram. In some situations, combining disulfiram with alcohol can produce dangerous and even fatal reactions. Disulfiram has never been popular with patients because of the noxious and unpleasant sensations that occur when disulfiram is combined with alcohol. The most frequent resolution to this discomfort has been to stop taking disulfiram.

Naltrexone's mechanism of action and side-effect profile is entirely different from that of disulfiram. Naltrexone is an opiate antagonist that blocks the mu-opiate receptors in the brain. In some individuals, this results in a reduction in the craving for alcohol and in the rewarding effects that alcoholics often feel when they drink alcohol. Unlike disulfiram, drinking while taking naltrexone does not result in an ill feeling. Naltrexone principally has gastrointestinal side effects. In particular, nausea and vomiting are the most common reasons for premature discontinuation of naltrexone. Occasional elevations in liver function tests may occur, and these blood tests should be monitored by practicing clinicians.

Although not all published research studies on naltrexone have found it to have an advantage over placebo in reducing excessive drinking, the majority of double-blind, placebo-controlled studies have reported positive outcomes in patients who took their medications daily. The advantage of naltrexone over placebo generally has been demonstrated because of the following reasons: a) fewer relapses, b) longer periods of abstinence, and c) a return to sobriety more rapidly after slips.

Other medications are being studied for their value in treating alcohol dependence. There has been a long-standing interest in treating alcohol dependence with serotonergic agents (e.g., serotonin agonists [buspirone], antagonists [ondansetron], and serotonin reuptake inhibitors [sertraline]). The literature has been inconsistent, but more recent research suggests that some of these types of medications can be effective in promoting abstinence in some alcohol subtypes. Pettinati and colleagues previously reported that sertraline (200 mg/day) over a 3-month period dramatically improved abstinence rates in type A alcoholics (i.e., sertraline vs. placebo rates: 53% vs. 16%, respectively) but not type B alcoholics (i.e., sertraline vs. placebo rates: 10% vs. 24%, respectively). One group of investigators reported that ondansetron (8 μg/kg/day) over a 3-month period resulted in better outcomes for early-onset (i.e., type B) but not late-onset (i.e., type A) alcoholics. Therefore, particular subtypes of alcoholics may exhibit a differential therapeutic response to specific kinds of serotonergic agents. Additional studies are needed to further establish and extend these exciting findings.

Acamprosate, which stimulates N-methyl-d-aspartate (NMDA) receptors, appears to ameliorate the negative effects of protracted alcohol withdrawal. Acamprosate has been approved in 24 countries around the world for the treatment of alcohol dependence. Currently, it is being studied in the United States in a national, multisite, randomized trial funded by the NIAAA. This study, called COMBINE, is comparing the combination of acamprosate and naltrexone with either medication alone and with placebo. These medications are being used in combination with one or two types of psychosocial interventions of different intensity levels. (The COMBINE study is described later in this chapter.)

COMBINING PSYCHOSOCIAL AND PHARMACOLOGICAL TREATMENTS FOR ALCOHOL DEPENDENCE

No one pharmacotherapy or psychosocial intervention has been proved to be a universally effective treatment for alcohol dependence. Similarly, data do not support the idea that combination treatment is the option for all patients. For example, some patients either do not want to take medication or are not interested in participating in psychosocial treatment, although these patient attitudes sometimes change over the course of monotherapy.

To date, the use of pharmacotherapy in treating alcohol dependence has always been given in the context of a psychosocial intervention. In part, this has occurred because few people believe that pharmacotherapy alone is an effective treatment for alcohol dependence. In addition, adherence to a medication regimen is improved when pharmacotherapy is supported by psychosocial treatment. In the next section, we summarize specific benefits in prescribing pharmacotherapy for alcohol dependence in the context of psychosocial interventions and the benefits of adding pharmacotherapy to psychosocial interventions to treat alcoholism. We also suggest that overlapping but potentially synergistic benefits may result from integrating psychosocial and pharmacotherapy treatments into one primary approach to treating alcoholism. Finally, we describe some models for treating alcoholism that are currently under investigation ; these models integrate pharmacotherapy and psychosocial treatments.

What Benefits Can Psychosocial Treatment Add to Pharmacotherapy?

It is unlikely that medication alone can benefit individuals with severe alcohol or drug dependence. Studies have demonstrated that many individuals with alcohol or drug dependence have problems in multiple areas, including medical, psychological, legal, employment, and social functioning. Some also have shown that the individual's functioning in these areas can improve if additional services or interventions that target these problems are provided. Additionally, medications alone cannot directly address complex dilemmas that many patients bring to treatment, such as a longing for intimacy or feelings of spiritual emptiness. Nonetheless, the kinds and levels of intensity of interventions that are needed for providing an effective pharmacotherapy need further study.

An additional major consideration when a pharmacotherapy is prescribed is medication noncompliance. Medication noncompliance is a universal phenomenon that diminishes the value of effective pharmacotherapy. For example, a consistently high rate of skipping medication doses can modify the profile of an otherwise efficacious treatment, resulting in its association with treatment failure. Medication noncompliance is not only a result of common forgetfulness but can also occur from intolerable medication side effects, negative attitudes toward pill-taking, a desire to experience euphoria, and reluctance to mix alcohol and medication. Response rates to efficacious pharmacotherapies will increase if proactive strategies are employed in the form of a psychosocial intervention to encourage patients to take their medication(s) as prescribed. As part of the COMBINE study, a psychosocial intervention called medical management (MM) was developed. MM includes methods to enhance medication compliance in treatments involving pharmacotherapy.

In part, this psychosocial intervention encourages open discussions between the clinician and patient about the importance of medication compliance in securing successful outcomes. (COMBINE and MM are described later.)

Finally, because addiction treatment traditionally has not included pharmacotherapy, patients being treated with medications may require added support when confronted with a community that may be opposed to treating addiction with medications. Such attitudes are changing, and people are generally more accepting of pharmacotherapy as an aid in addiction treatment (e.g., nicotine patch, gum, etc.). Nonetheless, education and reassurance from a professional clinician that pharmacotherapy is a viable aid in achieving abstinence from alcohol will likely continue to be required in treating alcohol-dependent patients.

What Benefits Can Pharmacotherapy Add to Psychosocial Treatment?

In regard to alcoholism, much as in other chronic illnesses, we now know that chemical changes in the brain are associated with long-term excessive drinking. Many researchers now believe the chemical changes associated with chronic drinking may play a role in intensifying craving during abstinence or in precipitating a rapid return to drinking. Some persons who have diabetes mellitus or hypertension, for example, can maintain health with only diet and exercise. Far more, however, require medications that "treat their chemistry" while they try to manage their illness with nonpharmacological strategies.

The number of patients who drop out of substance abuse treatment is uniformly high across various types of psychosocial treatments. Frequently, this occurs because patients cannot endure their intense craving for alcohol, or because they continue to drink while in treatment. For some patients, even a modest reduction in craving or drinking, which some pharmacotherapies may offer in the initial stages of treatment, may be sufficient to maintain them in treatment. In cases in which drinking may function as a maladaptive attempt to relieve, or escape from, anxiety or depression, medicines that reduce these symptoms may help individuals refrain from returning to drinking early in treatment.

Because psychosocial and pharmacological treatments can both contribute to the therapeutic response in the management of alcohol dependence, it is theoretically possible that patients who receive both types of effective treatment will derive added benefits or may benefit more rapidly than if they received either treatment alone. We also know that because alcoholism is a heterogeneous disorder, some individuals may respond better to either psychotherapy or pharmacotherapy. If the clinician cannot determine at treatment entry which of the two approaches will optimally benefit a particular patient, the clinician may increase the probability of treatment success by initiating both treatments together, allowing patients who may respond better to one of the interventions to succeed in treatment.

Is There a Synergistic Effect of Combining Psychosocial and Pharmacological Treatments?

The experiences described earlier illustrate how the integration of psychosocial and pharmacological interventions can enhance the effectiveness of either intervention alone. Pharmacotherapy can help correct derangements of brain chemistry, permitting some patients to reduce their depression, anxiety, and craving, and thus think more clearly, less encumbered by emotional highs and lows. Psychosocial interventions can increase motivational readiness, coping skills, self-esteem, and the quality of interpersonal relationships. Together, these treatments can have additive or potentially synergistic effects for some patients.

Synergistic effects of combination therapy occur when either one or both of the treatments are inherently improved and when additive algorithms cannot explain the benefits derived. In the earlier sections of this chapter, some of the examples described were clearly additive models in which more benefits were derived because more than one treatment was given (two are better than one). However, some of the benefits described are not additive but rather dependent on synergism derived from the integration of psychosocial interventions and pharmacotherapies. For example, better adherence to pharmacotherapy, which can occur because of concomitant psychosocial support, promotes better pharmacotherapy outcomes than those derived only from taking medication. Also, fewer concerns about intense craving and out-of-control drinking through the use of medication may allow patients to concentrate better on the content of psychosocial treatment sessions and, thus, derive more benefits from counseling.

Investigative Models Integrating Pharmacotherapy and Psychosocial Treatments

The COMBINE study is an NIAAA-funded clinical trial investigating the efficacy of combining medications and psychosocial treatment for alcohol dependence. The major goal of the COMBINE study, ongoing at the time this chapter was written, is to evaluate the efficacy of combining naltrexone and acamprosate with MM, with and without a combined behavioral intervention (CBI), in 1375 alcohol-dependent patients. These psychosocial treatments represent "minimum" and "maximum" interventions along a treatment continuum. Each patient receives 4 months of combined treatment and participates in 12 months of follow-up. In addition to the study of efficacy, COMBINE is examining the cost-effectiveness of the various combined interventions.

As part of the COMBINE study, a committee of investigators has defined the MM approach and produced a manual with patient and clinician materials for MM delivery. MM is designed to approximate a primary-care approach to alcohol dependence, with an emphasis on evaluations that focus on abstinence and overall health. As part of the MM intervention, the medical professional provides information about alcohol dependence and about the medications being used to treat the disorder. The MM clinician also is able to provide referrals to peer support groups. As part of the focus on medications, the MM clinician is instructed to be vigilant in assessing medication compliance by monitoring pill counts and having focused discussions with the patient about pilltaking. When noncompliance occurs, the MM clinician evaluates with the patients the reasons for missing or skipping medications and helps patients devise plans to enhance medication compliance in the future. Session structure varies according to the patient's drinking status and treatment compliance.

COMBINE investigators also developed CBI, and a manual for this treatment has been produced. The four phases of CBI are (1) enhancing commitment to change; (2) developing a treatment plan; (3) implementing selected treatment modules; and (4) maintaining and monitoring treatment plans. CBI was designed to incorporate some of the best features of available psychosocial therapies with proven efficacy for treating alcohol dependence. CBI includes motivational enhancement, cognitive behavioral therapy, and relationship enhancement therapy, and a significant other attends some of the sessions with the patient. In CBI, the number of sessions and types of modules are flexible, depending on the individual patient's readiness to change. In the COMBINE study, patients may have up to 20 CBI therapy sessions over a 16-week period.

OTHER CONSIDERATIONS: THE DUALLY DIAGNOSED PATIENT

The Epidemiologic Catchment Area Study and the National Comorbidity Study both confirmed that there is a frequent association between substance use disorders and psychiatric illnesses. As there are established pharmacotherapies for treating many psychiatric disorders (e.g., mood and anxiety disorders), pharmacotherapy is more frequently included as part of the treatment plan for alcohol-dependent patients who have a psychiatric disorder. Nonetheless, there are few established models for integrating pharmacotherapy and psychosocial interventions in treating psychiatrically ill alcohol-dependent patients. Furthermore, results of studies that treat depressed alcoholics with an antidepressant plus addiction counseling have not thus far been conclusive; some studies have shown that patients experienced improvement in both depression and substance use; others have reported mood improvement only, and a few have demonstrated no better results in mood or drinking outcomes than those produced by placebo. Increasingly, research attention has focused on the question of whether some dually diagnosed patients may benefit from two medications simultaneously (e.g., an antidepressant and an alcohol-specific drug such as naltrexone). Psychosocial treatment may require inclusion of not only addiction counseling but also focused strategies to reduce psychiatric illness. There are several NIAAA-funded ongoing investigations that are testing models for integrating several pharmacotherapies and multifocused psychosocial interventions for treating depressed alcoholics. Further studies, some supported by NIAAA and others by NIDA, are examining optimal strategies to treat substance-dependent patients who have schizophrenia, social phobia, posttraumatic stress disorder, and personality disorders.

FUTURE DIRECTIONS

Besides our continual exploration of new pharmacotherapies and psychosocial interventions to treat alcoholism, it is also important to investigate systematically whether outcomes can be enhanced or extended by integrating established efficacious forms of pharmacotherapy and psychosocial treatments for treating alcohol dependence. In addition, we need to determine whether benefits from combined therapy will be available for most alcoholic patients or for only specific subgroups (e.g., those with major depression). Currently, we have little evidence, if any, to guide us in selecting a combination regimen over a monotherapy. The NIAAA COMBINE project is only one model of integrating pharmacotherapies with psychosocial interventions, and this model is currently being tested in a national study for its potential merits. Future studies also are needed to evaluate alternative integrative models (e.g., concurrent vs. sequential combined treatments) and best delivery systems (e.g., primary care, psychiatric or psychological specialty practices, substance abuse treatment programs, etc.).

When combined treatments are examined, more studies will be needed to measure process variables that result from the integration of several treatment modalities. For example, studies need to quantify incremental benefits derived from the delivery of one modality of treatment vs. combined treatments. In addition, the field needs empirical demonstrations of synergistic results when interventions are combined. For example, it would be important to quantify how modest effects from one intervention could be enhanced when delivered in the presence of a complementary intervention.

In addition, we know little about how to prevent relapse once acute treatment for alcohol dependence is discontinued. For example, in treatment of patients with severe depression, pharmacotherapy is typically used as a maintenance strategy to prevent relapse after an acute treatment improvement has been achieved. Interestingly, one research team has shown that continuing a psychosocial intervention after discontinuing pharmacotherapy can extend the positive outcomes gained in treating alcoholism by combined interventions. Therefore, longer-term psychosocial treatment may be therapeutically beneficial even after active treatment with medication has been stopped.

Finally, researchers need to examine efficacy, modalities of treatment, and treatment intensity in the context of the cost of health care delivery (i.e., cost-effectiveness and cost-benefit analyses). As multiple interventions are applied, the cost of treatment delivery increases, sometimes substantially. However, alcohol dependence is a difficult disorder to treat acutely and recurs in a large proportion of the patient population. If outcomes can be enhanced significantly by combining treatments, increased treatment costs may be well justified. Further research is needed to establish the optimal combination of pharmacologic and psychosocial treatments for alcohol-dependent patients.

ACKNOWLEDGMENTS

The work was supported by grants from the National Institute on Alcohol Abuse and Alcoholism [R01-AA09544 to Dr. Pettinati; U10 AA11756 Cooperative Agreement with Drs. Pettinati and Weiss]; the National Institute on Drug Abuse [DA 00326 to Dr. Weiss]; and a grant from the Dr. Ralph and Marian C. Falk Medical Research Trust to Dr. Weiss.

We thank Dr. William Dundon and Donna Giles for technical assistance.

SUGGESTED READINGS

Carroll KM, Rounsaville BJ, Nich C, Gordon LT, Wirtz PW, Gawin F: One-year follow-up of psychotherapy and pharmacotherapy for cocaine dependence: delayed emergence of psychotherapy effects. Arch Gen Psychiatry 51:989–997, 1994.

Onken LS, Blaine JD, Boren JJ (eds.): Integrating Behavioral Therapies with Medications in the Treatment of Drug Dependence. Rockville, MD: NIDA Research Monograph 150:110–128. National Institute on Drug Abuse, NIH Publication No. 95–3899, 1995.

Pettinati HM, Volpicelli JR, Pierce JD Jr, O'Brien CP: Improving naltrexone response: An intervention for medical practitioners to enhance medication compliance in alcohol dependent patients. J Addict Dis 19: 71–83, 2000.

Volpicelli JR, Pettinati HM, McLellan AT, O'Brien CP: Combining Medication and Psychosocial Treatments for Addictions: The BRENDA Approach. New York: Guilford Press, 2001.

Weiss RD, Greenfield SF, Najavits LM: Integrating psychological and pharmacological treatment of dually diagnosed patients. In: Onken LS, Blaine JD, Boren JJ (eds.), Integrating Behavioral Therapies with Medications in the Treatment of Drug Dependence. Rockville, MD: NIDA Research Monograph 150: 110–128. National Institute on Drug Abuse, NIH Publication No. 95–3899, 1995.

Zweben A: Integrating pharmacotherapy and psychosocial interventions in the treatment of individuals with alcohol problems. J Soc Work Pract Addict 1:65–80, 2001.

14

EMERGENCY MANAGEMENT OF ALCOHOL ABUSE AND DEPENDENCE

Robert Swift

Alcohol use disorders, including intoxication, abuse, and dependence, are major causes of physical and behavioral morbidity and mortality and require emergency intervention. Studies conducted in hospital emergency department settings find that anywhere from 9% to 31% of all emergency room visits are associated with alcohol use. Alcohol also is involved with other drug use and abuse. The Drug Abuse Warning Network (DAWN), which monitors drug emergencies, reported that alcohol in combination with other drugs was mentioned in 34% (204,524) of emergency department drug episodes in the year 2000.

Alcohol use causes a considerable impact on health care and on society in general. Alcohol use is estimated to cause 100,000 excess deaths annually. Approximately 15% of all motor vehicle accidents and 50% of fatal crashes are estimated to be alcohol related. Liver cirrhosis accounts for 8% of all deaths, and one half of these are directly due to alcohol. The psychosocial impact of alcohol is also considerable. Survey data show that 15% of heavy alcohol users missed work because of illness/injury in the previous 30 days, and 12% of heavy users skipped work because they were drinking in the previous 30 days. Alcohol use is commonly associated with suicide, community and domestic violence, and child abuse. Total annual costs to the U.S. economy of alcohol abuse and dependence in 1998 were estimated to be $184.6 billion, with $26.3 billion incurred by health care costs.

Persons working in emergency settings are frequently required to deal with alcohol-related problems, and to evaluate, treat, and arrange disposition for persons who appear with alcohol-related emergencies. These include emergencies in which alcohol is the manifest problem, such as alcohol intoxication and alcohol withdrawal, and emergencies in which alcohol is contributory, such as trauma, psychiatric disorders, and medical problems stemming from chronic alcohol use. Patients who seek medical assistance for alcohol treatment may require the involvement of a significant number of social services. Particularly frustrating to both clinician and patient is the situation faced by a patient with profound social needs, such as homelessness, who is not eligible for medical treatment. In such a case, referral to social agencies may assist the patient, but there are many instances in which no assistance can be obtained.

EVALUATION OF PATIENTS

When a person has a medical or behavioral emergency, the most important initial action required is triage: the assessment of the immediate need, the level of care required by the condition, and direction or referral to appropriate services. Alcohol use always should be considered as a possible contributor to all conditions, given the strong association between problematic alcohol use and the development of a problem requiring emergency intervention. Assessing problem alcohol use is easy when individuals show obvious signs of intoxication and have the smell of alcohol on their breath. However, many people who have medical, surgical, or behavioral problems are identified only later as having problems with alcohol use. It is important to be aware not only of the amount of alcohol that may have been consumed at the particular time but also of the pattern of alcohol consumption. Patients are often reluctant to report drug and alcohol use out of fear of legal consequences or shame. Heavy chronic alcohol users are often resistant to believing that their use of alcohol may account for their problems.

Thus, all people in an emergency setting should be screened for alcohol (and drug) use as part of the initial evaluation and triage processes. Although no screening method is absolutely accurate in identifying people with problematic alcohol drinking, most methods have sensitivities and specificities in the range of 80% to 90%.

Screening for Alcohol Problems

Patients who are awake and responsive should be interviewed to determine the existence of an alcohol use history. Establishing a supportive clinical relationship is the best way to elicit information about alcohol and drug use. By expressing empathy and concern, the clinician is more likely to instill trust and obtain accurate information. Optimally, clinicians should conduct a detailed alcohol and drug history, perform a physical and mental status examination, order and interpret necessary laboratory tests, and meet with family or accompanying others to obtain additional information.

To obtain an alcohol use history, many clinicians routinely ask questions about quantity and frequency of use, such as "How much do you usually drink?" and "How often do you drink alcohol?" These questions usually are effective for detecting mild to moderate episodic alcohol use but have been shown to be less effective in heavy users. In determining problem use, it is more effective to explore whether the person has experienced deleterious social or behavioral consequences from alcohol or has poor control of its use. Furthermore, the quantity of alcohol consumed does not by itself make a diagnosis of alcohol abuse or alcohol dependence; rather, knowing the effects of alcohol on the individual's functioning is more important.

Several standardized interviews have been developed that distinguish those who have alcohol-use-related problems from those who do not. The CAGE Questionnaire is a four-item test that uses the letters C (cut down), A (annoyed), G (guilty), and E (eye opener) as a mnemonic. A "yes" answer on two or more of the questions shown in Table 14.1 raises suspicion for problematic alcohol use.

Another short screen for alcohol use, which has been shown to be effective in emergency settings, is the Rapid Alcohol Problems Screen (RAPS4). The RAPS4 questions four items associated with heavy alcohol consumption: "remorse," "amnesia," "perform," and "starter."

Other screening tests that have proved to be effective in emergency settings include the Brief Michigan Alcohol Screening Test (BMAST), a 10-item test that identifies heavy drinking through its

Table 14.1.   Brief Interview Screens Useful for Alcohol Problems in Emergency Settings

The C-A-G-E

Have you ever felt the need to Cut down on drinking (or drug use)?
Have you ever felt Annoyed by criticisms of drinking (or drug use)?
Have you ever had Guilty feelings about drinking (or drug use)?
Have you ever taken a morning Eye opener (or used drugs to get going in the morning)?

The Rapid Alcohol Problems Screen (RAPS4)

1. Remorse: During the last year, have you had a feeling of guilt or remorse after drinking?
2. Amnesia: During the last year, has a friend or family member ever told you about things that you could not remember you said or did while you were drinking?
3. Perform: During the last year, have you failed to do what was normally expected of you because of drinking?
4. Starter: Do you sometimes take a drink when you get up in the morning?

social and behavioral consequences, with a sensitivity of 90% to 98%. The Alcohol Use Disorders Identification Test (AUDIT), which was developed by the World Health Organization for a multinational project, and the Drinker Inventory of Consequences (DrInC), both of which have been shown to be effective in screening individuals and distinguishing problem drinkers from those who are not.

Patients who experience an altered mental status due to alcohol and drug intoxication or withdrawal may be incapable of providing an accurate history. In these circumstances, it is important to interview family members or acquaintances. It also is helpful to examine bottles or medications in the patient's possession.

There is an association between alcoholism and psychiatric disorders, including affective illness, schizophrenia, and anxiety disorders. Suicide attempts frequently occur in the setting of acute alcohol

Table 14.2.   Methods for the Determination of Recent Alcohol Consumption

Acute Consumption

Blood alcohol measurement
Urine alcohol measurement
Saliva alcohol measurement
Breath alcohol measurement

Recent Heavy Consumption

Gamma-glutamyl transferase (GGT)
Carbohydrate-deficient transferrin (CDT)
Mean corpuscular volume (MCV)

intoxication. A complete psychiatric evaluation is necessary for patients who appear to have significant psychiatric symptoms.

The Physical Examination

The physical examination of the patient provides important information about alcohol use and its medical manifestations. Patients who are acutely intoxicated with alcohol usually have the smell of alcohol on their breath as well as flushed skin and mental status changes consistent with intoxication. Cardiovascular and mental status changes may, however, depend on the blood alcohol level and the tolerance to alcohol. Chronic users with a high tolerance may appear only moderately intoxicated even at extremely high blood alcohol concentrations.

Even without signs of current intoxication, certain physical findings should always raise suspicion of recent alcohol consumption. Trauma to the head or that caused by accidents, fights, or self-affliction, often occurs in the setting of recent alcohol consumption. Heavy chronic alcohol use can produce telangiectasis of the facial region, facial edema, pancreatitis, and parotid gland enlargement. Hepatic enlargement and/or tenderness, palmar erythema, gynecomastia (in males), dilated abdominal veins, and hemorrhoids are all symptoms of cirrhosis. Chronic alcohol use can induce neurological abnormalities, including peripheral neuropathy, cerebellar dysfunction, and dementia. Mild to moderate alcohol users can have gastritis and systolic hypertension.

In addition to the physical examination, a complete mental status examination should be performed and should include tests of memory, concentration, abstract reasoning, affect, mood, and form and thought content. There is an association between alcoholism and psychiatric disorders, including affective illness, schizophrenia, and anxiety disorders. Suicide attempts occur frequently in the setting of acute alcohol intoxication. A formal psychiatric evaluation should be conducted in patients who appear to have significant psychiatric symptoms.

Laboratory Testing

There are a variety of laboratory methods that can be used to test objectively for the presence of alcohol in patients attending the emergency department. Because alcohol is dissolved in the body water compartment, it can be measured in essentially any body fluid, including blood, urine, saliva, vitreous fluid, and sweat. The concentration of ethanol in whole blood has become the standard system for measuring and reporting ethanol concentrations in the body. Most laws referring to alcohol specify that the proportion of alcohol in the whole blood be used to measure the level of intoxication. Blood alcohol level (BAL) or blood alcohol concentration (BAC) is calculated by using the weight of ethanol in milligrams and the volume of blood in deciliters. This yields a BAC that can be expressed as a proportion (i.e., 100 mg per deciliter or 0.100 g per liter) or as a percentage (i.e., 0.10% alcohol by volume). This system is almost universally adopted and is sometimes referred to as the "weight by volume" or "w/v" method. When ethanol concentrations are measured in other body fluids, such as saliva or urine, these are usually converted to blood alcohol concentrations for standardization purposes. Since the 1980s Breath measurement of ethanol has been used as a reliable estimate of blood ethanol concentration. Breath measurement relies on the property of ethanol to separate from blood into the inspired air. When air is inhaled deeply into the lungs and the breath is held briefly, ethanol vapor rapidly diffuses out of the pulmonary capillary blood into air in the alveoli and equilibrates with blood. Several handheld commercially available devices (Breathalyzer, Intoximeter) measure breath alcohol and report an equivalent BAC.

Many laboratory abnormalities associated with substance use disorders may be related to end-organ damage, vitamin deficiencies, and generalized malnutrition. In alcoholism, abnormalities observed on hematologic screening include leukopenia, thrombocytopenia, macrocytic and sideroblastic anemias, and target cells. Opioid users may have abnormal liver function tests and positive serology for hepatitis B, hepatitis C, or HIV.

Abnormal values on diagnostic laboratory tests sometimes are used to screen for alcohol use, but they are not absolutely reliable or specific. In heavy alcohol users, liver function tests such as aspartate aminotransferase (SGOT) and gamma-glutamyl transferase (GGT) may be abnormal; however, a significant number of heavy drinkers may have normal test values. Carbohydrate-deficient transferrin (CDT) has been found to be quite effective in detecting recent heavy drinking and has recently been approved by the Food and Drug Administration (FDA) for this purpose. The basis for the test is the inhibition by ethanol of sialic acid transfer to glycoproteins such as serum transferrin. Heavy drinking results in a reduced sialic acid content of transferrin, which is measured by the CDT test.

TREATMENT

General Considerations

To provide optimal treatment of substance use and dependence, the clinician must know about therapies for the acute management of intoxicated or withdrawing patients and must be familiar with options for long-term treatment and rehabilitation. A treatment plan should be practical, economical, and based on sound principles. In reality, the treatment of alcohol problems outside the emergency department setting usually depends on the protocols imposed by managed care organizations and third-party payers.

Brief Interventions

Effectively confronting patients with their alcohol or drug problems and then getting them into treatment requires special skills and techniques. Historically, physicians have felt poorly prepared to contend with addictive disorders. Since the early 1990s, several methods have been developed to help physicians successfully assess and intervene with patients. "The Physician's Guide to Helping Patients with Alcohol Problems," released by the National Institute on Alcohol Abuse and Alcoholism (NIAAA), presents several useful intervention methods.

Brief interventions, conducted in a supportive manner, are extremely effective in facilitating the patient's entrance into alcoholism treatment. The patient's presentation with an emergency provides a "teachable moment," when patients are more open to considering that their alcohol consumption is directly related to their current problem. Brief interventions can consist of just one session in the emergency department, which may take 10 to 30 minutes. During the session, the clinician provides education about substance use and dependence and negotiates a plan for cutting down or eliminating substance use. During the intervention, the patient is told that the use of alcohol and drugs poses a serious threat to health and well being; the evidence (historical or medical data) is pointed out in an objective and nonjudgmental manner. The clinician can explain that alcohol or drugs have affected the brain and central nervous system to the extent that the patient can no longer control their use and so may have lost sight of the negative effects that are occurring. Emphasis should be placed on the effects that alcohol has already had on the patient's health and the current problem. If appropriate, it is useful to compare the patient's excessive alcohol use with that of the general population, emphasizing that the amount of alcohol consumed is hazardous. During the intervention, the physician should be prepared for denials, excuses, and insincere promises to stop.

Blame for the problem should be placed not on the patient but on the alcohol or drug. However, the clinician should point out that even though the disease may not be the patient's fault, now that is the patient has been advised of the illness, getting effective treatment for the illness is *the patient's* responsibility. The patient and the clinician should jointly develop a contract, preferably written, which defines the treatment and the intervention plan. A formal means of assessment of effectiveness and follow-up should be part of the plan. Involvement of the patient's spouse, family, significant others, and employers may be helpful in bringing the individual into treatment. Should this type of presentation not be effective in getting the patient to agree to treatment, consultation with a specially trained addictive disorders specialist is recommended.

Treatment of Alcohol Intoxication and Withdrawal

Acute *alcohol intoxication* results in behaviors ranging from a euphoric and hyperactive state with affective lability to obtundation and coma. Because the chronic use of alcohol can produce significant tolerance, the blood alcohol level cannot be used as a sole determinant of physiological status. For alcohol-naïve patients, such as new college students, BACs in the 0.30 g/liter range can be fatal, whereas chronic drinkers, more tolerant of alcohol, can be awake and alert at the same BAC. Moreover, lesser amounts of alcohol can be fatal when coadministered with other sedative medications, owing to the synergistic effects. Thus, the clinician should tailor the treatment to the patient's clinical status.

Treatment of alcohol intoxication is essentially supportive. At lower levels of intoxication, treatment consists of observing, providing a safe environment, and addressing any behavioral problems. An alcohol level should be determined by using one of the several methods described earlier. Toxicological screening also is important, because alcohol is used in the context of other drugs. Patients should be kept well hydrated, and vomiting or other symptoms should be treated symptomatically. Serial alcohol levels should be determined, and the patient should not be discharged until the BAC is below the threshold for intoxication (usually 0.08 g/liter), and optimally not until the BAC is less than 0.04 g.

The management of behavioral problems caused by alcohol intoxication can be difficult in the emergency setting because of close quarters and busy staff. It is, however, as important as the medical management of the problem. Intoxicated patients have poor control of judgment and motor coordination and may injure themselves or others. Alcohol also can cause paranoia, anxiety, and behavioral disinhibition, including inappropriate anger and hostility. If possible, intoxicated patients should be observed constantly. Inappropriate behaviors should be addressed verbally, but, in some cases, physical or chemical restraints may be necessary. If suicidal behavior is associated with acute alcohol intoxication, patients should be assessed for suicide potential. Behavioral problems that threaten the patient or others and those which do not resolve as intoxication wanes should be evaluated by a psychiatrist or other behavioral health specialist.

At higher levels of intoxication, when there is significant sedation or obtundation, treatment consists of maintaining physiological homeostasis through support of vital functions. Ingestion of large amounts of alcohol can result in prolonged slowing of the respiratory rate, leading to respiratory acidosis, arrhythmias, cardiac arrest, and death. Thus, highly intoxicated patients with depressed respiration should be intubated, treated with a paralyzing agent if necessary, and transferred to an intensive care setting for close monitoring.

Disulfiram (Antabuse) is an irreversible inhibitor of the enzyme acetaldehyde dehydrogenase, and is used as an adjunctive treatment in selected alcoholics. If alcohol is consumed in the presence of disulfiram, the toxic metabolite acetaldehyde accumulates in the body, producing tachycardia, skin flushing, diaphoresis, dyspnea, nausea, and vomiting. This unpleasant reaction provides a strong deterrent to the consumption of alcohol. Death may occur, however, if a person using disulfiram consumes large amounts of alcohol, usually resulting from massive vasodilatation. Patients taking disulfiram who consume alcohol and become symptomatic require close monitoring of blood pressure and cardiac status.

Advances in pharmacotherapy for alcohol dependence have, however, provided several useful alternatives. Naltrexone, a mu-opioid antagonist, is FDA-approved for the treatment of alcohol dependence. Serotonergic agents, namely selective serotonin reuptake inhibitors and the serotonin-3 antagonist, ondansetron, have shown promise in treating various subtypes of alcoholism. Finally, the sulfamate-substituted fructopyranose, topiramate, also has been shown to be a promising medication for treating alcohol dependence. Establishing an excellent physician-patient relationship that facilitates exploration of these treatment alternatives is critical to maintaining compliance and optimizing treatment (see also chapter 12 in this book).

Patients who have *alcohol withdrawal syndrome* require evaluation of the severity of their withdrawal and may require behavioral or pharmacological intervention. Alcohol withdrawal is caused by the brain's adaptation to the chronic presence of a depressive drug. When alcohol is removed, the excitatory adaptations are unopposed by the sedative drug, and a state of central nervous system excitation occurs. Typically, the severity of alcohol withdrawal peaks at 1 to 3 days after cessation of alcohol use or after a significant reduction in use, and the duration is 5 to 7 days. Patients who have mild to moderate alcohol withdrawal may show tachycardia, diaphoresis, rapid tremor, and anxiety. Those with severe withdrawal show autonomic symptoms but also have confusion, disorientation, hallucinosis, and grand mal seizures. The severity of withdrawal depends on the amount and length of alcohol exposure, the presence of medical complications, and the psychological state of the patient. Current data suggest that less than 5% of individuals who undergo detoxification develop severe, life-threatening withdrawal delirium. The previous occurrence of withdrawal delirium or seizures in a patient is the best predictor of recurrence. An underlying illness, such as infection, trauma, or pain, can worsen the signs and symptoms of withdrawal. For example, an infection during withdrawal can predispose the patient to a change in mental status.

Treatment of the alcohol withdrawal syndrome includes correction of physiological abnormalities, hydration, nutritional support, and pharmacological therapy for the increased activity of the nervous system. The administration of sedative medications markedly attenuates the signs and symptoms of withdrawal and greatly reduces the possibility of withdrawal delirium and withdrawal seizures. Benzodiazepine derivatives are the treatment of choice, and their efficacy is well established by double-blind controlled studies. Benzodiazepines are minimally toxic and have anticonvulsant activity. A withdrawal scale such as the revised clinical institute withdrawal assessment for alcohol scale can be used for titrating the medication according to the severity of the withdrawal symptoms. For treatment of withdrawal, patients receive an initial oral or intravenous dose of a long half-life benzodiazepine (10 to 20 mg of diazepam or 50 to 100 mg of chlordiazepoxide) that is repeated every hour until the patient is sedated or has significantly decreased withdrawal signs and symptoms. A short-acting benzodiazepine, such as lorazepam or oxazepam, may be used and is indicated when elimination time for benzodiazepines is prolonged (e.g., with significant liver disease or in the elderly). Most patients show marked reduction in withdrawal signs and symptoms after several doses of medication. Patients administered long half-life benzodiazepines usually require little or no additional medication after a loading regimen. Patients with heavy sedative dependence or polysubstance dependence may, however, require additional medication to suppress withdrawal. Elderly patients and those with medical illnesses require close observation to ensure prevention of overmedication. In patients receiving calcium channel antagonists and adrenergic blockers, some signs of withdrawal, such as hypertension, tachycardia, and tremor, may be obscured.

Other medications, such as beta-adrenergic blocking drugs, anticonvulsants, and antipsychotics, are often administered to control withdrawal symptoms. Antiepileptic medications, such as carbamazepine, valproic acid, gabapentin, and topiramate appear effective in reducing most signs and symptoms of alcohol withdrawal and are widely used in European countries. When antiepileptic medications are used, patients are rapidly titrated to the blood levels that are therapeutic for seizures. It is useful to add benzodiazepines for breakthrough symptoms. Beta-adrenergic blockers, such as propranolol and atenolol, have been used as primary agents in the treatment of alcohol withdrawal, but they are most effective in reducing peripheral autonomic signs of withdrawal, and less so for central nervous system signs, such as delirium. Adrenergic-blocking drugs are particularly useful for controlling tachycardia and hypertension in patients with coronary disease. Neuroleptic medications, such as haloperidol or risperidone, are useful for treatment of hallucinosis and paranoid symptoms associated with withdrawal.

Alcoholics commonly suffer from poor nutrition and deficiencies in vitamins and minerals. Oral or parenteral thiamine (50 to 100 mg/day) should be administered to all alcohol users as soon as possible, and before the administration of glucose, to prevent the development of the ataxia, nystagmus, ophthalmoplegia, and mental status changes that are characteristic of the Wernicke-Korsakoff syndrome. Low magnesium is often present in alcoholics and may intensify withdrawal and predispose the patient to seizures. Magnesium levels should be obtained and deficits replaced with oral or intramuscular magnesium sulfate. Multivitamin supplements also are commonly administered. Diabetic alcoholic patients are subject to hypoglycemia, and glucose should be monitored and regulated.

Studies suggest that many alcohol-dependent patients may not require pharmacologically assisted detoxification. Even within a medical setting, many patients respond to "supportive care" and require little or no pharmacological intervention. However, those patients with a history of delirium tremens or seizures or the presence of medical or psychiatric comorbidities require inpatient detoxification and pharmacotherapy. Some authorities have expressed concerns that repeated, untreated alcohol withdrawal might worsen subsequent episodes because of kindling effects, and have suggested that all symptomatic withdrawing patients receive pharmacological treatment.

FOLLOW-UP TREATMENT

The goals of long-term treatment include maintaining a state of abstinence from alcohol and psychological, family, and social interventions to maintain recovery. These goals are best achieved through the patient's participation in a comprehensive treatment program, beginning after discharge from the acute care setting. If patients require hospitalization for treatment of a medical or surgical problem, a recommendation for alcohol treatment should be passed on to the accepting service. An alcohol treatment referral should be made for all patients who are discharged from the emergency setting. Although most treatment can be provided in an outpatient setting, halfway houses, therapeutic communities, and other residential treatment situations may be necessary to ensure an environment free of drugs and alcohol. Outpatient individual and group therapy for alcoholism is widely available within medical or psychiatric settings, or in freestanding alcohol treatment programs. An excellent resource that describes the types of alcoholism treatment is the *Handbook of Alcoholism Treatment Approaches: Effective Alternatives* authored by Hester and Miller (2002). Unfortunately, the type of follow-up treatment that is available for many patients depends on the ability to pay and the whims of managed care.

Many alcohol-dependent individuals have experience with Alcoholics Anonymous (AA). AA is an independent organization founded in 1939. Its only goal is to help individuals maintain a state of total abstinence from alcohol and other addictive substances, through group and individual interactions between alcoholics in various stages of recovery. Although there is a paucity of objective outcome data on the efficacy of self-help groups, these groups are described as being useful by many individuals. Often, hospitals are used as meeting sites by local AA groups, and psychiatric or medical inpatients may easily attend meetings. If the spiritual emphasis of AA is not consistent with the patient's beliefs, other self-help organizations, including Rational Recovery (RR) and the Secular Organization for Sobriety (SOS), may be considered.

Social support is an extremely important predictor of successful alcohol treatment. Alcohol use causes many family problems due to financial and emotional stress. Educating and counseling other family members about their role(s) in the patient's alcohol use and treatment are important factors in the avoidance of enablement and denial. Often, it is necessary to treat emotional distress, psychopathology, or substance use in other family members as well. Valuable emotional support and education for spouses and children may be provided by self-help organizations such as Al-Anon and Alateen.

As mentioned previously, several pharmacological agents have been shown to have efficacy as adjuncts in the treatment of alcohol dependence. Pharmacological agents to treat alcohol dependence should always be used as adjuncts in treatment, as part of a comprehensive program that addresses the psychological, social, and spiritual needs of the patient.

SUGGESTED READINGS

Cherpital C: A brief screening instrument for problem drinking in the emergency room: the RAPS4. Rapid Alcohol Problems Screen. J Stud Alcohol 61:447–449, 2000.

Hester R, Miller W (eds.): Handbook of Alcoholism Treatment Approaches: Effective Alternatives, 3rd Edition. Boston: Allyn & Bacon, 2002.

Johnson BA, Ait-Daoud N, Bowden CL, DiClemente CC, Roache JD, Lawson K, et al: Oral topiramate for treatment of alcohol dependence: a randomised controlled trial. Lancet 361:1677–1685, 2003.

Malcolm R, Myrick H, Brady KT, Ballenger JC: Update on anticonvulsants for the treatment of alcohol withdrawal. Am J Addict 10(Suppl):16–23, 2001.

Samet JH, Rollnick S, Barnes H: Beyond CAGE. A brief clinical approach after detection of substance abuse. Arch Intern Med 156:2287–2293, 1996.

Soderstrom CA, Smith GS, Kufera JA, Dischinger PC, Hebel JR, McDuff DR, et al: The accuracy of the CAGE, the Brief Michigan Alcoholism Screening Test, and the Alcohol Use Disorders Identification Test in screening trauma center patients for alcoholism. J Trauma 43:962–969, 1997.

Swift RM: Drug therapy for alcohol dependence. N Engl J Med 340: 1482–1490, 1999.

INPATIENT ALCOHOLISM SERVICES

William B. Lawson
Robert Mickey

WHEN HOSPITALIZATION SHOULD BE USED

Today there are numerous treatments for alcohol in the outpatient setting. These include therapeutic communities, outpatient centers, day hospitals, and partial hospital settings. Many studies have found few differences and more cost savings when outpatient services are compared with the same services provided in an inpatient setting. As a result, most care is now carried out in an outpatient setting. Detoxification is a service, however, that requires frequent assessments and specific treatments to prevent the complications of withdrawal. Consequently, detoxification now dominates inpatient care, although outpatient detoxification is widely used. Similarly, acute intoxication leading to unconsciousness or respiratory distress should be treated initially on an inpatient basis.

The following are widely accepted guidelines used to determine whether inpatient care is needed:

1. Patients with alcohol overdoses that cannot be treated in an emergency room or outpatient setting. These are the patients who are unconscious or have severe respiratory depression.
2. Delirium tremens. This is a life-threatening complication characterized by hallucinations and disorientation. The mortality rate when untreated has been estimated to be 20%. With treatment, the rate has been estimated to be as low as 1%. A past history of delirium tremens is also an important consideration in determining admission, because it suggests the likelihood of future episodes.
3. Individuals who have very heavy alcohol use and high tolerance. These individuals are at risk for a complicated withdrawal syndrome. In particular, their high tolerance may prevent the unwary clinician from recognizing these as high-risk individuals.
4. Individuals concurrently abusing other drugs. These patients may be at risk because the alcohol may interact with other agents by either masking a severe withdrawal, being exacerbated by other sedatives, or otherwise complicating the medical consequences.
5. Individuals who have a severe comorbid general medical disorder. Alcohol's effect on peripheral metabolism may worsen the outcome or complicate the diagnosis of numerous general medical conditions. Patients with severe cardiac disease may not be able to be adequately monitored in an outpatient setting.
6. Individuals who have a comorbid psychiatric disorder that endangers themselves or others. These include individuals with

suicidal ideation. Alcoholism is itself a risk factor for suicide and depression and can further complicate related conditions. Moreover, the disinhibition can worsen combativeness in psychotic individuals.

7. Individuals who have been documented as failing to benefit from a lesser restrictive environment including partial hospitalization or day treatment. These patients should also be considered for a residential or hospital setting that can safely provide the care they need.

8. Patients who have not responded to treatment in lesser restrictive settings. These individuals should be considered for outpatient care.

How Should the Newly Admitted Patient Be Acutely Managed?

1. The acutely intoxicated or withdrawing individual should have a detailed assessment that would include the following information:
   a. Detailed drinking history, including history of past treatments and complications
   b. Psychiatric and medical history
   c. Psychosocial history
   d. Physical examination and vital signs , including examination for volume status, dehydration, head injury, and tremulousness
   e. Laboratory tests: Liver function tests, electrolytes, breathalyzer, urine drug screen

2. If acutely intoxicated individuals are unconscious, they require appropriate monitoring, hydration, and nutrition. Conscious individuals also require reassurance and maintenance in a supportive environment. External stimulation should be decreased when medically possible, and staff should be encouraged to provide frequent information for reality orientation. There should be adequate hydration and nutrition.

3. Acute withdrawal may be characterized by two of the following DSM-IV criteria: nausea and vomiting, tremor, sweating, anxiety and irritability, agitation, skin sensations, heightened sensitivity to light and sound, headache, and problems with concentration and orientation. The general pattern of acute withdrawal is as follows:
   a. Symptoms of withdrawal occur within the first 4 to 12 hours after substantial reduction or cessation of drinking.
   b. Peak withdrawal symptoms after 48 hours include risk of seizures. Seizures can occur from 24 hours to 5 days after drinking ceases.
   c. Delirium tremens can occur between 48 and 96 hours after withdrawal begins.
   d. Uncomplicated withdrawal may last only 72 hours.
   These time frames may be difficult to ascertain because the patient is a poor historian or because the history is absent.
   Other drug abuse or comorbid medical conditions may also affect these time frames.

4. Acute treatment requires reduction of central nervous system (CNS) irritability and restoration of physiological balance.
   a. Benzodiazepines are often used to eliminate CNS irritability. Loading doses of chlordiazepoxide, 200 to 400 mg, or diazepam, 20 to 40 mg, have been used, and they can then be given in divided doses every 2–4 hours. Shorter acting agents, such

as oxazepam or lorazepam, may be used. They have the further advantage of being less toxic in the patient with severe hepatotoxicity. A whole host of other agents, with probably greater risk and more cross tolerance, have been used, including barbiturates, chloral hydrate, and paraldehyde. Beta blockers and clonidine have been used as well for mild cases of withdrawal, but they have little efficacy in preventing seizures.

b. Thiamine should be given to prevent neurological complications including the Wernicke-Korsakoff syndrome, neuropathies, and dementia. Without treatment, these syndromes may have a profound effect on morbidity. Wernicke's encephalopathy is characterized by ophthalmoplegia, ataxia, and confusion. Ocular abnormalities include nystagmus, eye muscle palsies, and pupillary abnormalities. The mortality rate is 20% if untreated, and recovery is incomplete in 40% of causes. Eighty percent of these patients develop Korsakoff's syndrome or alcohol amnestic disorder. The individual develops anterograde and retrograde amnesia that is permanent in half the cases. Cerebellar ataxia and dementia may also occur.

c. Fluids should be administered depending on whether the patient is dehydrated or volume loaded, both of which are common.

d. Sometimes antipsychotics are necessary for treatment of patients with severe withdrawal symptoms complicated by hallucinosis, delusions, or combativeness, which may be a part of withdrawal or of underlying psychiatric illness. Haloperidol has been the traditional treatment of choice because of its relative lack of potential for side effects and sedation and because of its availability in multiple forms for administration. Intramuscular forms of atypical antipsychotics such as olanzapine and ziprasidone may make these agents the treatments of choice, because they have little or no extrapyramidal side effects. Antipsychotics should not be used as adjuncts to benzodiazepines because they are not particularly effective for treating withdrawal.

5. Maintenance treatment includes ongoing observation and tapering of benzodiazepines or other sedatives, with instructions to the staff to restart or increase the dose if symptoms re-emerge. As the patient's sensorium clears, some programs institute psychological or educational counseling.

What Is the Discharge Process?

In this era of shortened length of hospital stay, care must be taken to ensure that the withdrawal process is stable and complete. If the patient is being referred to a therapeutic community, day treatment center, or partial hospitalization facility, the release may take place at an earlier point in the process than if the individual is discharged to a treatment program with limited opportunities for observation. Ideally, psychotherapeutic treatment should be started before discharge so that continuum can be maintained after discharge. Thus, starting treatment before discharge may have an added benefit. More often than not, limited opportunities for continuum of care may exist, and it is important for the staff to ensure medical and psychiatric follow-up if necessary. Twelve-step programs, motivational programs, and cognitive/behavioral approaches have been shown to be effective in alcohol treatment. There is evidence that inpatient care may increase their effectiveness.

Because medical conditions are often comorbid with alcohol dependence, adequate provision should be made for follow-up services. Complications of chronic alcohol use include cirrhosis of the liver, various gastrointestinal disorders including gastritis and ulcers, increased risk of hepatic and gastrointestinal cancers, cardiomyopathy, and other cardiovascular disorders. Female patients run the risk of having an unborn child develop fetal alcohol syndrome if abstinence is not achieved. Although alcohol is not a direct risk factor for AIDS, it is associated with high-risk behavior that can lead to AIDS. Consequently, every effort should be made to educate the patient about the complications of ongoing abuse.

Psychiatric symptoms are often seen with alcohol abuse and withdrawal. Some are the direct consequence of alcohol effects on the brain; these tend to resolve. Hallucinosis, delusional states, and combativeness often resolve after withdrawal. Symptoms indistinguishable from major depression that are seen with withdrawal do resolve. However, the epidemiological studies show that comorbid psychiatric disorders occur very commonly with alcohol dependence, and it may be difficult to distinguish a comorbid condition from the alcohol complication. Depressive symptoms may take up to 4 weeks to resolve. Because antidepressants may require 2 or more weeks to show efficacy, the provider may have to start treatment before an alcohol depressive syndrome starts to resolve. An approach used to distinguish these patients is to determine whether they have a prior history of major depression unrelated to periods of alcohol use and/or a strong family history of affective disorder. In the alcoholic patient, use of tricyclic antidepressants is discouraged, and selective serotonin reuptake inhibitors are encouraged because of their safer side-effect profiles.

Over half of bipolar or schizophrenic patients may develop alcohol or substance dependence. Bipolar affectively disordered patients, in particular, may be misdiagnosed as having alcohol dependence associated with depression. Treatment with antidepressants may precipitate a manic episode or rapid cycling. Care should be taken in identifying these patients. The use of antimanic agents, such as lithium or valproate, should be monitored with care.

Psychotic symptoms may not resolve for 12 weeks in some patients, which sometimes causes difficulty in making the diagnosis of schizophrenia. Atypical antipsychotics are recommended because of their safety profile. Treatment programs focusing on comorbidity are effective in these normally noncompliant patients. Most studies show that integrated treatment (i.e., treatment programs for alcohol abuse and mental disorders presented as a single program) is more effective than concurrent (i.e., alcohol treatment presented simultaneously but separately with mental illness treatment) or sequential treatment, in which one treatment follows the other. Since comorbidity often extends the length of stay, instituting an integrated treatment program for these patients before discharge may be desirable.

Often, there are social complications connected to alcohol use. These include employment problems, marital and family difficulties (including domestic violence), and a host of legal difficulties ranging from driving offenses to problems resulting from the disruptive behavior that occurs with acute intoxication. The inpatient stay offers an opportunity to begin resolution of these difficulties, but it has the additional complication of a financial strain and time lost from a job if the individual is working. Child care issues arise if the patient is a single parent and these cause more family stresses. Homelessness may also be a serious consequence for individuals with comorbid conditions. Social services on the inpatient unit can play a key role on the treatment team by beginning to address these issues before discharge. The stay in the inpatient unit can be an opportunity for family or couple therapy to begin and for a spouse or other family member to become acquainted with support groups. Initiating supportive work and job counseling while the patient is still receiving inpatient care has been found to improve outcome.

In conclusion, inpatient care may be necessary for some individuals with alcoholism. A detailed medical and psychiatric evaluation is necessary. Current pharmacotherapies can improve withdrawal outcomes. Initiation of various interventions before discharge can improve the transition to outpatient care.

SUGGESTED READINGS

Goodwin DW, Gabrielli WF Jr. Alcohol: clinical aspects. In: Lowinson JH, Ruiz P, Millman RB, Langrod JG (eds.), Substance Abuse: A Comprehensive Textbook, 3rd Edition. Washington, D.C.: American Psychiatric Press, Inc., 1997, pp. 142–148.

Gottheil E, McLellan AT, Druley KA: Length of stay, patient severity and treatment outcome: sample data from the field of alcoholism. J Stud Alcohol 53:69–75, 1992.

Institute of Medicine. Broadening the Base of Treatment for Alcohol Problems. Washington, D.C.: National Academy Press, 1990.

Nace EP: Inpatient treatment of alcoholism: a necessary part of the therapeutic armamentarium. Psychiatr Hosp 21:9–12, 1990.

Vogel PA, Eriksen L, Bjornelv S: Skills training and prediction of follow up status for chronic alcohol dependent inpatients. Eur J Psychiatry 11:51–63, 1997.

NETWORK THERAPY

Marc Galanter

Network therapy is designed to bring addicted patients to a successful recovery in office-based treatment. It is defined as an approach to rehabilitation in which specific family members and/or friends are enlisted to provide ongoing support for the treatment goals and to promote attitude change in the patient. This approach augments modalities such as individual therapy, pharmacotherapy, or 12-step programs, and its goal is the achievement of abstinence from alcohol with effective relapse prevention.

THE RATIONALE

Most health professionals are ill prepared to help alcoholic or drug-abusing people achieve recovery, even though addicted individuals and their families regularly turn to them for help. Furthermore, few alcoholic people are willing to go to 12-step programs such as Alcoholics Anonymous (AA) until they have endured their illness for a long time, and most drop out of AA before becoming involved. Two pointed questions inevitably arise: How can we engage and treat the alcoholic individual more effectively? How can we make treatment more efficient?

Over the past few years, inpatient rehabilitation facilities for substance-abusing patients have been offering increasingly limited lengths of stay. These programs are useful because they terminate the patient's access to drugs and create a safe environment for detoxification and education, but they often disrupt supportive family and social ties when patients are hospitalized. They also do not allow patients to deal with drinking cues in their home environment. It is, therefore, reasonable to support rehabilitation of patients by means of the social ties available in their own community.

In enhancing the effectiveness of ambulatory therapy, an individual's immediate network may include spouse, friends, or family of origin, and perhaps a friend from work. Components of this network are, therefore, members of the natural support system that usually operates without professional involvement. If they can be brought to act constructively and in concert, the strength of their social influence can serve as a therapeutic device.

ADDRESSING THE PROBLEMS OF RELAPSE AND LOSS OF CONTROL

To understand a psychosocial therapy that uses network support, we must first define the target problem clearly and then consider how the network bears on it. From a clinician's perspective, the problems of *relapse* and *loss of control*, embodied in the criteria for substance dependence in DSM-IV of the American Psychiatric Association, are central to the difficulty of treating addiction. Because alcoholic patients are typically under pressure to *relapse* into drinking, they are seen as poor candidates for stable attendance at treatment sessions; moreover, they tend to drop out of treatment precipitously. *Loss of control* has been used to describe the addicted individual's inability to reliably limit consumption once an initial dose is taken.

These clinical phenomena are generally described anecdotally, but they can also be explained mechanistically by recourse to the model of conditioned withdrawal, which relates to the psychopharmacology of dependency-producing drugs. It helps explain the spontaneous appearance of alcohol craving and relapse. Drugs of dependence such as alcohol typically produce compensatory responses in the central nervous system at the same time that their direct pharmacological effects are felt, and these compensatory effects partly counter the drug's direct actions. Thus, if an opioid antagonist is administered to an addicted subject who is maintained on morphine, latent withdrawal phenomena are unmasked. Similar compensatory effects are observed in alcoholic subjects who are maintained on alcohol; they evidence evoked response patterns characteristic of withdrawal while they are still clinically intoxicated. These latent phenomena can serve as conditioned stimuli to alcohol-seeking or drug-seeking behavior.

Withdrawal feelings, and hence craving, can be elicited by cues previously associated with the alcoholic's use of alcohol. Thus, an alcohol dose itself can serve as a conditioned stimulus for enhancing craving, as can the alcoholic's usual drinking context. Exposure to the smell of liquor in a bar can precipitate the "need" to drink, just as seeing the paraphernalia for injecting heroin can lead a heroin-addicted individual to relapse.

The conditioned stimulus of alcohol use, or an environmental trigger, or even the affective state regularly associated with drinking can all lead directly to alcohol-seeking behavior before alcoholic individuals consciously experience withdrawal feelings. They may then automatically seek out alcohol on experiencing anxiety, depression, or narcissistic injury, all of which may have become conditioned stimuli.

Often modulations in mood state are the conditioned stimuli for drinking, and the substance-abusing individual can become vulnerable to relapse through a reflexive response to a specific affective state. Such phenomena are described clinically as *self-medication*. Such mood-related cues, however, are not necessarily mentioned spontaneously by the patient in a conventional therapy because the triggering feeling may not be associated with a remembered event, and the drug use may itself avert emergence of memorable distress. Here is an example of this phenomenon:

In the course of his therapy, an alcoholic lawyer found that his drinking had often been precipitated by situations that threatened his self-esteem. After 6 months of sobriety, he had a relapse that was later examined in a network session as follows: Immediately before his relapse, he had received a report that his share of the firm's profits would be cut back, which he took to be evidence of failure. He reported that he had felt humiliated and then very anxious, a state previously associated with turning to alcohol. Without weighing the consequences, he went out to purchase a bottle of liquor, returned to his office, and began drinking. He said that he had not thought to control this behavior at the time.

This example helps to explain why relapse is such a frequent and unanticipated aspect of addiction treatment. Exposure to conditioned cues, ones that were repeatedly associated with drinking, can precipitate reflexive drug craving during the course of therapy, and such cue exposure can also initiate a sequence of conditioned behaviors that lead addicted individuals to relapse unwittingly into drug use. This leads to patients who have very limited capacities to control consumption once a single dose of drug has been taken.

APPLICATION TO TREATMENT

What, then, can serve as a minimally noxious aversive stimulus that would be specific for the conditioned stimuli associated with drug craving, thereby providing a maximally useful learning experience? Specific techniques have been developed to address this need. A self-report schedule can be used to assist patients in identifying the cues, situations, and moods that are most likely to lead to alcohol craving. Through *relapse prevention* techniques, patients are taught strategies for avoiding the consequences of the alcohol-related cues they have identified.

This approach can be introduced as part of a single-modality behavioral regimen, but it also can be used in a supportive network context. By means of *cognitive labeling*, drinking cues are associated with readily identified guideposts to aid the patient in consciously averting the consequences of prior conditioning. Similarly, guided recall can be employed to explore the sequence of antecedents of given episodes of craving or drinking "slips" that were not previously clear to a patient. These approaches can be applied concomitant with an examination of general adaptive problems in individual counseling.

Having examined the need for identifying drinking triggers, we can now consider the use of network therapy. Family treatment for alcohol problems has been shown to support superior outcomes for treatment, enough that the modal approach is often said to involve family members. Indeed, the idea of the therapist's intervening with the patient's family and friends to start treatment was introduced in the concept of the "intervention," one of the early ambulatory techniques in the addiction field. In this approach, family and friends are brought together to confront the alcoholic and insist that treatment begin. More broadly, the availability of ongoing social support for patients can contribute to a positive outcome.

The Couple as a Network

A cohabiting couple provides an initial example of how the naturally occurring social network can be used to develop a secure basis for rehabilitation. Couples therapy for addiction has been described in both ambulatory and inpatient settings, and a favorable marital adjustment is associated with a diminished likelihood of dropout and a positive overall outcome. For example, the use of disulfiram has yielded relatively little benefit overall when it is prescribed for patients to take on their own. This agent is only effective insofar as it is ingested as instructed, typically on a daily basis. Alcoholic patients who forget to take required doses are likely to resume drinking in time, and such forgetfulness often reflects the initiation of a sequence of conditioned drug-seeking behaviors.

The involvement of a spouse in observing the patient's consumption of disulfiram yields a considerable improvement in outcome because it allows for introduction of a system of monitoring. Patients alerted to taking disulfiram each morning by this external reminder are less likely to experience conditioned drug seeking when exposed to addictive cues and are more likely to comply with the dosing regimen on subsequent days.

The technique also helps to clearly define the roles in therapy for both the alcoholic patient and the spouse. Spouses need not monitor drinking behaviors they cannot control; nor do they actively remind the alcoholic patient to take each disulfiram dose; they merely notify the therapist if they do not observe the pill being ingested on a given day. Decisions on managing compliance are then allocated to the therapist, thereby avoiding entanglement of the couple in a dispute over the patient's attitude and compliance.

Other behavioral devices demonstrated to improve outcome could be incorporated into the couples therapy format. For example, setting the first appointment as soon as possible after an initial telephone contact can improve the outcome by undercutting the possibility of an early loss of motivation. Spouses can also be engaged in history taking at the outset of treatment to minimize the introduction of denial into the patient's initial presentation. The initiation of treatment with such a regimen is illustrated in the following case:

After an alcoholic man was referred for treatment, the psychiatrist initially engaged both the patient and his wife in an exchange on the telephone so that all three could plan for the patient to remain abstinent on the day of the first session. They agreed that the wife would meet the patient at his office at the end of the workday on the way to the appointment. This encounter would ensure that cues presented by the patient's friends, who might be going out for a drink after work, would not lead him to drink. In the session, an initial history was taken from the patient and his wife, allowing the wife to expand on ill consequences of the patient's drinking, thereby avoiding his minimizing of the problem. The patient's recent medical examination had revealed no evidence of relevant organ damage, and the option of initiating treatment with disulfiram at that time was discussed. The patient, with the encouragement of his wife, agreed to take his first dose that day and to continue under her observation. Subsequent sessions with the couple were dedicated to dealing with implementation of this plan, and concurrent individual therapy was initiated.

The Network's Membership

Networks should ideally consist of a number of members so as to achieve maximal support. Once the patient has come for an appointment, the technician undertakes the establishment of a network with active collaboration from the patient. The two, aided by those parties who join the network initially, must search for the right balance of members. The therapist must carefully promote the choice of appropriate network members because the network will be crucial in determining the context of the therapy. This process is not without problems, and the therapist must think strategically to avoid conflicts that may occur among network members, and particularly to avoid inclusion of substance abusers who could undermine an abstinence orientation.

The Network's Task

The therapist's relationship to the network is one of a task-oriented team leader rather than a family therapist oriented toward restructuring relationships. The network is established to implement a straightforward task, that of aiding the therapist to sustain the patient's abstinence. It must be directed with the same clarity of purpose as a task force in any effective organization. Competing or alternative goals, such as meeting the psychological needs of the network members, must be prevented from interfering with the primary task; if other needs are indicated, a member can be referred for treatment in another context.

Unlike family members involved in traditional family therapy, network members are not led to expect symptom relief or self-realization. This approach prevents the development of competing goals for the network's meetings. It also protects the members from having their own motives scrutinized, and thereby supports their continuing involvement without the threat of an assault on their psychological defenses. Since network members have volunteered to participate, their motives must not be impugned, and their constructive behavior should be commended. Network members should be acknowledged for the contribution they are making to the therapy. Network members have a counterproductive tendency to minimize the value of their contribution. The network must, therefore, be structured as an effective working group with good morale. The following example helps to illustrate this point:

A woman was engaged in a family-held business, except when her alcohol problem led her into protracted binges. Her father, brother, and sister were prepared to banish her from the business but decided first to seek consultation. The father was a domineering figure who intruded in all aspects of the business, evoking angry outbursts from his children, and they often reacted with petulance. The situation came to a head when the patient's siblings angrily petitioned the therapist to exclude the father from the network 2 months into the treatment, and the father then implied that he might compromise his son's role in the business. The father's potentially coercive role, however, was an issue that the group could not easily handle. The father could not deal with a situation where he was not accorded sufficient respect, and there was no real place in this network for directly addressing the father's character pathology. The therapist therefore supported the father's membership in the group, pointing out the constructive role he had played in getting the therapy started. The children then became less provocative as the group responded to the therapist's expectation of civil behavior.

Some Specific Techniques

Anxiety-reducing tactics can be used in the network to avert disruptions and promote cohesiveness. These include setting an agenda for the session and using didactic instruction. A framework is provided for each session by starting out with the patient's account of events related to cue exposure or substance use since the last meeting. Network members are then expected to comment on this report to ensure that all members are engaged in a mutual task with correct, shared information. As the following example shows, their reactions to the patient's report are also addressed:

An alcoholic man began one of his early network sessions by reporting a minor lapse into drinking. His report was disrupted by an angry outburst from his older sister. She said that she had "had it up to here" with his frequent unfulfilled promises of sobriety. The clinician addressed this source of conflict by explaining in a didactic manner how behavioral cues affect vulnerability to relapse. This didactic approach helped to defuse the assumption that relapse is easily controlled and relieved consequent resentment. Members were then led to plan concretely with the patient how he might avoid further drinking cues in the period preceding their next conjoint session.

Patients undergoing detoxification often experience considerable anxiety. The expectation of distress, coupled with conditioned withdrawal phenomena, may cause patients to balk at completing a detoxification regimen. In individual therapy alone, the clinician would have little leverage on this point. When augmented with network therapy, however, the added support can be invaluable in securing compliance.

The network serves other practical ends. Patients are strongly inclined to deny drinking problems during relapse. The network may be the only resource the clinician has for communicating with a relapsing patient and for assisting in reestablishing abstinence. Consider the following example:

A patient relapsed into drinking after 6 months of abstinence. One of the network members consulted with the psychiatrist and then stayed with the patient in his home for a day to ensure that he would not drink. He then brought the patient to the psychiatrist's office along with the other network members to reestablish a plan for abstinence.

The Use of Alcoholics Anonymous

The use of AA is desirable whenever possible. One approach is to tell patients that they are expected to attend at least two AA meetings each week for at least 1 month to become familiar with the program. Some patients are easily convinced to attend AA meetings. Others may be less compliant. The therapist should mobilize the support network as appropriate to continue pressure for the patient's involvement with AA for a reasonable trial. It may take a considerable period of time, but, ultimately, patients may experience something of a conversion wherein they adopt the 12-step ethos and express a commitment to abstinence, a measure of commitment rarely observed in patients who experience psychotherapy alone. When this occurs, the therapist may assume a less active role in monitoring the patient's abstinence and keep an eye on the patient's ongoing involvement in AA. Conversely, if after 1 month of meetings the patient is quite reluctant to continue, and if other aspects of the treatment are going well, nonparticipation in AA may have to be accepted.

Contrasts with Family Therapy

Like family and group therapy, network therapy brings several people together to address a behavioral and psychological problem. Approaches vary among practitioners of group and family modalities because therapists may focus on the individual patient or try to shape the family or group overall. In the network, in contrast, the focus is always on the individual patient and the addictive problem. In network therapy, unlike systemic family therapy, the practitioner avoids focusing on the patient's family history in the network sessions themselves, because involvement in family conflicts can be disruptive to the network's primary task of helping the therapist maintain the patient's abstinence. Such a focus would establish an additional agenda and set of goals, potentially obliging the therapist to assume responsibility for resolving conflicts that are not necessarily tied to the addiction itself. Family and interpersonal dynamics can be addressed individually with patients at their own sessions.

A technique of family therapy that bears considerable similarity to the network format is the *strategic family approach.* As in network therapy, this approach focuses directly on the current problem rather than on the dynamics of the family system. Treatment is begun with a careful examination of the nature of the symptoms, their time course, and the events that take place as they emerge. As in other behaviorally oriented therapies, the focus is a relatively narrow one, and an understanding of behavioral sequences associated with the problematic situation is of primary importance. This identification of circumstances surrounding the problem's emergence can be likened to ferreting out conditioned cues that lead to the addicted subject's sequence of drug use. Both strategic family therapy and the network approach assume that these circumstances will suggest options for bringing about the problem's resolution.

RESEARCH ON NETWORK THERAPY

Network therapy is cited by the American Psychiatric Association Practice Guidelines for Substance Use Disorders as an approach used to facilitate adherence to the clinician's treatment plan. In this regard, three studies that were carried out by the New York University team illustrate its use. In one, the feasibility of training naive therapists was demonstrated. Residents with no previous outpatient treatment experience were taught to apply network therapy to cocaine-addicted patients. Over three quarters of their patients succeeded in establishing a network. The patients achieved urine toxicology results similar to those reported in the medical literature who had undergone treatment by experienced professionals in the field.

Another study was conducted in a community-based addiction treatment clinic. Counselors working in this outpatient setting were able to learn how to apply network therapy and incorporate it into their 12-step-oriented treatment regimens. When network therapy was added to counselors' ongoing care, it was found to enhance treatment outcome, as measured by urine toxicologies. This study supported the utility of transferring the network technology into community-based settings.

Another study illustrated ways in which psychiatrists and other professionals could be offered training in network therapy by a distance learning method using the Internet, a medium that offers the advantage of not being fixed in either time or location. The sequence of material presented on an Internet web site (med.nyu.edu/substanceabuse) was divided into didactic "sessions," each followed by a set of questions, with a hypertext link to download relevant references. The course took about 2 hours to complete, and the large majority of professionals who took it gave a positive evaluation to its use in their practices.

APPLICATION PROTOCOL FOR NETWORK THERAPY

This section summarizes the main points to be observed in treatment.

Who Needs Network Therapy?

- Individuals whose problems are too severe for the network approach in ambulatory care include those who cannot stop their drinking even for a day or comply with outpatient detoxification.
- Individuals who can be treated with conventional therapy and without a network include those who have demonstrated the ability to moderate their consumption without problems.

Start a Network as Soon as Possible

- It is important to see the alcohol-abusing patient promptly because the window of opportunity for openness to treatment is generally brief.
- If the patient is married, the spouse should be engaged early on, preferably at the time of the first telephone call. The clinician should point out that addiction is a family problem. The therapist can enlist the spouse in ensuring that the patient arrives at the therapist's office with a day's sobriety.
- In the initial interview, the exchange should be framed so that a good case is built for the grave consequences of the patient's addiction, and this should be done before the patient can introduce a system of denial. In this way, the therapist does not put the spouse or other network members in the awkward position of having to contradict a close relative. Then the clinician must make it clear that the patient needs to be abstinent, starting now.
- When seeing an alcoholic patient for the first time, the clinician should plan for the patient to take disulfiram in the office at the first visit. The patient should continue taking disulfiram under observation of a network member.
- At the first session, the clinician should make arrangements for a network to be assembled, generally involving a number of the patient's family members or close friends.
- From the first meeting, clinicians should consider whatever is necessary to ensure sobriety until the next meeting, and that should be planned with the network. Initially, the plan might consist of the network's immediate company and a plan for daily AA attendance.
- People who are close to the patient, who have had a long-standing relationship with the patient, and who are trusted should be included. Members with substance problems should be avoided because they will let the network down when their unbiased support is needed.
- The group should be balanced. A network composed solely of the parental generation, of younger people, or of people of the opposite sex should be avoided.
- The tone should be directive. The therapist must give explicit instructions to support and ensure abstinence.

Three Priorities in Running the Ongoing Therapy

1. *Maintaining abstinence.* The patient and the network members should report at the outset of each session any events related to the patient's exposure to alcohol and drugs. The patient and network

members should be instructed on the nature of the relapse and plan with the therapist how to sustain abstinence. Cues to conditioned alcohol seeking should be examined.

2. *Supporting the network's integrity.* The patient is expected to make sure that network members keep their meeting appointments and stay involved. The therapist sets meeting times explicitly and summons the network for any emergency, such as relapse; and does whatever is necessary to secure membership stability if the patient is having trouble doing so.

3. *Securing future behavior.* The therapist should combine any and all modalities necessary to ensure the patient's stability, such as a consistent, alcohol-free residence; avoidance of substance-abusing friends; attendance at 12-step meetings; compliance in taking medications such as disulfiram or an agent like naltrexone to reduce craving; and ancillary psychiatric care.

Also, the patient should meet with the clinician as frequently as necessary to ensure abstinence, perhaps once a week for 1 month, every other week for the next few months, and every month or every other month by the end of 1 year. Individual sessions run concomitantly. Make sure that the mood of meetings is trusting and free of recrimination. Explain issues of conflict in terms of the problems presented by addiction rather than getting into personality conflicts. Once abstinence is stabilized, the network can help the patient plan for a new drug-free adaptation.

Ending the Network Therapy

Network sessions can be terminated after the patient has been consistently abstinent for at least 6 months to 1 year. This should be done after discussion with the patient and network of the patient's readiness for handling sobriety.

An understanding is established with the network members that they will contact the therapist at any point in the future if the patient is vulnerable to relapse. The therapist can also summon the members. Before termination, these points should be made clear to the patient in the presence of the network, but they also apply throughout treatment.

SUGGESTED READINGS

Galanter M: Network Therapy for Addiction: A New Approach, Expanded Edition. New York: Guilford Press, 1999.

Institute of Medicine. Broadening the Base of Treatment for Alcohol Problems. Washington, D.C.: National Academy Press, 1990.

Johnson VE. Intervention: How to Help Someone Who Doesn't Want Help. Minneapolis: Johnson Institute Books, 1986.

Marlatt GA, Gordon J (eds.): Relapse Prevention: Maintenance Strategies in the Treatment of Addictive Behaviors. New York: Guilford Press, 1985.

Steinglass P, Bennett L, Wolin SJ. The Alcoholic Family. New York: Basic Books, 1987.

Treatment Settings

PRIMARY HEALTH CARE SETTINGS

Patrick G. O'Connor
David A. Fiellin

In a national survey, approximately two thirds of American adults reported that they used alcoholic beverages (liquor, wine, or beer). A considerable number of individuals in the United States experience problems because of their drinking. These problems result in significant morbidity and mortality and result in more than $100 million in health care costs and economic losses in the United States. Alcohol use disorders are among the most prevalent medical problems in the U.S. general population—the prevalence of alcohol abuse and dependence is estimated to be between 7.4% and 9.7% among Americans, and the lifetime prevalence of these disorders is even higher.

Since alcohol use results in medical and other health problems, the prevalence of alcohol use disorders is higher in most health care settings than it is in the general population. For example, the prevalence of alcohol abuse and dependence in general outpatient and inpatient medical settings has been estimated to be between 15% and 40%, respectively. These data strongly support the need for physicians to screen all patients for alcohol use disorders. Early recognition and treatment have been shown to be critical in helping to prevent the long-term sequelae of alcohol use.

The spectrum of drinking behaviors associated with potential or actual alcohol problems encountered by physicians in primary care settings extends from "at-risk" or "hazardous" drinking to "harmful" or "problem" drinking leading to a diagnosis of alcohol abuse or alcohol dependence. At-risk and hazardous drinkers are considered to be in danger of alcohol-related consequences either because of their level of consumption or because of comorbid conditions. "At-risk" drinking is defined by the National Institute on Alcohol Abuse and Alcoholism (NIAAA) as more than 14 drinks per week or more than 4 drinks per occasion in men younger than 65 years of age and more than 7 drinks per week or more than 3 drinks per occasion in women and in all individuals aged 65 years and older. "Harmful" and "problem" drinkers exhibit physical or psychological harm from alcohol consumption. Criteria for the more severe conditions of alcohol abuse or alcohol dependence are provided in the DSM (Diagnostic and Statistical Manual)-IV of the American Psychiatric Association.

Primary care physicians are in a unique position to identify and treat patients with at-risk drinking and alcohol problems. Studies suggest that the lifetime prevalence of at-risk drinking and alcohol abuse may be as high as 35%, and the frequency of problem drinking may be as high as 10% in primary care settings. The NIAAA and other experts have indicated that primary care physicians can be instrumental in initiating therapy and providing advice on further treatment options for patients with, or at risk for, alcohol problems.

Research has demonstrated convincingly that primary care physicians can effectively screen and diagnose problem drinking in their patients. In addition, the role of primary care physicians in providing direct treatment for their patients has become increasingly demonstrated in a variety of studies. This chapter reviews the state of the art of screening and treatment for alcohol problems in primary care settings.

SCREENING AND DIAGNOSIS

Information gathered from the history, physical examination, and laboratory tests is generally needed to provide a complete picture of the extent of alcohol problems in affected patients.

History

Primary care physicians need to ask all patients about current and past alcohol use. "Do you currently or have you ever used alcohol?" quickly identifies those patients who are not lifetime abstainers and who require further screening. Those who answer "yes" to this question should proceed through further questioning. In addition, given the importance of family history as a risk factor for alcohol problems, it is important to ask all patients about alcohol use in their families.

Among patients who use alcohol, the next step is to obtain a detailed history regarding quantity and frequency of current and past alcohol use. Quantity and frequency questions should be asked to determine both current and past alcohol use. These include the following questions: What type or types of alcoholic drinks (beer, wine, spirits) do you consume? How much do you usually drink on a typical drinking day? Do you ever drink more than your usual amount and, if so, how much? These questions establish a patient's "typical" drinking pattern and identify "at-risk" and "binge" drinking.

The screening instruments include the standardized questionnaires that have been developed to detect alcohol abuse and dependence. The CAGE questionnaire and the AUDIT screening instrument are the two instruments that have been examined most extensively in primary care settings. The CAGE questionnaire includes the following four questions: Have you ever felt that you should *C*ut down on your drinking? Have people *A*nnoyed you by criticizing your drinking? Have you ever felt bad or *G*uilty about drinking? Have you even taken a drink first thing in the morning (*E*ye-opener) to steady your nerves or get rid of a hangover? The CAGE is scored by giving one point for each positive response to the four questions with a range of possible total scores from 0 to 4. This instrument is designed to detect lifetime abuse and dependence and does not distinguish between lifetime problems and current problems. The CAGE has been demonstrated to have a sensitivity of 43% to 94% and a specificity of 70% to 97% when a cutoff score of greater than or equal to 2 is used to indicate a "positive" result.

The Alcohol Use Disorders Identification Test (AUDIT) contains 10 questions that cover quantity and frequency of alcohol use, drinking behaviors, adverse psychological symptoms, and alcohol-related problems. Unlike the CAGE questionnaire, the AUDIT was designed to identify hazardous (e.g., at-risk) drinking and harmful (e.g., alcohol use that results in physical or psychological harm) drinking and focuses on recent (current to past year) drinking behaviors. Each question is scored from 0 to 4, and a total score of greater than or equal to 8 is considered to be a positive result.

Once these steps are taken, the next step is to assess specific areas in suspected or known problem drinkers to get more detailed information about patients with potential alcohol problems. The diagnostic criteria of alcohol abuse and dependence should be assessed, and a detailed review for evidence of alcohol-related medical, psychiatric, behavioral, and social problems should take place. Use and abuse of other substances is highly prevalent and should also be assessed among people with alcohol problems.

Physical Examination and Laboratory Studies

Patients who drink excessively require a detailed physical examination and selected laboratory studies. The physical examination needs to be thorough and complete given the wide variety of systems that can be adversely affected by the use of alcohol—especially the neurological, cardiac, and gastrointestinal/hepatobiliary systems. The examination should focus particularly on systems identified in the history where problems may exist.

Laboratory studies can be useful for patient assessment in known or suspected drinkers but need to be used selectively. Potentially useful tests include liver enzyme and function tests, mean corpuscular volume (MCV), and carbohydrate-deficient transferrin. Routine assessment of liver enzymes is warranted to identify evidence of ongoing alcoholic hepatitis in patients with alcohol problems.

TREATMENT APPROACHES IN PRIMARY CARE

There has been an increasing body of evidence that supports an active role for primary care physicians in the care of patients with alcohol problems. Providing treatment—either directly or by referral to specialized services—logically follows the process of screening and diagnosis of alcohol problems. When provided directly in primary care settings, treatment approaches can include counseling and, possibly, the use of medications to prevent relapse to alcohol use. Patients in primary care settings who are appropriate for treatment based probably include those who are at-risk drinkers or those problem drinkers who do not have severe alcohol dependence and substantial alcohol-related comorbidities (e.g., active/unstable psychiatric disease). More complex patients with alcohol problems generally require specialized alcohol treatment programs and/or specialists (e.g., psychiatrists).

Counseling Strategies in Primary Care

Counseling-based nonpharmacologic treatment strategies have been studied extensively for the care of patients with, or at risk for, alcohol problems. These approaches are based on the principles and processes of behavioral change and typically involve the type of counseling commonly used by primary care physicians.

Brief Interventions

The approach most intensively studied in the primary care setting is the use of "brief interventions." Initially developed for the treatment of tobacco dependence, brief interventions employ simple counseling techniques that apply to a wide variety of primary care clinical situations. Although there are a variety of brief intervention approaches that have been studied in primary care, they all have some characteristics in common. These counseling sessions are short (5 to 20 minutes) and focused, incorporating four components. These include motivational techniques, feedback about the problems associated with alcohol use, discussion of the adverse effects of alcohol, and setting drinking limits. They are typically considered to be appropriate as primary therapy for at-risk or nondependent problem drinkers. Along with counseling, brief interventions often include the provision of educational handouts (examples are available from the National Institute on Alcohol Abuse and Alcoholism web page—*www.niaaa.nih.gov*).

Several randomized trials have evaluated the efficacy of brief interventions in the United States, Europe, and elsewhere. Two systematic reviews that examined the efficacy of brief interventions for nondependent drinkers in a variety of health care settings documented that the majority of randomized trials demonstrate a benefit of these approaches (vs. a control intervention). One analysis calculated a pooled odds ratio of 1.95 (95%confidence interval = 1.66 to 2.30) for decreased drinking after a brief intervention compared with no intervention.

A more recent systematic review, focused exclusively on brief intervention approaches studied in primary care settings, demonstrated that these approaches were similarly effective in primary care. Four major randomized trials were identified in primary care, including one based in the United States, one in the United Kingdom, one in Australia, and one performed in 10 countries by the World Health Organization (WHO). The studies performed in the United States and the United Kingdom had uniform findings in demonstrating the efficacy of standardized brief interventions among heavy and problem drinkers in primary care. Subjects in the intervention groups attended a brief interview with their physician that covered alcohol consumption and evidence of alcohol-related problems. They then received educational materials and a "prescription" to cut their drinking down to specified levels, whereas control subjects received no advice concerning their drinking. These brief interventions demonstrated a reduction in alcohol consumption at a level of 5 to 10 drinks per week, and a dose-response effect was seen in those subjects who received more intensive therapy. The U.S. study was performed in several community-based primary care practices in Wisconsin and was designed to be generalized to typical primary care settings. Subjects in the intervention showed improvement in major drinking behaviors (e.g., drinks per week, binge-drinking episodes), but those in the intervention group also experienced decreased hospitalization (in men).

The Australian and WHO studies have produced less uniform results with these interventions. The Australian study compared three groups: a full brief intervention, a 5-minute single session, and a drinking assessment only. At 6 and 12 months, this study showed significant overall reductions in alcohol consumption for all patients. However, this study failed to demonstrate a difference between treatments in the percentage of patients who reported drinking above recommended "safe" levels. The WHO study involved 10 countries, including Costa Rica, Australia, the United Kingdom, Norway, Mexico, Kenya, Bulgaria, the Soviet Union, Zimbabwe, and the United

States, and enrolled 1661 nondependent heavy drinkers. These subjects were recruited from a variety of health care settings, including primary care, and were randomly assigned to one of three treatment arms: (1) a 15-minute brief counseling group, (2) a 5-minute simple advice group, and (3) an untreated control group. Men in the intervention group in this study were demonstrated to have significant improvements in some drinking behaviors, whereas women in both the intervention and control groups improved.

Despite the generally positive findings from these studies, the methods used may somewhat limit the utility of their application. The enrolled subjects had a spectrum of alcohol problems, including problem drinkers and excessive drinkers, and, in some cases, it was not clear whether patients with alcohol dependence were excluded in all cases. In addition, although they were generally similar, the components and intensity of the brief interventions varied across studies. For instance, in one study, the intervention included a single physician who delivered a warning without follow-up, whereas another provided up to three follow-up visits; in addition, the use of ancillary treatments varied across studies. In some cases, the interventions required specialized training for study physicians that might not be routinely available in primary care. Finally, follow-up rates that ranged between 58% and 93% suggest that retention may limit overall effectiveness. Despite these limitations, the overwhelming evidence that brief interventions can result in decreased alcohol consumption in primary care and other health care settings supports their widespread use in primary care.

Referral to Specialty Services

Patients with alcohol dependence and more complex alcohol-related comorbidities are generally more appropriate for treatment in specialized alcohol treatment settings and at Alcoholics Anonymous facilities. It is important for primary care physicians to be familiar with the principles and components of these programs as well as the process of patient referral. A study of counseling approaches in alcohol treatment programs—Project MATCH (Matching Alcoholism Treatments to Client Heterogeneity)—examined three specific treatment strategies: cognitive behavioral coping skills therapy (CBT), motivational enhancement therapy (MET), and 12-step facilitation therapy (TSF). Although the therapies were found to be equivalent in the 1726 study subjects with alcohol abuse or dependence, the fact that all three treatments produced a significant and sustained reduction in drinking outcomes from baseline to follow-up should be quite encouraging to both primary care physicians and their patients. For example, at 3-year follow-up, the median percent days abstinent for the outpatient group was 86% for the prior 90-day period, with 29% of the group reporting complete abstinence.

Pharmacologic Agents to Prevent Relapse

Research on medications to prevent relapse has resulted in three medications that are widely used in the U.S. and Europe—disulfiram, naltrexone, and acamprosate. As of early 2003, only disulfiram and naltrexone were approved by the Food and Drug Administration for the prevention of relapse in alcohol dependence, whereas acamprosate has been studied extensively in Europe. Each of the three drugs has been studied in specialty settings; however, little is known about their effectiveness in primary care settings. More recent and ongoing research may, however, shed light on their utility in primary care.

Disulfiram

Disulfiram prevents alcohol use by the potential of an adverse reaction to the consumption of alcohol (including: flushing, nausea, vomiting, diarrhea) in those who take it. Although research on its broad application to patients with alcohol dependence has failed to convincingly demonstrate its effectiveness, it has been shown to be helpful in carefully selected patients. These include patients who are highly motivated and receive disulfiram in a structured and supervised treatment setting. Thus, its use in primary care is unproved.

Naltrexone

Naltrexone hydrochloride, approved in 1994 for the treatment of alcohol dependence by the U.S. Food and Drug Administration, acts as a specific mu opioid antagonist and is thought to block the effects of alcohol-induced increases in endogenous opioid activity. Naltrexone may decrease alcohol use by blunting alcohol's pleasurable effects and suppressing craving in alcohol-dependent patients. Due to its effects on opioid receptors, naltrexone is contraindicated in patients who are currently receiving, or withdrawing from, any opiates. It is also contraindicated in patients with liver failure or significant hepatitis, although it has been demonstrated to lessen liver enzyme abnormalities in patients with mild elevations because of its impact on drinking.

Two initial placebo-controlled randomized trials demonstrated the efficacy of naltrexone combined with psychosocial counseling in alcohol-dependent patients. Both trials provided naltrexone, 50 mg/day, for a 12-week period, in combination with group therapy or individual counseling in specialized alcohol treatment settings. A combined analysis of these studies documented that 54% of patients who received naltrexone remained abstinent, in comparison with 31% who received placebo. Each trial also demonstrated significant decreases in the proportion of days when drinking occurred and scores on assessments of craving in the naltrexone-treated groups. A subsequent study of patients enrolled in one of these studies showed that after the 12-week course of naltrexone was completed and the medication was stopped, the benefits of naltrexone faded over time—suggesting that a 12-week course of naltrexone may not be sufficient.

Several additional studies of naltrexone have confirmed its effectiveness in specialized alcohol treatment settings. However, its use in primary care settings has been the subject of only a few completed and ongoing studies. In a pilot study, 29 alcohol-dependent patients received both naltrexone (50 mg/day) and seven brief counseling sessions (similar to those used in brief intervention studies) administered by primary care practitioners. In a within-patient pretreatment and post-treatment analysis, significant differences in the proportion of days in which total abstinence was maintained (37% vs. 89%, $p < 0.001$); days abstinent from heavy drinking (49% vs. 97%, $p < 0.001$); drinks per drinking occasion (9.5 vs. 2.5, $p < 0.001$), and change in serum gamma-glutamyl transferase (GGT) (68 vs. 45, $p < 0.001$) were documented.

This study led to a larger randomized clinical trial that occurred in two phases: Phase I—initial naltrexone treatment, and Phase II—naltrexone maintenance. In Phase I (10 weeks in duration), patients were all treated with naltrexone (50 mg/day) and were randomized to receive it in one of two models: primary care management (PCM) or specialized treatment using cognitive behavioral therapy (CBT). As with the pilot study described earlier, the counseling received in the PCM group was brief and administered by primary care providers. The CBT group received individualized therapy from a psychotherapist. Treatment outcomes for both groups were similar, suggesting that naltrexone therapy and brief counseling may be feasible and effective in primary care settings. In Phase II (24 weeks in duration), patients from the two treatment groups from Phase I (PCM and CBT) were randomly assigned to continue naltrexone therapy or placebo while continuing to receive their initially assigned counseling approach. Interestingly, the results from this phase of the study demonstrated that continued use of naltrexone was helpful in PCM but not in CBT. This suggests that longer term (greater than10 to 12 weeks) naltrexone therapy might be particularly useful in primary care settings.

Acamprosate

The precise mechanism of action of acamprosate is uncertain but appears to be related in part to its effects on the excitatory glutamate system. As with naltrexone, the mechanism of action of acamprosate is postulated to include a reduction of craving. The recommended daily dosage is 1.3 to 2 grams/day in divided doses. Its most common side effect is diarrhea, and it is contraindicated in pregnant or breast-feeding women and in those with impaired renal function or severe hepatic failure.

Four major randomized clinical trials examined the efficacy of acamprosate in the treatment of alcohol dependence—primarily in specialized alcohol treatment settings. All four trials demonstrated increased abstinence rates in patients receiving acamprosate compared with those who had placebo. Although the overall outcomes of these trials were roughly similar to those of studies of naltrexone, these studies followed patients for a longer period of time—up to 1 year. In one study, at 48 weeks, the mean absolute abstinence rate was 43% in the acamprosate group and 21% in the control group ($p = 0.005$).

Other Pharmacologic Approaches to Prevent Relapse

A variety of other medications have been studied for relapse prevention in alcohol dependence. These include selective serotonin reuptake inhibitors, 5-HT$_3$ antagonists (e.g., ondansetron), other serotonergic agents, gamma-amino butyric acid/glutamate compounds (e.g., topiramate), and dopaminergic agents. Also, there is ongoing research examining the effectiveness of combinations of medications (e.g., naltrexone plus acamprosate and ondansetron plus naltrexone) in the treatment of alcohol problems. A combined approach, like that used for the treatment of hypertension and diabetes, makes sense given the differing mechanisms of action of various drugs and may be well suited for primary care.

SUGGESTED READINGS

Fiellin DA, Reid MC, O'Connor PG: Screening for alcohol problems in primary care: a systematic review. Arch Intern Med 160:1977–1989, 2000.

Fiellin DA, Reid MC, O'Connor PG: New therapies for alcohol problems: application to primary care. Am J Med 108:227–237, 2000.

Ninth Special Report to the United States Congress on Alcohol and Health. U.S. Department of Health and Human Services, 1997.

O'Connor PG, Schottenfeld RS: Patients with alcohol problems. N Engl J Med 338:592–602, 1998.

O'Malley SS, Rounsaville BJ, Farren C, Namkoong K, Wu R, Robinson J, O'Connor PG: Initial and maintenance naltrexone treatment for alcohol dependence using primary care vs specialty care: a nested sequence of 3 randomized trials. Arch Intern Med 163:1695–1704, 2003.

The Physician's Guide to Helping Patients with Alcohol Problems: National Institute on Alcohol Abuse and Alcoholism. Bethesda, MD: The National Institutes of Health, 1995.

REHABILITATION PROGRAMS

Gantt P. Galloway
Douglas Polcin

Selection of an appropriate rehabilitation program for an alcoholic is an essential first step in designing a treatment program. This selection requires both knowledge of the characteristics of treatment programs and consideration of individual patient factors.

Rehabilitation programs vary widely with respect to intensity, duration, program philosophy, and whether they are residential or outpatient. A variety of systems have been designed to match patients to treatment settings, and although the evidence base is limited, one of the best developed is the American Society of Addiction Medicine's Patient Placement Criteria. Patient characteristics used in this system to determine appropriate referrals fall into six categories:

1. Acute intoxication and/or withdrawal potential

Acute intoxication and substantial withdrawal potential are indications that inpatient treatment (see Chapter 15) should be considered. Physiologic monitoring and pharmacotherapy address the goals of ensuring patient safety and reducing discomfort, which may improve acceptance of early recovery and engagement with treatment.

2. Biomedical conditions and complications

As with intoxication and withdrawal, medical conditions that require intensive monitoring or treatment will require an inpatient setting.

3. Emotional, behavioral or cognitive conditions and complications

Comorbid psychiatric conditions should be treated in a setting where the staff is trained in their management and appropriate medications can be used. Although many treatment programs are able to effectively treat mild to moderate Axis I and Axis II psychiatric disorders, more severe conditions (e.g., schizophrenia, depression with psychotic features, and unstable borderline personality), call for selection of a program that has specialized capabilities with respect to comorbidity.

4. Readiness to change

Readiness to change is one of the more difficult criteria to evaluate and incorporate into treatment planning. The lack of awareness of the need to change is an indicator of severity; at the same time, it may translate functionally into a resistance to more intensive treatment modalities. To avoid increasing the patient's resistance to treatment, it may be necessary to make a recommendation that incorporates the patient's denial that intensive treatment is needed. If such a compromise is made, it is important to secure the patient's agreement that a more appropriate level of care will be employed in the event of unsuccessful initial treatment.

An understanding of the stages of change as they relate to motivation to quit is very helpful when this decision is discussed with a patient. In a very short time, a precontemplator (a patient who does not present a motivation to change and does not see drinking as having adverse consequences) can become a contemplator (a patient who has begun to recognize some of the problems associated with drinking but is not at the point of making specific plans to change), and a contemplator can take action by means of a successful interview technique. Even in a very brief interview, knowledge of the starting point can help physicians take patients through the appropriate steps for their stage of change.

5. Relapse, continued use, or continued problem potential

High likelihood of continued drinking is an indication of the need for a more intensive program, such as inpatient or residential treatment. Consequences of continued drinking, such as danger to self or others and criminal justice sequelae, should also be evaluated when the physician is assessing the appropriate level of care for the patient. Severity of dependence (see Chapter 5 for assessment methods) and response to prior treatment are factors to be considered when evaluating the likelihood of continued drinking.

6. Recovery/living environment

Environmental factors can play a key role in relapse and recovery. If the patient's environment is sufficiently hostile to recovery (e.g., living with a drinking spouse or homelessness), residence in a sober environment during treatment may be required to achieve and maintain abstinence. On the other hand, if the patient is living in an environment supportive of recovery, there are advantages to outpatient treatment. For example, the patient's work environment and family life do not need to be interrupted while the patient engages in a plan for recovery.

THERAPEUTIC COMMUNITY TREATMENT

Therapeutic communities (TCs) are highly structured, intensive, residential programs. Over the past three decades, community-based TCs have been frequent referral sources for alcoholics and addicts in the criminal justice system. In recent years, some TCs have worked within prison systems to begin providing services to inmates while they serve their sentences. Lengths of treatment vary from 6 months to several years. Alcoholics who are most appropriate for TC referral are those with extensive criminal justice histories, antisocial behaviors, severe alcoholism, or concurrent drug addiction.

The therapeutic elements of TCs include confrontation of antisocial and dysfunctional behaviors associated with alcoholism, social support and encouragement to develop a sober lifestyle, and intensive work on the underlying emotional issues that drive drinking. Patient behaviors that are pro-social and recovery-oriented are rewarded, and antisocial behaviors and violations of program rules are discouraged. The philosophy is that the TC environment must mandate behavioral changes before patients are able to engage in productive counseling.

Treatment modalities usually include individual, group, family, and psychoeducation workshops. However, recovery skills in the TC are practiced constantly. Stress and conflict during daily activities such as meals, cleaning, recreational activities, or unstructured time in the program offer opportunities for patients to practice coping with conflict and emotions without resorting to substance use. The problems that patients experience during daily interactions often reveal issues that require attention in group sessions and individual counseling. TCs use a phase or stage system that rewards patients and gives them more responsibility as they progress in their treatment. Early phases of treatment focus on helping patients adapt to the structure, rules, and expectations of the program. Consequences for rule violations and rewards for program compliance are particularly important. Staff and senior patients develop strategies that help new patients make a connection with the community and establish supportive relationships with peers. New patients initially may have a "peer buddy" who explains the program and provides emotional support and encouragement. Typically, patients in the early phases of treatment do not receive home passes and only leave the facility accompanied by staff. Although patients do work on the emotional issues that drive their addiction, that is not the primary focus. Compliance with program expectations and a strong connection to the community is necessary before intensive emotional work can begin.

During the middle phases of treatment, patients typically focus intensively on the core emotional issues that underlie their addiction, which may include physical and sexual abuse, dysfunctional family of origin, trauma resulting from the use of alcohol, and psychiatric disorders such as depression and anxiety. Patients with severe psychiatric disorders such as schizophrenia, chronic mood disorder, disabling anxiety, or frequent suicidal gestures would not be considered appropriate for most TCs. The intensity of most TC environments and the level of confrontation can exacerbate symptoms in patients who exhibit substantial psychiatric instability.

In the middle phases of treatment, patients also may begin brief, structured visits to their homes. Discussion of patients' experiences during home visits can help promote counseling work on emotional issues that need attention. As a rule, there is a "client government" or "council," generally composed of patients who have made a transition into a specific phase of treatment (i.e. "senior peers"). The client government is responsible for monitoring daily operations of the program such as cooking, cleaning, and consequences for violation of program rules. In addition to work on emotional issues, patients in the middle phases of treatment take on increased responsibility in the milieu, such as positions in the client government.

The final phases of treatment focus on assumption of increased responsibility in the program, such as becoming a senior peer, and transitioning back to the community. When senior peers provide assistance to newcomers in the program, they solidify what they have learned about recovery and increase their self-esteem. The status of a senior peer and the role modeling that they are expected to provide newcomers reinforces the progress they have made up to that point. Making the transition back into the community entails being sober while dealing with real world situations such as finding a job and a place to live. At this time, patients spend a considerable amount of time in the community and confronting high-risk situations that trigger urges to drink. These situations offer transitioning patients excellent opportunities to practice relapse prevention skills and to discuss in their counseling sessions how they handled those situations. As these individuals spend more time at home, unresolved family issues may become more prominent, and these can be addressed in family counseling as well as in individual and group counseling sessions.

Historically, TCs have emphasized a peer-oriented approach, and many of the staff have been graduates of the programs in which they received therapy. Now, many TCs employ a variety of licensed and certified counselors as well as mental health professionals. Some have psychiatrists and other medical personnel to attend to the medical and psychiatric needs of patients that otherwise could go unmet or that might require coordination with outside resources. Although there is still an emphasis on consistency and structure in treatment, there tends to be a bit more flexibility. Some patients may receive more confrontation than others, and some may receive specialized services within the TC, such as treatment for abuse issues, HIV services, or psychoeducation about specific matters that women or minority groups deal with in recovery. In general, these changes have made TCs more responsive to the needs of subgroups of patients, such as dual diagnosis, women's issues, minority concerns, and concurrent HIV infection.

RESIDENTIAL RECOVERY PROGRAMS

Residential treatment programs are licensed intensive treatment centers with professional staff trained to deal with a wide range of issues experienced by alcoholics. Residential programs both resemble and differ from TCs. Like TCs, they are conducted in residential settings providing patients a clean and sober place to live while they initiate abstinence. Also like TCs, they teach respect and a sense of responsibility as well as foster relationship and recovery skills, and they offer opportunities to practice recovery skills during ordinary daily activities such as managing conflicts with peers or completing house maintenance chores. There is also an emphasis on peer relationships, particularly when senior peers help facilitate the recovery of newcomers. However, these elements are less formalized than in TCs, and residential recovery programs have less of an emphasis on phases of treatment that are associated with increased responsibilities and autonomy. Finally, many residential recovery programs employ a type of patient government, often called a "resident's council," to manage daily operations and make recommendations to staff about program operations.

There are major philosophical differences between TCs and residential recovery programs. Residential programs tend to be of shorter duration, ranging from about 3 months to 1 year. Some combination of individual, group, and family counseling is offered, although these services are not used as frequently and intensively less as those in TCs. Residential recovery programs employ a "social model" philosophy of recovery that relies heavily on the 12-step program of Alcoholics Anonymous; this program is also reflected in their counseling interventions. Patients are usually expected to attend a minimum number of 12-step meetings per week, and 12-step meetings are often held at the program site.

Residential programs may follow a medical model or work in cooperation with a physician. TCs are usually opposed to medical assistance with sobriety. Although there is some emphasis on adhering to a program structure, there are fewer program requirements and more autonomy than are available in TCs. Patients have a less intensive treatment regimen and are expected to make the transition into the community sooner. There tends to be less emphasis on daily behavior monitoring of patients, resulting in less focus on rewards and consequences for specific behaviors, although there are consequences for major program violations such as drug use.

Although TCs involve intensive daily treatment until patients are in the latter phases of therapy, many patients in residential recovery programs are employed shortly after entering the program. In some cases, patients may be required to find employment because they contribute financially to the maintenance of the program. Residential recovery programs are, therefore, more likely to facilitate integration into the community earlier than TCs, and TCs are more likely to provide the intensive monitoring, structure, and therapy for the emotional issues that fuel alcoholism.

In general, patients with serious criminal justice histories, antisocial behaviors, failures in previous treatment, and severe levels of alcoholism are more appropriate for TCs. Probation and parole officers often find the intensive 24-hour monitoring in TCs appropriate for more severe cases. Residential social model programs may be more suitable for patients who have a history of successful employment, are amenable to 12-step recovery, less problems with antisocial behavior, fewer treatment failures, and relatively less severe histories of alcoholism. Whether a TC or a residential treatment program is selected for a patient, it is essential that there is a plan for step-down care after discharge (i.e., outpatient treatment, clean and sober housing, or both). Although the term "aftercare" is sometimes used, alcoholism is a chronic disease much like essential hypertension, and should be treated or monitored on a lifelong basis.

Like TCs, residential recovery programs have a history of hiring staff in recovery and de-emphasizing professional treatment within the program. However, TCs tend to hire clients who graduate from the program, whereas residential recovery programs look primarily for staff who are familiar with 12-step recovery. Although some programs still eschew professional services within the program, others hire licensed or certified mental health and addiction professionals as well as medical and psychiatric consultants. Integration of professional services into some residential recovery programs has occurred in part as a response to demands for increased accountability from funding sources. It is essential to determine in advance whether the cost of a treatment facility includes all needed services, including step-down care.

DAY TREATMENT AND STRUCTURED OUTPATIENT PROGRAMS

Outpatient modalities can be characterized as day treatment programs or structured outpatient programs. The main difference is that day treatment programs are somewhat more intensive, meeting 3 to 5 days per week for several hours. Structured outpatient programs may meet as little as 1 or 2 hours per week. Managed care funding of treatment supports outpatient care because it is less expensive than inpatient care, and studies have shown that many patients, particularly those with good social support and only mild or moderate addiction severity, can be effectively treated in outpatient settings.

In addition to being heterogeneous with respect to intensity, outpatient programs vary widely with respect to treatment approach, which can include psychoeducational training, cognitive-behavioral modification, motivational enhancement, supportive care, and 12-step facilitation. Many programs require some degree of documented attendance at Alcoholics Anonymous meetings. It appears that programs that minimize confrontation achieve greater success; this is especially pertinent to outpatient programs, where barriers to dropping out of treatment are minimal.

Outpatient programs are most appropriate for patients who have indicators for high likelihood of a good outcome: (1) gainful employment, (2) strong family support, and (3) absence of mental illness. Some outpatient programs take place in facilities that can easily integrate a variety of medical and psychiatric services into alcoholism treatment. "Broad-based" outpatient programs offer individual, group, family, and vocational counseling while still emphasizing peer support and 12-step recovery. Usually, at least some of the staff are in recovery and participate actively in 12-step programs. However, not all outpatient programs are based within multiservice settings, and those that are not must refer to outside agencies for a variety of services (e.g., medical, detoxification, psychiatric care, vocational training).

There are many advantages to receiving treatment in an outpatient facility. First, individuals who are employed are able to keep their work positions without disruption and are able to keep their addiction and recovery private. Second, family life is less disrupted and patients are able to maintain familial roles. Third, if sobriety is established while the patient lives in the community, there is no need to generalize recovery skills from a residential or inpatient program to the community in which the patient resides. In the outpatient setting, patients develop and maintain sobriety in the presence of relapse triggers, life stresses, and social relationships that they continue to face. Fourth, costs are substantially lower than those of inpatient or residential treatment facilities, and most necessary services can be obtained on an outpatient basis.

There are also limitations to the effectiveness of outpatient treatment. Patients who are residing in environments with many cues for drinking may find recovery difficult because of the social rewards and encouragement to use alcohol. In addition, patients with high levels of severity, a history of treatment failure in outpatient settings, a propensity toward engaging in high-risk behaviors, extensive medical or psychiatric problems, or extensive criminal justice histories may require the containment and support of residential or inpatient settings.

SOBER LIVING HOUSES

Characteristics of the social environment have a strong impact on drinking and treatment outcome. Family, friends, and workplace peers can influence drinking in several ways. They can promote alcohol consumption, support abstinence or moderation, influence the problems associated with alcohol, or facilitate entry into treatment.

Assessment Variables
Patient Preference
Diagnosis
Course of Illness
Prior Treatment Response
Family History
Mental Status

Matching Variables
Intoxication/Withdrawal
Biomedical Conditions
Psychological Conditions
Relapse Potential
Treatment Readiness
Environmental Status

Modifying Variables
Age: Adolescent or Geriatric
Gender
Sexual Orientation
Culture/Language/Ethnicity
Religion
Service Availability/Access
Financial Resources
Health Care Professional?
Childcare/Eldercare
Patient Preference

PLACEMENT

➤ **Assessment Variables** form the first level of data for input to decision rules.

➤ **Matching Variables** are the specific data elements that are then required for multidimensional matching to a discrete level of care.

➤ **Modifying Variables** may be used to modify the level of care determination based on intervening factors that exist within the patient or treatment system.

One way for alcoholics to ensure that their social environment promotes abstinence is to become a resident of a sober living house.

Sober living houses, also known as 12th step, Oxford, or clean and sober houses, are low-cost, alcohol-free, and drug-free residences for individuals who are attempting to establish or maintain sobriety. The philosophy of recovery in sober living houses is based on a social model that emphasizes peer support, attendance at Alcoholics Anonymous meetings, and a democratic form of government. Although sober living houses became popular in certain regions as a way of helping individuals with alcohol problems shortly after World War II, they are still not widely known or extensively used by treatment professionals. Nonetheless, the aforementioned factors plus the low cost and substantial negative consequence of relapse—eviction—are all compelling reasons why sober living housing may be an important adjunct to the substance abuse treatment system.

Sober living houses vary greatly in terms of physical characteristics and implementation of the social model philosophy. Some are small two-bedroom or three-bedroom houses, and others are large, encompassing entire apartment complexes, single-room occupancy hotels, or multiple smaller houses. Some residences are highly democratic and have few house rules, whereas others are more structured and have house managers who monitor resident compliance with house expectations. Regardless of size or level of structure, most sober living houses have several common characteristics. Unlike formal rehabilitation programs, sober living houses do not provide group counseling, referrals to community resources, on-site Alcoholics Anonymous meetings, structured daily activities, or a maximum length of stay. They do not have paid staff. Although residents in sober living houses are usually encouraged to attend Alcoholics Anonymous meetings, there are only three basic obligations: no use of alcohol or drugs, adherence to house rules, and prompt payment of rent.

Sober living houses could play a more important role in the continuum of recovery services. They could be especially helpful in providing sober housing for the large number of homeless individuals who have alcohol problems. Homeless individuals are especially unlikely to establish sobriety unless housing issues are addressed, although sober living houses also are appropriate for many other alcoholics. Sober living houses can be used as transitional placements for patients who are completing residential treatment, as clean and sober residences for those participating in outpatient or day treatment services, and as placements for probationers and parolees. As sober living houses are low in cost compared with inpatient and residential alternatives, they may be an option for a broader range of patients.

SELECTING AND LOCATING A PROGRAM

Knowledge of the different types of rehabilitation programs is an essential step in formulating an effective treatment plan for an alcoholic. With this knowledge in hand, the next step is to consider how

Fig. 18.1. Variables to be considered in patient placement. (Modified from Gartner L, Mee-Lee D. The Role and Status of Patient Placement Criteria in the Treatment of Substance Abuse Disorders. Rockville, MD: U.S. Department of Health and Human Services, 1995, p. 36.)

these programs compare with each other and what factors influence the choice of a program for a given patient.

A variety of patient-specific factors may affect the acceptability and likely efficacy of a treatment program for a given patient. Do patients have family members who play a significant role in their lives and who could be involved in treatment? If so, a program that has a family treatment component should be selected. Do patients have a strong religious orientation? If so, it may be appropriate to consider a religious-based treatment program. Similarly, some patients may feel more comfortable in a single-gender program or a program that has experience with gay, lesbian, bisexual, or transgender patients. (Figure 18.1 provides a summary of factors to be considered in the placement of patients.

Within the categories presented above, especially day treatment and structured outpatient care, programs may vary considerably with respect to program rules and treatment approach. For example, some programs prohibit use of detoxification medications, psychiatric medications, or both, and are, therefore, not appropriate for patients in need of such treatment. Even if a program permits the use of psychiatric medications, it is important to consider whether it can provide adequate support, either alone or in combination with another treatment provider, for a patient with a comorbid condition.

Some programs rely on a confrontational approach, which may be appropriate for criminal justice or antisocial patients in a TC setting. However, there are strong contraindications for using confrontational approaches with other patients, such as dual-diagnosis patients or those with a history of physical or sexual abuse, for whom a supportive approach is indicated.

If the patient has had prior treatment experiences, evaluation of these may provide insight into optimal treatment placement. Failure to achieve sobriety in a prior treatment episode should lead to consideration of a higher level of care or a treatment program that addresses specific issues associated with the failure of the prior treatment episode.

Finding a Treatment Program

Once the general characteristics of treatment programs have been considered in light of the specifics of the patient's circumstances, there remains the issue of selection. One way to find treatment programs is to use online listings (e.g., *http://www.findtreatment.samhsa.gov/facilitylocatordoc.htm*, *http://www.soberrecovery.com/*, and *http://www.oxfordhouse.org/*). Consulting with colleagues and telephoning or visiting local treatment programs are also invaluable ways of familiarizing oneself with the local options available for patients.

SUGGESTED READINGS

De Leon G: Residential therapeutic communities in the mainstream: diversity and issues. J Psychoactive Drugs 27:3–15, 1995.

Dodd MH: Social model of recovery: origin, early features, changes, and future. J Psychoactive Drugs 29:133–139, 1997.

Mee-Lee D, Shulman GD, Fishman M, Gastfriend DR, Griffith JH (eds.):

ASAM Patient Placement Criteria for the Treatment of Substance-Related Disorders (ASAM PPC-2R). Chevy Chase, MD: American Society of Addiction Medicine, 2001.

Miller WR, Rollnick S: Motivational Interviewing: Preparing People to Change Addictive Behavior. New York: Guilford Press, 1991.

Polcin DL: Sober living houses: potential roles in substance abuse services and suggestions for research. Subst Use Misuse 36:301–311, 2001.

ALCOHOL AND THE WORKPLACE

Richard A. Rawson
Ruthlyn Sodano
Patricia Marinelli-Casey

Why a chapter on alcohol and the workplace? What makes the connection between alcohol use and employment, vocational issues and/or workplace settings a substantial enough topic to warrant a dedicated chapter in this textbook on alcohol use and alcoholism? Are alcohol-related problems influenced by employment status or type of occupation? Does employment status/occupation play a role in recovery from alcoholism? Are there unique factors concerning how alcohol problems are prevented, identified, and treated that are specific to the workplace? Have alcohol-workplace issues influenced the broader array of practices and policies concerning societal positions on substance abuse and workplace and health care?

The goal of this chapter is to address a range of questions concerning the relationship between problem alcohol use and employment and the workplace. There is a substantial body of research that demonstrates that presence or absence of employment, type of employment, and characteristics of the work environment are meaningfully related to the likelihood of problem alcohol use. Similarly, for individuals in recovery from alcohol misuse/alcoholism, relapse to alcohol use influences and is influenced by employment status. It is widely accepted in treatment settings that a comprehensive treatment plan must include considerations of employment and occupational development.

Few domains have been as influential in developing a societal response to alcohol use and misuse-related problems as the workplace. Programs developed during the 1940s and 1950s in industrial settings have provided the foundation for some of the most innovative alcohol identification and treatment referral processes in use today and contributed to the referral base for many of the early alcoholism treatment programs. Employee Assistance Programs (EAPs), which initially focused solely on alcohol use and misuse, have established a clear presence in the worksite as employee advocates and ombudsmen on a variety of physical health, mental health, disability, and substance abuse-related topics in the workplace. As a result of the efforts associated with the development of EAPs, the vast majority of employers in theUnited States have explicit, written policies and practices for addressing a wide range of behavioral and health-related issues, including, but not limited to, substance abuse. The early efforts to find a way to constructively address the problem of alcohol use in the workplace have led to the creation of an entire human service system within the workplace.

ALCOHOL USE AND EMPLOYMENT: A BRIEF BACKGROUND

The relationship between employment and alcohol use/misuse is an excellent case study for demonstrating the difference between an association and a causal relationship. There are a number of associations that suggest that being employed is linked to less alcohol use and better performance in treatment and successful recovery from problem alcohol use. For example, individuals who are unemployed have higher rates of heavy alcohol use than those who are employed; patients who are retained in substance abuse treatment longer are more likely to be employed than those who drop out of treatment prematurely; and individuals who have relapsed during their recovery are more likely to be unemployed (62% vs 40%) and more likely to have changed jobs (44% vs 12%) than those who have not relapsed. Certainly, it is logical that having a job should contribute to positive self-esteem and, consequently, provide an improved opportunity for an individual to master the challenges of achieving recovery from alcohol use disorders.

However, the relationship is not as simple as the formula: Get a job and stay sober. Nor is it the converse: Stop drinking and become employed. Employment and problem alcohol use have a more complex relationship. In fact, the amount of research on this topic is limited with regard to problem alcohol use and employment, whereas, in contrast, the literature is extensive (and much more clear-cut) on the topic with regard to illicit drug use and employment. A group of investigators demonstrated that there were specific aspects of work environments that were associated with higher rates of relapse to alcohol use during a 2-year follow-up period. Compared with "remitted" individuals, "relapsed" individuals were more likely to have been in jobs with high stress (e.g., high demands, low autonomy, tedium, and group conflict) and jobs with higher amounts of physical discomfort (e.g., heat, noise, humidity, fumes, and cold). Further, they reported that individuals who have supportive families are less sensitive to job-related stresses that influence alcohol relapse than individuals without family support. In short, there are characteristics of the job and the person's support system that determine how a specific job will affect, and be affected by, problem alcohol use.

From an overall policy and treatment planning perspective, however, there is little question that improved employment status of individuals is generally consistent with lower rates of problem alcohol use. Methods for improving employment status as part of a strategy for supporting alcohol treatment goals may require a range of vocational activities. Not all individuals who enter the alcohol recovery process are job ready, even for the most rudimentary employment. Many do not know how to obtain employment or prepare for a successful job interview. Some individuals in early recovery have few ideas regarding the types of occupational activities for which they would be well suited. Others have never been employed and have no understanding of basic principles of expected work performance responsibilities. Finally, individuals with obstacles to gaining employment (e.g., parents with preschool-aged children, physically handicapped and/or learning disabled individuals) may not have any skills for overcoming these barriers to employment. In short, there are numerous challenges to matching persons who are attempting to successfully sustain their recovery from problem alcohol use with the correct employment/vocational guidance. For this reason, the development of specific strategies for assisting recovering people with employment challenges has become an important component to comprehensive alcohol recovery treatment planning.

ALCOHOL USE AND EMPLOYMENT: TREATMENT AND VOCATIONAL SERVICES

Individuals who enter treatment for problem alcohol use frequently have an array of problems in addition to their use of alcohol. One of the leading substance abuse treatment assessment tools, the Addiction Severity Index (ASI), assesses seven domains of functioning, one of which is employment. Among clients admitted to publicly funded treatment programs, the employment domain is frequently assessed as an area of substantial need. Once a determination is made that employment/vocational services are a needed component of the treatment plan, it is important to ascertain whether the individual has clearly identified job skills and interests that make appropriate employment possible once alcohol use and other acute problems have been addressed. With patients who have good employment histories and job-seeking skills, there may be little need for extensive assistance by treatment staff in this area. A far more common scenario, particularly in publicly funded programs, is that many patients do not have adequate skills to immediately address their vocational/employment needs, and the necessary first step is to conduct a vocational assessment.

Vocational Assessment

It is rare for community treatment programs to have vocational specialists or licensed psychologists with the skills and training required to conduct a complete vocational assessment. Frequently, alcohol and drug abuse counselors are called on to complete initial assessments, which is generally an appropriate first step. A recent Substance Abuse and Mental Health Services Administration (SAMHSA) publication, "Integrating Substance Abuse Treatment and Vocational Services," provides an excellent resource for guiding counselors through the process of assessment by giving them clear instructions on when more specialized expertise is required. One of the most emphasized points in the SAMHSA manual is that it is important for treatment programs to have close working collaborative relationships with local agencies or professionals who specialize in vocational assessment and placement. Although it is desirable to build these skills into substance abuse treatment organizations, a significant number of patients require the expertise, skills, and resources of professional vocational experts. It is not unusual to find that some patients in substance abuse treatment have struggled throughout their lives with vocational and employment issues that have resulted from undiagnosed psychological limitations and learning disabilities. Many local resources in this area can be identified through the extensive referral assistance network affiliated with the U.S. Department of Labor (www.dol.gov) and with each state's employment agency.

To initiate an effective program for addressing these needs, it is necessary to conduct a systematic assessment of the individual's functional capabilities and limitations. In short, an assessment of these areas consists of reviewing whether the individual has the basic essential resources and skills needed to enter the workforce (e.g., housing, transportation, reading skills, social interaction skills) and determining whether there are any obvious physical, psychological, or social limitations that would preclude initiating an employment search. The next level of assessment can often benefit from the use of the extensive array of vocational and interest assessment inventories accessible at state departments of rehabilitation.

Once an assessment has been completed, the plan for a vocational placement has to accommodate a large number of idiosyncratic considerations. Many substance abuse patients have poor job-seeking skills and can benefit tremendously from the use of strategies presented in workshops for job seekers. Frequently, special employment opportunities are funded by the U.S. Department of Labor for certain groups, including individuals with disabilities (State Departments of Rehabilitation Services), persons (primarily women) who are enrolled in welfare to work programs (wtw.doleta.gov), veterans (Department of Veterans Affairs), and individuals on probation and parole..

ALCOHOLISM AND THE WORKPLACE: A BRIEF BACKGROUND

Throughout the mid-20th century, as psychiatry, psychology, and self-help movements were beginning to shape the future definition of treatment for alcoholism, industrial programs established in workplace settings were evolving to identify employees with alcohol-related problems and find ways to help them stay in the workforce. Much of the impetus for this movement came about during World War II when the extremely high demand for industrial workers brought a group of individuals into workplace settings who, under normal circumstances would not have been considered employable. Furthermore, the shortage of workers in industrial settings during this period made it important to retain as many employees as possible. Hence, employers initiated the industrial alcoholism programs as a way of sustaining workforce involvement of individuals with alcohol-related problems.

After World War II, these industrial alcoholism programs continued, often as informal alliances between an employer's staff doctor and employees who were members of Alcoholics Anonymous. Throughout the 1950s and 1960s, the number of these programs increased, as did the influence of their referrals to the early alcoholism treatment programs. The passage of the Hughes Act in 1970 and the creation of the National Institute on Alcoholism and Alcohol Abuse (NIAAA) were promoted and supported by the cadre of physicians and leaders in the growing number of industrial alcoholism programs. In fact, during the early years of NIAAA, one of its major priorities was to disperse occupational specialists throughout the United States to help establish programs in workplaces that would identify and help employees with alcohol-related problems. This effort formed the foundation of the current EAP movement.

The recognition and acceptance by industry leaders of alcoholism as a treatable disorder that can be productively addressed and remedied with professional and peer assistance was a critically important step in the perception of alcoholism as a health care problem and not a moral failing. Industry program doctors and personnel directors worked to extend health insurance coverage for alcoholism treatment further reinforcing the claim that alcoholism was a health care issue. Acceptance of this position was a critical step in building the financial resources necessary to support early commercial treatment centers. Without the leadership of the industrial alcoholism program leaders and later the EAP leadership, the private treatment system would not have burgeoned as it did in the 1980s. Furthermore, the tremendous expansion in the number of EAPs, from 5000 to over 20,000 during the decade of the 1980s was a direct consequence of the workplace alcoholism programs initiated in the 1940s and 1950s.

ALCOHOLISM AND THE WORKPLACE: THE CURRENT SITUATION

Alcoholism continues to affect a large portion of the population of the United States, and the majority of these adults at risk for alcohol problems are in the workforce. In 2000,rates for current alcohol use were 57.3% for full-time employed adults aged 18 years and older, compared with 49.1% of their unemployed peers. However, binge rates and heavy alcohol use rates were somewhat higher for unemployed persons than for full-time employed persons. In a 1997 national survey, heavy drinking (indicated by consumption of five or more drinks per occasion on 5 or more days in the previous 30 days) by full-time employees approached 7.6%. There is evidence from the 1992 NIAAA National Longitudinal Alcohol Epidemiologic Survey that some occupations have higher rates of alcohol use than others. For example, approximately 57% of executives and military personnel report being current drinkers (more than 12 drinks in the past year), whereas only about 20% of household domestic workers report being current drinkers. Similarly, the percentage of individuals reporting being heavy drinkers differs across occupations: 28% of laborers/equipment cleaners report being heavier drinkers (1 or more ounces of alcohol per day), whereas only about 11% of technical specialists and administrative workers report this heavy rate of alcohol use.

Society pays a substantial price for the damage associated with alcohol use. The big picture of economic cost for alcohol abuse and dependence in the U.S. was estimated at $148 billion for 1992. This estimate includes the cost of health care services (treatment, prevention, and support) at $18.820 billion, losses in productivity (from illness and premature death) at $106.997 billion, and additional costs associated with alcohol-related crime and motor vehicle crashes at $22.204 billion. In 1995, productivity losses alone that were attributed to alcohol were estimated at $119 billion.

In addition to the aforementioned formal productivity costs cited are the workplace costs associated with problem alcohol use and related behaviors, which are much more difficult to estimate. For example, the frequency of being "hung over" at work has been positively correlated with the frequency of feeling sick at work, sleeping on the job, and having problems with job tasks or coworkers. In another similar study, it was found that drinking on the job, problem drinking, and the frequency of getting drunk in the previous 30 days were positively associated with absenteeism, being tardy for work or leaving early, poor quality and quantity of work, and arguments with coworkers. Compared with other employees, alcohol and substance abusers have four times as many accidents, three times as many absences, three times as many health claims, five times as many workers' compensation claims, and only two thirds of the productivity of fellow employees. Up to 40% of industrial fatalities and 47% of industrial injuries can be linked to alcohol consumption and alcoholism.

The work environment may foster several factors that contribute in the first place to alcohol use and related problems among employees. Several studies have linked increased drinking with lower job satisfaction and higher job stress. Additionally, greater alcohol use has been associated with decreased faith in management and lower involvement with, and commitment to, the job. However, further research is needed to clarify the causality of this relationship, because some workers may have difficulty coping with normal job situations because of excessive drinking.

Drinking behavior also is influenced by worksite culture, which is often intimately connected with the specific occupation of the workers. One author found that in regard to drinking behavior, workers were differentially socialized according to their occupational choice. In a study of a large manufacturing plant where drinking was prevalent, 852 salaried and hourly workers completed a survey that asked questions about alcohol use and beliefs. It appeared that drinking was a reflection of an organized culture that had developed around alcohol use, and the culture in turn tolerated and encouraged the presence of alcohol-related behavior.

Although blue-collar workers generally have higher rates of alcohol abuse, other sectors of employment should not be overlooked. Directors of large companies were found to have a death rate from liver cirrhosis that was 22 times higher than the normal rate. Physicians show comparatively high rates of problem alcohol use. Microcultures of heavy drinking also exist in upper management.

WORKPLACE RESPONSES TO ALCOHOL USE-RELATED PROBLEMS

Clearly, it is to the advantage of both the employee and the employer for the behavior and consequences associated with alcohol use to be detected early. For the employer, it is advantageous to reduce the number of on-the-job accidents and prevent serious losses from occurring in association with quality or quantity of job output. There also is the motivation to retain otherwise productive employees, especially where there is a substantial investment in job training. For the employee, preventing the loss of a job is crucial for preserving mental health as well as social and financial well-being. If alcohol abuse is allowed to destroy the employee's ability to work, the employee will be removed from the labor market, abandoned to struggle alone with alcoholism, and left to face a daunting series of obstacles in trying to regain employment. Allowing alcoholic behavior to worsen benefits no one. As the workplace exercises control over an individual's continued employment, it possesses unique leverage in terms of being able to motivate and effect behavior change. Additionally, the workplace presents the opportunity for earlier intervention than if the progression of alcoholic behavior would continue until employment was lost.

How, then, does a workplace deal with this dilemma? First, the problematic alcohol-using employee must be identified. In instances of serious alcohol dependence, an individual often displays visible job performance deterioration that is evident to supervisors. Nevertheless, without the proper training and knowledge, supervisors can unwittingly and inappropriately become caught up in counseling the employee. This places undue responsibility on the supervisor, and the level of care that alcoholic employees need may not be met. Employees also may be reluctant to open up to supervisors who have the authority to discipline and fire them. A far better and more effective option is for supervisors to have available a system whereby the employee can be referred for evaluation and referral to treatment without loss of job, benefits, or confidentiality. The level of communication between such a program and the employee's place of work would need to be open to such a degree that the employer could be confident that the employee would be making progress while feeling safe in the level of confidentiality granted.

Employee Assistance Programs

EAPs grew out of this unique need in the workplace as was recognized during the period of the industrial alcoholism programs. EAPs have helped to diffuse the stigma of admitting to alcohol-related problems because EAPs now assist people not only with substance abuse problems but with a multitude of other difficulties. At present, EAPs are often managed by clinical professionals who place emphasis on marital, legal, financial, and family problems. Since the early 1980s, employers have been trying to find ways to more effectively manage their behavioral health care expenditures. For many companies, EAPs have become an important component of managed behavioral health care..

EAPs provide the workplace with access to professional assistance regarding alcohol problems. This assistance covers various aspects of helping employees with developing or established alcoholism by means of identification, intervention, motivation, referral, and follow-up. Secondly, there is a set of written policies and procedures to coordinate this function with the overall working structure of the workplace. Variations in the program's structure are functions of the size of the workplace (e.g., places of employment with more than 3000 employees are cost-justified in having an internal EAP) and of the geographic distribution of employees.

Functions of an EAP

PROCESS OF IDENTIFICATION: The first step in implementing EAP policy concerning problem alcohol use in the workplace is to develop expertise in detecting individuals who are affected. Often, a troubled worker's supervisor is in the best position to notice the problem. To perform this function adequately, supervisors require training in the behavioral and physical signs of alcohol abuse that relate to job performance. There are a numerous signs of alcohol abuse, such as the following: (I) The employee may start to come in to work late or call in sick; while on the job, the employee may appear disoriented, have poor concentration, and show declining quality of performance and quantity of output; often, there is a marked change in mood or lability of mood, and relationships with coworkers also may begin to deteriorate. One or two of these signs alone may not be indicative of alcohol abuse or drug use, but if multiple signs emerge and develop into a pattern over time, the supervisor should consider the possibility of a substance abuse problem. Depending on the personnel policy of the workplace, more active responses may include (1) consultation with the EAP; (2) a direct discussion of the problem with the troubled employee in concert with the EAP; and/or (3) asking the employee to take a breath alcohol or urine test. Generally, however, the supervisor is primarily responsible for taking action regarding deteriorating job performance by facilitating contact between the employee and the EAP. Mandating an employee to seek EAP services is often seen as a last resort and is often not a legal option.

INTERFERENCES WITH SUPERVISOR DECISIONS AND POLICY IMPLEMENTA-TION: There are specific factors that affect a supervisor's decision to take appropriate action or ignore the behaviors indicative of problem alcohol use. Personal background influences decision-making, and supervisors who have had personal previous experience with drugs and alcohol are more tolerant of alcohol-related problems in the workplace. There also may be personal issues hindering a confrontation of the problem, such as anxiety about encroaching on a coworker's private problems. One study found that supervisors were fearful of making a false accusation, which resulted in stress and a more cautious approach. Rather than risk making a false accusation and experiencing the stress of addressing the ensuing emotional issues, the supervisors were more comfortable with increasing their level of tolerance. This was especially true if safety was not an issue. Supervisors tended to be less tolerant if there was a safety risk. This study also found that supervisors often believed they were undertrained and overburdened in implementing policy. They did not feel confident in their ability to correctly apply policy, felt a lack of support from administration, and doubted the confidentiality of the EAP.

The implementation of EAP policy is further hampered by the stigma attached to the belief that the EAP serves only serious abusers of alcohol and substances and is not a general resource for health promotion. This stigma is often part of the culture permeating the workplace, which is one of the most influential factors affecting supervisor use of the EAP. If the supervisor is operating in an environment that avoids communication or has a general negative view of the EAP, increased tolerance of alcohol-related problem behaviors will be a likely result.

Workplace culture can breed tolerance (or intolerance) of alcohol and substance abuse in several ways. Different occupations often have different drinking norms. New employees are socialized into these cultures, and, furthermore, occupations that traditionally condone heavy drinking attract job seekers who are likely to engage in these behaviors in the first place. The culture of the management that oversees workers in high-risk occupations is a key factor in addressing drinking excess in the workers. One research team evaluated the apparent effects of two distinct managerial cultures on the drinking behaviors of workers. One setting had a hierarchal management design typical in the United States, where norms of drinking before and during work shifts are permissive. The other setting was a Japanese model transplanted to the United States, in which policies regarding use of alcohol were more strictly enforced. The Japanese model clearly predicated more conservative drinking norms than the traditional hierarchical U.S. model, and workers in this environment reported substantially less drinking.

In a somewhat different vein, supervisors' interactions with policy makers and enforcers as well as upper management influence the level of tolerance of problem drinking behavior. One study found that this interactive policy was seen as straining relations with the human resources (HR) department. Often, policy toward employee drinking and other problem behaviors is covered only during a supervisor's orientation or in seminars that review employee benefits, including health insurance and other matters. This informational type of training aims to increase knowledge about formal policy such as drug testing, discipline guidelines, and counseling. Although this information is important, this strategy does little to integrate the key points of policy into the supervisor's culture; instead, it contributes to feelings of being overwhelmed and undertrained by the HR department. In the absence of additional training and skill development, many supervisors have the cynical view that policy is merely a way for the HR department to cover legal liability requirements.

Belief systems in which trust and security are strong greatly facilitate the process of EAP policy implementation. As shown in one survey, team member and supervisor support for EAPs increased workers' beliefs that the EAP could help them with a drinking problem. A fitting illustration of the importance of worker support for the EAP is found in unionized working cultures. We found that hourly union workers were more likely than salaried workers in the same company to use EAP services. This was likely attributable to the union's respect and backing of EAPs as well as contract provisions, which lent a sense of security to those who choose to take advantage of EAP services. Those responsible for contract administration were found to be highly influential in developing the feeling among union workers that the program was their own and would protect troubled employees from discipline when they sought help. In contrast, salaried personnel displayed more concern, fear, and reluctance about employing the services of the EAP.

To successfully incorporate programs such as the EAP, it is important that the existing social support in the work environment is used. Additionally, a positive regard for the EAP among workers (starting with supervisors) needs to be cultivated by means of effective training. Among a large sample of manufacturing employees, belief in EAP efficacy had the largest effect on stated likelihood to use an EAP. Strategies that demonstrate an increase in knowledge and support for EAPs in the general workplace population should be capitalized on as an opportunity to intervene in the destructive habits of problem drinking.

TRAINING: Effective supervisory training programs are often integrated with the company's EAP. The training aims to increase knowledge about formal policy such as alcohol/drug testing, discipline guidelines, and available counseling for those who need help through the EAP. Training also should incorporate an increase in supervisors' awareness of the importance of alcohol abuse prevention and their pivotal role in this effort. Policy should be seen as a useful tool for enhancing the safety and well-being of all members of a work group.

Success of the program depends in large part on the social environment of the workplace and, more specifically, the role of supervisors in this environment. One author has documented several psychosocial factors that predict whether supervisors will intercede with an employee in need of help. Factors include a feeling of closeness with workers, support from upper management for helping employees, and positive belief systems around the act of helping. Supervisors are much more likely to talk with troubled employees when an ethos of helping exists.

To improve the responsiveness of supervisors, the first step is to ensure that they find their own supervisors to be approachable. Next, because of the prevailing pattern of approaching others to discuss worker problems rather than contacting the EAP, it may be of use to integrate the EAP into such conversations. Disseminating information about EAP services may help to dispel the view that the EAP is a "last resort." Additionally, it may be helpful for supervisors to discuss the reasons for their tolerance and to help create an awareness of other options that are available, such as talking to the EAP or a supervisor as a means of coping with difficult situations instead of raising tolerance. Open discussion regarding tolerance may assist supervisors in differentiating formal and appropriate use of policy from use that is informal and perhaps inappropriate. Group discussion centered on problems related to interacting with troubled employees may also serve to allay anxiety and improve the usefulness of the EAP. This strategy is based on constructive confrontation models and promotes exploration rather than avoidance of stressors. Role-playing is also very effective in reviewing tips and guidelines for dealing with workers who have alcohol-related problems. A well-rounded supervisory-training program, as detailed here, does much to increase the likelihood of communication with the company's EAP. It decreases fear of the workplace grapevine, strengthens the belief that the EAP is vested in protecting employee confidentiality, and improves attitudes toward help-seeking and supervisors responsiveness to a troubled employee.

Program Services for Referred Employees

Initial contact between the troubled employee and the assistance program may come about mainly through either (1) a referral from the employee's supervisor based on deteriorating job performance and strong indications of alcohol abuse, or (2) through a recommendation or self-referral on the part of the employee. Typically, the initial contact is completely confidential. However, if employees are required to meet the stipulations of the program, they may choose to sign a release-of-information statement to confirm that they are taking part in treatment; in this way, participation can be confirmed and used by the company as a condition for continued employment. The information shared with the employee's supervisor is limited to details regarding compliance with the treatment plan.

The treatment plan is based on participation in both individual and group therapy. Alcoholics Anonymous support groups are often an integral part of the therapy along with participation of the employee's family. Continued alcohol and drug testing is often used as an objective measure of the employee's progress. If the employee's degree of abuse warrants more intensive services, the EAP may provide a reference to an inpatient hospital or a more comprehensive day program. These recommendations are typically made when it is clear that the afflicted individual does not have a network of social support to succeed in a less structured environment.

EAPs can be viewed as gatekeepers to mental health-related services and benefits. The EAPs often establish discounted fee arrangements with providers of therapy and hospital-based treatment programs covered under the company's insurance plan. They have good relationships with these providers to facilitate an appropriate treatment plan for the individual employee. The combined product of these EAP services should result in effective treatment with cost savings for the employee and the employer as well as the insurance carrier and/or managed care plan.

As relapse rates for substance users are notoriously high, monitoring of the employee should continue long after the treatment phase is completed. The recommended length of continuing care monitoring is usually between 6 months and a year. An effective continuing care program should employ a clinical consultant from the EAP to maintain contact with the recovering employee. For this period, the consultant should facilitate the drafting of a new contract between the worker and the employer that includes ongoing alcohol and drug testing, continuing contact with the EAP, and participation in support groups or other forms of therapy. Contact should happen on a predetermined schedule to assess whether there are any signs of deterioration in the employee's recovery. The consultant is responsible for spotting a need for additional services or a need for change in the current contract. Without divulging details, the consultant continues to communicate with the worker's supervisor in a joint effort to monitor and inform the employee of progress from a quality-of-work perspective.

Models of Service

When EAPs are being researched, the first decision a company faces is whether to develop an internal program or to contract with an external vendor. As stated earlier, companies with more than 3000 employees would be cost-justified in establishing their own EAP. An internal EAP is staffed by qualified professionals who are employed directly by the company and vested in making the program an integral part of the company. In contrast, external EAPs are individuals or firms that provide services to the company on a contractual basis. These providers are usually compensated on a per-capita basis, with a set fee per employee per month. Some providers charge a subscription fee, which covers crisis-line services, training, and printed materials plus an additional fee for each case seen. Finally, some providers charge a straight fee for a service or charge on an hourly basis.

There are benefits and disadvantages to having an internal program rather than an external program. As part of the company, the internal EAP is more apt to appreciate the mood of the workplace and "the company approach" to different types of problems. Managers and supervisors are more likely to use an internal EAP when dealing with troubled employees. However, the employees may be more suspicious of an internal program, seeing it as an extension of management and not as a confidential resource. The opposite is true of external programs, with supervisors using them less and employees viewing them more favorably. However, it appears that workers still take greater advantage of services provided by an internal EAP. Finally, external programs may offer more depth of services than a smaller internal program.

The actual model of EAP services is selected by the company based on the number of sessions to be completed by the EAP. The models range from a telephone-only consultation to one to three, one to five, or one to eight person-to-person sessions. All models should provide a process that includes intake, assessment, brief counseling, consultation, referrals, and follow-up. The EAP should be competent to handle a wide variety of problems that may arise for employees rather than just alcohol and substance abuse. Other areas may include family difficulties; child/elder care; financial, psychological, and career issues; and critical incident debriefings.

In a survey of 6400 employees who had used EAP services in 84 worksites, alcohol-related problems were twice as likely as other types of problems to have received supervisory referrals. Individuals with alcohol-related problems may be reluctant to come forward, and this reluctance can prevent the timely address of these problems. Furthermore, an alcoholic employee intent on avoiding the issue may manipulate supervisors. Supervisors should strive to consult with the EAP at the first indications of an alcohol problem to clarify their role, discuss how to handle the situation, and learn how to work with the EAP for the good of the troubled employee.

Supervisors need to recognize that the EAP cannot be used as a tool for punishment. If an employee decides not to work with the EAP, this may not be used as grounds for dismissal. The supervisor needs to collaborate with the EAP to identify work-related criteria for continued employment. These criteria should then be discussed with the employee. At the time of the referral, the confidentiality of the EAP should be stressed, and the employee should be made aware that the only information that will be shared is whether on not the worker had contacted the EAP and whether cooperation with the EAP has been demonstrated. Whatever the decision regarding the use of EAP services, it should not be held against employee. Building trust in EAPs in the workplace is a crucial factor in creating an effective program.

Effectiveness of Employee Assistance Programs

There is a paucity of research on the effectiveness of EAPs. Nevertheless, some studies clearly lend support to the capability of EAPs in reducing alcohol problems in the workplace. The provision of careful post-treatment monitoring by the EAP appears to reduce rates of relapse. For example, in one study, 325 workers were referred to an EAP for alcohol or other substance abuse problems. They were assigned to one of two conditions: standard care (consisting of assessment and treatment) and standard care plus 1 year of follow-up with a counselor. The group that received follow-up counseling fared better than the group that did not, with 15% fewer relapses resulting in hospitalization, and 24% lower alcohol-related and substance-related health benefit claims.

Future Challenges

With the rising costs of health care and the onslaught of health maintenance organizations, today's EAP professional faces the difficulty of finding treatment resources that best meet the needs of the alcohol-abusing employee while also keeping the cost low. EAPs are entrusted to ensure that employees receive quality services from referrals they make. Research is needed to assess which programs and strategies are most effective in addressing alcohol problems in the workplace. The professionals in EAPs need to keep up with the demographic and technological advances that have such a large impact on industry and workers, and to continue to strive to understand

and fulfill the needs of the employee balanced with the needs of the employer.

SUGGESTED READINGS

Bennett JB, Lehman WE: Supervisor tolerance-responsiveness to substance abuse and workplace prevention training: use of a cognitive mapping tool. Health Educ Res 17:27–42, 2002.

Delaney W, Grube JW, Ames GM: Predicting likelihood of seeking help through the employee assistance program among salaried and union hourly employees. Addiction 93:399–410, 1998.

Donahoe TL, Johnson JT, Taquinoa MA: Self-disclosure as a predictor of EAP supervisory utilization. Employee Assistance Q 14:1–10, 1998.

Hopkins KM: Supervisor intervention with troubled workers: A social identity perspective. Hum Rel 50:1215-1238, 1998.

Roman PM, Blum C: Employee assistance programs. In: Galanter M, Kleber HD (eds.), Textbook of Substance Abuse Treatment. Washington, D.C.: The American Psychiatric Press, 1994, pp. 369–383.

Roman PM, Blum TC: The workplace and alcohol problem prevention. Alcohol Res Health 26:49–57, 2002.

ALCOHOL TREATMENT IN THE CRIMINAL JUSTICE SYSTEM

James W. Cornish
Douglas B. Marlowe

Alcohol use is implicated in approximately 40% to 50% of crimes committed in the United States. In national surveys conducted by the Bureau of Justice Statistics, more than 35% of state prison inmates and 25% of state jail inmates self-reported being under the influence of alcohol at the time of their offense, and roughly an additional 15% of prison and jail inmates reporting being under the influence of alcohol in combination with illicit drugs. These figures appear to be relatively stable across various offense categories. Whether used alone or in combination with other drugs, approximately 40% of state inmates reported being under the influence of alcohol during the commission of a violent offense; approximately 35% reported being under the influence of alcohol during the commission of a theft or property offense; and approximately 55% reported being under the influence of alcohol during the commission of a "public-order" offense such as driving while intoxicated or disorderly conduct. Importantly, about one quarter of these state inmates reported experiencing three or more positive symptoms on the CAGE (Cut down, Annoyed, Guilty, Eye-opener) questionnaire, which is consistent with a history of alcohol abuse or dependence.

These staggering figures apply not only to incarcerated populations but also to individuals under correctional supervision in the community. Almost 40% of offenders sentenced to community probation reported having used alcohol at the time of their offense, representing approximately 40% of probationers convicted of a violent crime, 19% of probationers convicted of a theft or property crime, and 75% of probationers convicted of a public-order offense. Roughly 25% of these state probationers reported three or more positive responses on the CAGE, consistent with a history of alcohol abuse or dependence. Similarly, 42% of individuals released on parole after a state prison sentence reported having used alcohol at the time of their offense, and approximately 25% of those state parolees reported symptoms of alcohol dependence on the CAGE.

ALCOHOL TREATMENT WITHIN THE CRIMINAL JUSTICE SYSTEM

National data from the Bureau of Justice statistics indicate that approximately one half to two thirds of alcohol-abusing offenders receive *some* form of substance abuse treatment while they are incarcerated or on probation. For instance, in 1997, 45% of inmates who were binge drinkers before their arrest, and 46% of inmates who were characterized as being alcohol-dependent according to the CAGE, reported attending some form of alcohol treatment during their current incarceration. Similarly, among probationers in 1995, approximately 50% of binge drinkers and 65% of alcohol-dependent individuals reported receiving some form of alcohol treatment during their current probationary sentence. It is important, however, to note that most of these services were self-help or peer-counseling groups as well as educational or drug-awareness programs. Less than 20% of binge drinkers and alcohol-dependent inmates received formal substance abuse treatment services, and less than 5% received intensive ambulatory substance abuse treatment services or segregated residential services. Further, only 8% of jail inmates reported participating in any form of substance abuse treatment, which is likely due to the relatively brief intervals of detention in jails.

The most commonly offered substance abuse intervention in jails and prisons is participation in standardized educational groups, which typically deal with such topics as the pharmacology of drug and alcohol use, progression from substance use to dependence, impact of addiction on the family, treatment options, and HIV/AIDS risk reduction. Although educational groups could potentially be useful as an early intervention strategy for youthful offenders, the research data uniformly indicate that they have virtually *no* effect on drug use or criminal recidivism among adult offenders.

Many prisons and jails also offer psychoeducational substance abuse counseling groups, which commonly focus on enhancing inmates' intrinsic motivation for change, improving their communication and problem-solving skills, teaching relapse prevention skills, practicing drug-refusal strategies, and developing community-based aftercare plans. A 1999 meta-analysis of studies of illicit drug users found *no* effect of these types of drug-focused group counseling interventions on subsequent drug use or criminal recidivism. Unfortunately, no effort could be made in that meta-analysis to control the *quality* of the counseling groups or to isolate the effects of particular types of interventions such as motivational enhancement therapy or relapse prevention therapy, which have been shown to produce positive effects in nonoffender populations. Moreover, no effort was made to evaluate the effects of providing needed aftercare services to those offenders after their release from prison. Greater promise was shown in that meta-analysis for self-help groups such as Alcoholics Anonymous or Narcotics Anonymous; however, there were too few scientifically acceptable studies of Alcoholics Anonymous or Narcotics Anonymous to reach any definitive conclusions.

To date, the most consistent evidence of success among incarcerated offenders has been obtained from in-prison therapeutic community programs. Although most of the extant therapeutic community research has focused on illicit drug abusers, many of the same general principles are likely to apply to alcohol-abusing offenders as well. Unlike traditional "milieu" therapies, which are run by professionally trained correction staffs, therapeutic communities are predominantly peer-administered programs. Inmates in therapeutic communities are segregated from the general inmate population. The peers exert substantial influence over each other by confronting negative personality traits, sanctioning inappropriate behaviors, rewarding positive behaviors, and providing mentorship and positive camaraderie. Clinical interventions commonly include confrontational encounter groups, process groups, and community meetings.

Several long-term evaluations have indicated that therapeutic community services must be provided along the full "prisoner reentry" continuum, ranging from in-prison treatment to work-release treatment to continuing outpatient treatment. In virtually all studies, in-prison therapeutic community treatment without aftercare had *no* appreciable effect on substance use or return-to-custody rates. However, offenders who completed a work-release therapeutic community program exhibited significant reductions of roughly 10 to 20 percentage points in return-to-custody rates and drug use over a 3-year follow-up. Moreover, these effects were enhanced for individuals who completed a continuum of services from in-prison through work-release therapeutic community treatment. Completion of both in-prison and work-release components was associated with a large reduction of 30 to 50 percentage points in new arrests and returns to custody over 3 years. It is important to recognize, however, that many of these studies used systematically biased comparison samples such as offenders who refused or dropped out of the interventions. This is likely to have overestimated the magnitude of the positive outcomes because it restricted the analyses to the most successful cases.

Regardless, the results of these evaluations underscore the critical importance of providing care services for offenders after release from prison. Generally speaking, treatment gains in institutional settings such as jails or prisons fail to generalize to the community at large and are lost within a relatively brief time. In-prison treatment does, however, confer certain benefits. Studies reveal that involvement in in-prison treatment significantly increases the likelihood that an offender will subsequently enter and remain in a care program after release from prison. It is possible that in-prison services may enhance offenders' motivation for change or may prepare them to make optimal use of substance abuse treatment services once they are in the community or in a transitional-release setting. What is clear, however, is that it is not sufficient merely to provide offenders with a referral to a community-based treatment program. It is essential to prepare them for what to expect, to facilitate the referral by transferring the necessary paperwork and clinical information to the referral source, and to follow-up to ensure that the offender has, in fact, completed the treatment referral.

PRINCIPLES OF EFFECTIVE CLINICAL INTERVENTIONS

Research reviews and meta-analyses have identified several factors that appear to characterize effective treatment programs for offenders. Outcome studies indicate that intensive treatment interventions appear to be best suited for high-risk offenders such as those who have an earlier age of onset of substance use or criminal activity, more severe criminal or substance use patterns, and previously failed experiences in treatment. Low-risk offenders, on the other hand, generally perform equally well when exposed to low-intensity interventions, and they may even perform somewhat worse when exposed to intensive interventions in an antisocial milieu. It is possible that for certain low-risk offenders, the mere fact of being incarcerated or having a run-in with the law may be sufficient to reduce their substance use or criminal recidivism. Moreover, requiring them to have increased contacts with more severe offenders in a treatment program, and having treatment interfere with their other family and employment obligations, could cause them to perform worse over the long-term.

Counseling interventions governing structured behavioral or cognitive-behavioral interventions generally appear to be superior to insight-oriented or nonstructured process interventions for offenders. In fact, treatments that are designed to improve offenders' self-esteem, or to address underlying symptoms of anxiety or depression, have been associated with *worse* outcomes in some studies. The best results have been obtained from programs that focused on restructuring clients' distorted antisocial cognitions, correcting their erroneous assumptions about the motives of others, and teaching adaptive problem-solving, communication and coping skills. Moreover, programs that effectively apply basic behavioral principles of operant conditioning have been associated with the best outcomes. In the most successful programs, for instance, clinicians have been in a position to immediately and reliably detect clients' accomplishments and infractions in the program, and to apply positive rewards for desired behaviors and negative sanctions for undesired behaviors. For instance, the most effective programs regularly monitor substance use through random, weekly Breathalyzer assessments and urinalyses. Negative results are met with contingent rewards such as reduced monitoring requirements, reduced criminal sanctions, or goods and services that support a productive lifestyle. Positive results, on the other hand, are met with contingent sanctions such as loss of privileges, increased counseling requirements, or a return to detention.

DIVERSION PROGRAMS

A number of diversion programs are available that may offer substance-abusing offenders an opportunity to complete a regimen of community-based treatment *in lieu of* receiving a criminal conviction or incarceration. For instance, many jurisdictions offer first-time or second-time offenders, including those charged with public order offenses and criminal driving while intoxicated, an opportunity for accelerated rehabilitative disposition. Offenders in accelerated rehabilitative disposition are typically placed on probation with substance abuse treatment as a mandatory condition of probation. The current criminal charges are commonly held in abeyance pending completion of treatment. If offenders satisfactorily complete the prescribed regimen, the record of their criminal charges may be expunged. This would entitle the individuals to respond truthfully on an employment application or similar document that they have not been charged with a drug- or alcohol-related offense, at least as this pertains to the current arrest episode.

Much of the available research on diversion programs has involved studies of illicit drug abusers, a substantial proportion of whom abuse alcohol as well. Statewide studies generally reveal that 50% to 70% of drug-abusing probationers fail to comply with their conditions of probation, including attendance at substance abuse treatment and drug testing. Partly as a result of these poor compliance rates, intensive supervised probation programs were developed to reduce probation officers' caseloads and to increase their resources for monitoring and intervening with offenders. The intensive supervised probation programs typically involve multiple weekly contacts with offenders and may include unscheduled drug testing, surprise home visits, and strict requirements for offenders to seek or maintain schooling or employment and complete community service obligations.

Evaluation studies reveal that intensive supervised probation programs are paradoxically associated with seemingly *worse* outcomes for offenders in terms of more technical violations and returns to custody. This is likely due to the fact that more intensive monitoring of offenders in these programs leads to a greater and more reliable detection of infractions. Unfortunately, many intensive supervised probation programs have tended to emphasize their monitoring and sanctioning functions at the expense of their rehabilitative mandate. As a result, they often have not been effective in "brokering" probationers' referrals to treatment and ensuring their continued engagement in treatment.

Under the rubric of what was originally termed "Treatment Alternatives to Street Crime"—now renamed "Treatment Accountability for Safer Communities"—hundreds of case management agencies were founded across the country to identify and refer substance-using offenders (mostly illicit drug abusers) to community-based treatment, to monitor offenders' progress in treatment, and to report compliance information to appropriate criminal justice authorities. Early evaluations concluded that these programs were effective at identifying substance abuse problems among offenders and making appropriate treatment referrals. Moreover, clients involved with the criminal justice system tended to remain in treatment significantly longer when they were under Treatment Accountability for Safer Communities supervision. An evaluation of five large and representative programs found, however, that effects on substance use and criminal recidivism were mixed. Drug use was reduced for program clients in three of the five sites, and criminal activity was reduced in only two of the sites. Moreover, the magnitudes of the positive findings were generally modest and confined to high-risk offenders. This suggests that the effects of Treatment Accountability for Safer Communities programs depend on how well the case managers carry out their roles.

The available evidence suggests that the most effective diversionary strategy for substance-abusing offenders is one that *integrates* substance abuse treatment services with close monitoring by criminal justice authorities and immediate and consistent consequences for offenders' noncompliance with treatment. The clearest example of such an integrated strategy is drug courts. These specialized courts were developed primarily for handling illicit drug abusers; however, many new forms of "problem-solving courts" are now being developed based on the drug court model, including courts for driving while intoxicated, mental health courts, and dependency courts for child abuse and neglect cases.

Drug courts provide nonviolent drug offenders with the opportunity to have their criminal record expunged contingent on completion of a *judicially supervised* course of drug treatment, case management, urinalysis monitoring, and ongoing status hearings before the judge in court. In drug courts, defendants are generally required to plead guilty or "no contest" to the charges as a precondition of entry into the program. Therefore, if the offender is terminated from the program for noncompliance with treatment or unremitting drug use, conviction and disposition are a relative formality. In addition, entry criteria for drug courts require clients to agree to be subject to specified slates of interim sanctions and rewards that may be applied by the judge in response to infractions and accomplishments in the program. For example, failure to attend a counseling session or the provision of a drug-positive urine specimen might be met with increased counseling requirements, fines, community service, or a brief interval of detention.

Reviews of nearly 100 drug court evaluations indicate that an average of 60% of drug court clients complete a year or more of treatment and roughly one half graduate successfully from the program. This compares quite favorably with typical retention rates in community-based drug treatment programs, where roughly 70% of probationers drop out or attend irregularly within 2 to 6 months. In largely uncontrolled or quasi-experimental studies, drug court clients have also demonstrated greater reductions in drug use, criminal recidivism, and unemployment compared with drug-abusing offenders on standard probation or intensive probation.

These data suggest that integrating substance abuse treatment with court supervision is a promising strategy for dealing with an otherwise recalcitrant population. As noted earlier, however, intensive interventions such as drug courts may be best suited to higher risk offenders, such as those with an earlier age of onset of substance abuse, prior failed experiences in substance abuse treatment, or comorbid antisocial personality disorder. Less intensive diversionary programs such as Accelerated Rehabilitative Disposition may be equally well suited to first-time offenders who have relatively uncomplicated substance abuse histories.

DETERRENTS TO DRIVING WHILE INTOXICATED

It is estimated that approximately 40% to 45% of traffic accidents and traffic fatalities in the United States are alcohol related. Although the majority of individuals arrested for driving while intoxicated do not repeat the offense, between approximately 20% and 35% of such individuals do go on to become repeat offenders by driving while intoxicated. Efforts to identify client-level risk factors for driving while intoxicated recidivism have generally produced mixed findings, with the resulting classification algorithms often being too complicated to be useful in clinical practice. For instance, to obtain efficient classification rates for high-risk vs. low-risk driving while intoxicated offenders, it is generally necessary to take several variables into account simultaneously, such as subjects' educational attainment, age at first arrest, number of prior driving while intoxicated convictions, blood alcohol concentration at time of arrest, and scores on such instruments as the CAGE or Minnesota Multiphasic Personality Inventory-2 MacAndrews Alcoholism Scale. Moreover, the optimal cut-off scores for these variables tend to shift from sample to sample, making reliable predictions very difficult for new programs.

A number of strategies oriented to public safety have been attempted to deter motorists from driving while under the influence. These include mandatory fines, community service requirements, or minimum jail sentences for offenders convicted of driving while intoxicated; mandatory intervals of license suspension after a criminal conviction for any designated alcohol-related or drug-related offense; and "administrative" license revocations for individuals who have not been formally convicted of a criminal offense. Meta-analyses generally reveal statistically insignificant to "small" success rates for these types of law enforcement policies, ranging from 1% to 17% reduction rates in driving while intoxicated recidivism.

Adding treatment or remedial components on top of license revocation generally reduces driving while intoxicated recidivism rates by an additional 7 to 10 percentage points. Unfortunately, as in most outcome studies with substance abusers, research has generally failed to identify specific types or modalities of treatment that may have effects relatively superior to those of other interventions, and has also failed to identify specific client-treatment matching effects.

The majority of driving programs for those convicted of driving while intoxicated tend to provide standard regimens of educational groups, covering such topics as the effects of alcohol on one's driving ability as well as victim impact statements and depictions of accident scenes. When administered alone, such educational groups have limited utility. However, their effects may be substantially enhanced when the educational sessions are combined with structured counseling interventions that teach practical strategies for avoidance of driving while intoxicated, such as blood alcohol concentration discrimination training, behavioral self-control training, and relapse prevention skills. Referrals to self-help groups are also commonly made; however, the unique effects on outcomes of self-help participation have not been reliably isolated or disaggregated from standard treatment interventions. It is also important to recognize that most studies have used relatively short follow-up windows of 6 months to 2 years, leaving open the question of whether the effects of programs to eliminate driving while intoxicated may diminish after termination of monitoring and license reinstatement.

GENERAL ALCOHOL TREATMENT PRINCIPLES

For the most part, substance abuse treatment for criminal justice clients is administered outside of prison. Persons within the criminal justice system should be evaluated and treated in the same manner as other substance abusers who are entering treatment. It is crucial to conduct a comprehensive evaluation to determine the physical and psychological status of a person before treatment to ensure that all substances of abuse are assessed and that all medical and psychological problems are identified. Persons targeted for treatment must have thorough medical and substance abuse histories, alcohol and drug screens, complete physical examinations, and appropriate laboratory studies. The results from the baseline evaluation are used to develop a treatment plan that is individualized and comprehensive. Because many substance abusers coadminister several substances, it is possible that a person may require treatment for two or more dependencies. For criminal justice clients, it is important for the treatment provider to discuss the treatment plan with the official responsible for the legal supervision of the client such as a parole or probation officer. In most situations, the criminal justice officer and the treatment team work together with respect to the client's participation and attendance at substance abuse treatment sessions. Treatment team members use the treatment plan as both a problem list and a reference by which to measure treatment progress.

Alcohol Detoxification

This is a process, initiated by the discontinuance of drinking, whereby alcohol is cleared from the body by natural metabolism and the major organ systems regulate to an alcohol-free state. Alcohol abstinence may be voluntary, as with entry into treatment or forced as a consequence of incarceration. Usually, within a day of discontinuing alcohol, most alcoholics experience symptoms of the alcohol withdrawal syndrome. The symptoms range from mild, manifested by headaches and irritability, to severe, such as seizures and even death. About 5% of alcoholics experience severe, life-threatening symptoms. Benzodiazepine therapy is safe, effective, and the treatment of choice for the prevention and treatment of alcohol withdrawal symptoms. Treatment typically lasts for 5 to 7 days, during which patients receive medication coupled with the replacement of fluids, electrolytes, and vitamins as required. Unfortunately, it is difficult to precisely determine which persons will develop severe symptoms. Consequently, medical supervision of detoxification is recommended for chronic drinkers who discontinue the regular intake of alcohol. In the criminal justice system, it is important to identify alcoholics who are newly incarcerated because they may be at risk of suffering alcohol withdrawal symptoms.

Relapse Prevention

Most treatments of alcohol dependence have involved self-help groups such as Alcoholics Anonymous or psychosocial therapies. Self-help groups such as Alcoholics Anonymous can offer important support for recovering alcoholics. The groups are based on a 12-step method of recovery and are composed of individuals interested in helping themselves lead alcohol-free lives. Participants are frequently reminded of the benefits of maintaining abstinence and the consequences of relapse. The newly recovering person is often assigned a sponsor who is an individual in the group with a prolonged time in an alcohol-free lifestyle. The sponsor presents a good role model for a person in recovery. Members may attend meetings as frequently as necessary. Self-help groups are also available to non–drug-abusing family members to help them understand the addictive process and how family dynamics can affect the recovering family member.

Psychosocial therapies are usually provided in rehabilitation programs, inpatient or outpatient programs, or therapeutic communities. Psychotherapy is a process that aims to identify inappropriate interpersonal processes and to develop strategies to correct these interpersonal problems. Cognitive-behavioral therapy emphasizes the identification of risky situations and the development of skills for coping with the cravings to consume alcohol. Motivational enhancement therapy focuses on techniques that help people to initiate meaningful actions to modify addictive behaviors. Research has shown that different psychotherapies have similar treatment effects. The National Institute on Alcohol Abuse and Alcoholism sponsored a study, Project Match, to compare the efficacies of three different types of psychosocial treatment for alcoholism: 12-step facilitation therapy, cognitive-behavioral therapy, and motivational enhancement therapy. Data from this large study involving 952 subjects show no significant difference for any one type of therapy; each therapy produced an abstinence rate of 60% for 12 to 15 months after enrollment.

A main focus for pharmacotherapy has been to augment the success rate over that of psychosocial treatments alone. Medication therapies have been targeted at specific problems that occur during a treatment program for alcoholism: alcohol detoxification, relapse prevention, and symptoms of coexisting psychiatric disorders.

In alcohol detoxification (see earlier), the symptoms of alcohol withdrawal syndrome can be prevented and treated with benzodiazepine medication. Pharmacotherapies used in relapse prevention include an alcohol-sensitizing agent or anticraving medications. Disulfiram was the first medication approved by the Food and Drug Administration (FDA) as a pharmacotherapy for alcohol dependence. Disulfiram inhibits alcohol dehydrogenase, an enzyme that is key to the metabolism of alcohol. In treated persons, a disulfiram-alcohol reaction causes an accumulation of acetaldehyde that produces noxious symptoms such as tachycardia, facial flushing, hypotension, nausea, and vomiting. These alcohol-sensitized symptoms strongly discourage the drinking of alcohol. The efficacy of disulfiram is diminished because patients often stop taking it. Administering disulfiram under the direct supervision of a treatment professional or family member may enhance medication compliance.

In 1994, the FDA approved naltrexone as a treatment for alcoholism that prevents relapse to drinking. Naltrexone is an opioid receptor antagonist that has been found to reduce alcohol preference in several animal models. Subsequent clinical studies showed that detoxified, naltrexone-treated subjects had reduced alcohol craving and relapse to drinking. Naltrexone-treated subjects appear to have blunted response (neither pleasant nor unpleasant) to consumed alcohol. As of 2002, 13 of 15 published controlled studies of naltrexone (or nalmefene, which is another opioid antagonist) show significant effects for the medication. Although the majority of the evidence favors the efficacy of naltrexone, not all studies have been positive. There are other promising anticraving medications that are in clinical trials. Acamprosate was developed in Europe as a medication that decreases the desire to drink alcohol. It has several actions, including an effect that reduces postalcohol neuronal excitability. Acamprosate is approved in Europe, and despite the negative U.S. multicenter trial, further studies are ongoing to establish its efficacy in the United States. In a recently published European study, the combination of naltrexone and acamprosate appears promising. The 5-HT_3 receptor antagonist ondansetron has been reported as effective in reducing alcohol consumption in early-onset alcoholics. The combination of naltrexone and ondansetron has also been reported as an effective treatment for early-onset alcoholics.

CONCLUSIONS

Although substance abuse treatment has been shown to be potentially effective in both criminal justice system and non-criminal justice system populations, the sad truth is that the vast majority of alcohol-using and drug-abusing offenders do not receive treatment services, or they receive minimally effective interventions such as participation in educational-counseling or peer-counseling groups. Efficacious medications such as naltrexone for alcoholics or methadone for opiate abusers are almost wholly unavailable to criminal justice system populations. Medications are not used because they have not been included as part of the available services to criminal justice clients. Moreover, very few correctional programs employ adequately trained professional clinicians, administer structured behavioral or cognitive-behavioral interventions, or provide meaningful access to essential aftercare services.

The reasons for this are varied. A significant reason for these omissions of treatment in criminal justice populations has been the long-standing emphasis on apprehension and punishment. Part of the problem is fiscal. It is very difficult to convince correctional administrators that the short-term costs of providing effective treatments for offenders will produce longer term cost savings. Moreover, any realized cost savings typically do not translate into direct benefits for the correctional institution itself. For example, prison beds are fixed costs that may not yield immediately identifiable savings from fewer alcohol-related re-arrests. The problem is also partly political. Many correctional officials and members of the public are resistant to the notion that alcohol dependence may be a treatable "disease." Instead, many people focus on the fact that the disorder typically *begins* with a repetitive pattern of voluntary misconduct. As such, there is little sympathy for "coddling" offenders by providing them with treatment. Many individuals bristle, in particular at the notion of giving medications to offenders, which may be viewed as too costly or as merely "substituting one drug for another."

Finally, there seems to be a pervasive perception on the part of many law enforcement officials and members of the public that substance abuse treatment really *does not* work. Failing to recognize that addiction commonly follows a chronic, relapsing course similar to that of hypertension or diabetes, many people view high rates of relapse after completion of substance abuse treatment as evidence that offenders "do not really want to get better."

It is essential for alcohol abuse treatment providers and researchers to better educate the public and policy makers about the nature of alcohol abuse and dependence. It is particularly important to marshal convincing evidence for the positive effects of formal alcohol treatment services for offenders, to differentiate effective from non-effective interventions, and to shed light on the chronic nature of this condition. Otherwise, offenders will continue to receive ineffective or below-threshold treatment for a serious and complicated disorder, and will continue to cycle in and out of the criminal justice system, and in and out of a life of crime.

SUGGESTED READINGS

Belenko S: Behind Bars: Substance Abuse and America's Prison Population. New York, NY: National Center on Addiction and Substance Abuse at Columbia University, 1998.

Kirby KC, Schmitz JM, Stitzer ML: Integrating behavioral and pharmacological treatments. In: Johnson BA, Roache JD (eds.), Drug Addiction and its Treatment: Nexus of Neuroscience and Behavior. Philadelphia, PA: Lippincott-Raven, 1997, pp. 403–419.

Leukefeld CG, Toms F, Farabee D (eds.): Treatment of Drug Offenders: Policies and Issues. New York, NY: Springer, 2002

Marlowe DB: Effective strategies for intervening with drug abusing offenders. Villanova Law Review 47:989–1026, 2002.

Taxman FS: Unraveling "what works" for offenders in substance abuse treatment services. National Drug Court Institute Review 2(2):93–134, 1999.

Wells-Parker E, Bangert-Drowns R, McMillen R, Williams M: Final results from a meta-analysis of remedial interventions with drink/drive offenders. Addiction 90:907–926, 1995.

AURICULAR ACUPUNCTURE IN ALCOHOL TREATMENT

Michael O. Smith
Patricia Culliton
Claudia Voyles

Acupuncture is currently used in the treatment of addiction by approximately 1500 treatment programs worldwide. Clinical evidence supports that auricular acupuncture is effective in ameliorating acute and long-term withdrawal and craving symptoms associated with alcohol addiction. Treatment programs use acupuncture as a foundation for later psychosocial recovery. It is a nonverbal, nonthreatening, first-step intervention that has an immediate calming effect on patients. Initial participation in a program with acupuncture has been found to improve patients' overall treatment retention and to facilitate their subsequent involvement in the therapeutic process. This chapter describes the practical use and research findings relating to acupuncture for alcohol treatment.

Trained clinicians needle three to five ear acupuncture points in patients who are seated for 40 to 45 minutes in a large group room This method facilitates the convenient treatment of a substantial number of patients to be at the same time. Acupuncture is integrated with conventional elements of psychosocial rehabilitation. Other core concepts reflected in many acupuncture-based programs include a supportive, nonconfrontational approach to counseling; emphasis on participation in an AA program early in the treatment process; reduced need to screen for "appropriate" patients; use of herbal "sleep mix"; willingness to work with court-related agencies and other agencies; and a tolerant, informal, family-like atmosphere.

As a safe, cost-efficient and effective adjunctive procedure, acupuncture has gained increasing acceptance from agencies that are responsible for overseeing alcohol treatment. The federal Center for Substance Abuse Treatment (CSAT) has held two consensus conferences that will result in publication in 2003 of a treatment improvement protocol on the integration of acupuncture in addiction treatment.

Alcohol treatment clinicians can easily and effectively learn the protocol in a 70-hour training program that emphasizes clinical apprenticeship. Each acupuncture detoxification specialist (ADS) can provide about 15 treatments per hour in a group setting under the general supervision of a licensed acupuncturist or other health professional, qualified according to local regulations. This arrangement allows acupuncture to be integrated with existing services in a flexible and cost-effective manner, increasing access and improving clinical relationships within the treatment milieu. Programs that address alcoholism along the continuum of care may successfully integrate acupuncture. Characteristically, acupuncture proves a very valuable tool for treating special populations, including criminal justice-involved patients, women, adolescents, and patients with concomitant mental disorders.

Acupuncture is a major component of the ancient tradition of Chinese medicine. Acupuncture was used by numerous 19th century U.S. practitioners, including Sir William Osler. In the early 1970s, American interest was renewed when relations with China were reopened. In the United States, most states have acupuncture licensing laws, many of which include exemptions allowing clinical staff with proper training in addiction treatment to provide a limited acupuncture protocol. Acupuncture consists of stimulation of specified locations on the surface of the body, which alters and improves bodily function. Acupuncture points are physiologically distinct from the immediate environment; they have less electrical resistance and, therefore, greater electrical conductivity. The points are warmer than the surrounding area by 0.1 to 0.2 fractions of a degree.

Needling is the most convenient and efficient means of stimulating acupuncture points. Acupuncture needles are stainless steel shafts of varying lengths and thicknesses. Acupuncture needles are provided in convenient sterile packages. Most Western facilities use the needles once and discard them, although needles may be cleaned, sterilized, and reused as is the case with surgical equipment.

Needles are inserted with a brief but steady movement. The procedure is nearly painless and causes rapid onset of a gratifying sense of relaxation. On first exposure, most patients express fear of the pain of needle insertion and are confused by the idea that little needles can cope with their big problems. This fear is easily overcome by letting prospective patients observe the actual treatment process.

Patients may notice local paresthesia effects such as warmth and tingling. Patients may feel quite sleepy after each of the first several treatments. This reaction is part of the quiet recovery process and passes readily. Rarely in alcohol treatment, patients experience a "needling reaction" of syncope, which resolves when the needles are removed.

EARLY DEVELOPMENT OF ACUPUNCTURE USE FOR SUBSTANCE ABUSE

Acupuncture treatment for drug and alcohol problems was primarily developed at Lincoln Hospital, a city-owned facility in the impoverished South Bronx. The Lincoln Recovery Center is a state-licensed treatment program, which has provided more than 500,000 acupuncture treatments in the past 28 years. Dr. Yoshiaki Omura was the consultant who began the program in 1974, initially applying electrical stimulation to the lung point in the ear for opiate detoxification. Patients reported less malaise and better relaxation in symptom surveys. Reduction in opiate withdrawal symptoms and prolonged program retention were noted with twice daily treatments.

Gradually, the ear acupuncture protocol was expanded by adding the "shen men" spirit gate), a point which is well known for producing relaxation. During a developmental process that extended over several years, other ear points were tried on the basis of lower resistance, decreased pain sensitivity, and clinical indication. Electric stimulation was discontinued. Dr. Michael Smith of Lincoln added the "sympathetic," "kidney," and "liver" points to create a basic five-point formula. Traditional Chinese theory associates the lung with the grieving process; the liver with resolving aggression; and the kidney with will power and rebirth.

From the point of view of Chinese theory, using a single basic formula for such generally depleted patients is appropriate. In traditional Chinese medicine, the lack of a clam inner tone in a person is described as a condition of "empty fire" (xu huo), because the "heat" of excess symptoms burns out of control when the calm inner tone is lost. It is easy to be confused by the "empty fire" that many alcoholics exhibit and to conclude that the main goal should be the sedation of excess symptoms. Alcoholics themselves use this approach by choosing to drink. Acupuncture helps patients with this condition to restore inner control. It is a supportive rather than a suppressive process.

CONTROLLED RESEARCH

H. L. Wen of Hong Kong was the first physician to report successful treatment of addiction withdrawal symptoms. He observed that opium addicts who received electro-acupuncture as postsurgical analgesia experienced relief of withdrawal symptoms. A number of controlled studies have been conducted since, using various modified versions of the National Acupuncture Detoxification Association (NADA) ear point formula. Two placebo-design studies provide strong support for use of acupuncture as a treatment for alcoholics. One research team studied 54 chronic alcohol abusers randomly assigned to receive acupuncture either at NADA ear points or at nearby point locations not specifically related to alcohol. Subjects were treated in an inpatient setting but were free to leave the program each day. Throughout the study, experimental subjects showed significantly better outcomes regarding their attendance and their self-reported need for alcohol. Significant differences favoring the experimental group were also found regarding: (1) number of self-reported drinking episodes, (2) self-reports of effectiveness of acupuncture in removing the desire to drink, and (3) number of subjects admitted to a local detoxification unit for alcohol-related treatment. These findings were later replicated by the same authors who used a larger (n = 80) sample over a longer (6-month) follow-up period. In the treatment group, 21 of 40 patients completed the 8-week treatment period compared with 1 of 40 controls. Significant differences favoring the experimental group were again noted. Researchers found a 52% retention rate for the experimental group of alcoholism patients compared with 2% for placebo patients. Placebo subjects self-reported more than twice the number of drinking episodes reported by experimental subjects. The number of experimental subjects was less than half that of the placebo subjects who were readmitted to the local hospital alcohol detoxification unit during the follow-up period.

Ear acupuncture charts indicate that all areas on the anterior surface of the ear are identified as active treatment locations. Use of a "placebo" or "sham" acupuncture technique is actually an effort to use *relatively* ineffective points in contrast to the conventional use of totally ineffective sugar pills in pharmaceutical trials. Sham points are usually located on the external helix or rim of the ear, although there is no consensus about the level of effectiveness of this procedure. The alcoholism studies described earlier used subjects highly prone to failure; therefore, they may have achieved a more effective demonstration of the difference between active and sham points.

These same authors purported to replicate their earlier studies in a recent trial. In this study, they found no statistically significant differences between groups receiving conventional treatment and various acupuncture groups, although the subjects reported decreased desire for alcohol. The 2002 study differs from the 1989 study in significant ways: (1) the average number of acupuncture treatments in the more recent study was 38% of the number of treatments given to the full-retention group in the previous study (10 rather than 26); and (2) acupuncture was embedded as a voluntary component in an extensive, mandatory, psychosocial protocol in the more recent study, whereas attendance at only two AA meetings per week of was required in the previous study. Each of these differences would be likely to reduce the potential impact of acupuncture in the recent study.

CLINICAL APPLICATIONS

Acupuncture detoxification programs report substantial reduction in recidivism rates. The Hooper Foundation (a public detox facility in Portland, Oregon) cited a decrease in recidivism from 25% to 6% in comparison with the rate in the previous year, when acupuncture was not used. The Kent-Sussex Detoxification Center (a state-run facility in Ellendale, Delaware) reported a decrease in recidivism from 87% to 18%.

The Substance Abuse Recovery program (Flint, Michigan) noted that 83% of a group of 100 General Motors employees were drug-free and alcohol-free a year after entering an acupuncture-based treatment program. Most of these patients had reported prior attempts at treatment and frequent relapses. All of the subjects in the 17% failure group had made fewer than five program visits. Seventy-four percent of the success group continued to attend AA and NADA meetings after completing the treatment program. Treatment protocols specifically designed for adolescents, such as those of the Alcohol Treatment Center in Chicago and a Job Corps-related program in Brooklyn, have shown retention rates comparable with those of adult programs.

Directors of the acupuncture social setting of the detoxification program conducted by the Tulalip Tribe at Marysville, Washington estimate a yearly saving of $148,000 resulting from fewer referrals to hospital programs. Inpatient alcohol detoxification units typically combine acupuncture and herbal sleep mix with a tapering benzodiazepine protocol. Patients report few symptoms and better sleep. Vital signs of these patients indicate stability and hence a much lower use of benzodiazepines. One residential program in Connecticut noted a 90% decrease in use of Valium over several years' time when only herbal "sleep mix" was added to the protocol.

Retention of alcohol detoxification patients at the Hooper Foundation increased by 50% when acupuncture was added their program in 1988. Some alcoholics who receive acupuncture actually report an aversion to alcohol. The Woodhull Hospital in Brooklyn reported that 94% of the patients in the acupuncture supplement group remained abstinent compared with 43% of the control group who received only conventional outpatient services. In general, acupuncture-based programs report improved engagement and retention of patients, a decreased number of discharges against medical/program advice (American Medical Association/American Psychiatric Association), increased completion rates, and improved client indicators of health and well-being.

Acupuncture treatment is generally made available to patients 5 to 6 days per week. Morning treatment hours seem to be more beneficial. Active patients receive treatment three to six times per week. The duration of acupuncture treatment depends on many factors. Inpatient programs should stress the use of acupuncture at the beginning of treatment for detoxification and stabilization and before discharge to alleviate separation anxiety. Outpatients typically receive acupuncture on an active basis for 1 to 3 months. About 10% of these outpatients choose to take acupuncture for more than 1 year if possible. Acupuncture is not primarily a "dose"-related phenomenon as is pharmaceutical treatment. Acupuncture more appropriately represents a qualitative service comparable to a school class or psychotherapy session. Acupuncture offers a support for relapse prevention. Relapsing patients are often able to continue to be involved in acupuncture even if they are no longer constructive participants in psychotherapy.

A wide range of patients can be accepted for the initial stage of treatment because there is no verbal motivational requirement. In addition, acupuncture is effective for a wide range of psychological states. Ambivalent streetwise patients find the acupuncture setting almost impossible to manipulate. The setting is so soothing and self-protective that even extremely antisocial people are able to fit into it. Problems relating to language and cultural differences are diminished. For new patients, frequent acupuncture treatments permit the gradual completion of assessment on a more accurate basis. Patients can be evaluated and triaged according to their ongoing response to treatment rather than merely on the basis of an interview.

The tolerant, nonverbal aspect of acupuncture facilitates retention during periods when the patient would otherwise be ambivalent, fearful, or resentful within a more intense verbal interpersonal setting. Ear acupuncture makes it easy to provide outpatient treatment on demand, without appointments, while patients are being acclimated to the interpersonal treatment setting.

Patients gradually develop respect for the values of the treatment process. Those same patients may be unable or unwilling to share their crises and failures verbally until they have time to reach more solid ground. In the acupuncture setting, time is an ally.

Acupuncture has many characteristics in common with the 12-step program (AA). It uses the group process in a tolerant, supportive, and present-time oriented manner. Participation is independent of diagnosis and level of recovery. Both approaches are simple, reinforcing, nurturing, and conveniently available. The emphasis on being responsible for oneself is common to both systems. In practice, acupuncture provides an excellent foundation for 12-step recovery. Patients seem less fearful and more receptive when they first enter the meetings. Acupuncture reduces "white-knuckle sobriety" considerably. There is less guarding and greater ability to support each other warmly. The increased ability to use 12-step meetings provides more stable support for continuing treatment on an outpatient basis and cultivating a clean and sober lifestyle.

PSYCHOSOCIAL MECHANISMS OF ACTION

It is essential to understand acupuncture's psychological and social mechanisms of action to use this modality effectively. Acupuncture has an impact on the patient's thoughts and feelings that is different from that of conventional pharmaceutical treatments. Later, we discuss how the use of acupuncture has a valuable and profound impact on the dynamics of the treatment processes as a whole. We should emphasize that acupuncture for the treatment of alcoholism is provided in a group setting. The new acupuncture patient is immediately introduced to a calm and supportive group process. Patients describe acupuncture as a unique kind of balancing experience: "I was relaxed but alert." "I was able to relax without losing control." Patients who are depressed or tired say that they feel more energetic after acupuncture treatment. This encouraging and balancing group experience becomes a critically important basis for the entire alcohol treatment process.

The perception that a person can be both relaxed and alert is rather unusual in Western culture, which customarily associates relaxation with somewhat lazy or spacey behavior and alertness with a certain degree of anxiety. The relaxed and alert state is basic to the concept of health in all Asian culture. Acupuncture encourages a centering, focusing process that is typical of meditation and yoga. Therapists report that patients are "able to listen" and "remember what we tell them." Restless, impulsive behavior is greatly reduced. On the other hand, discouragement and apathy are reduced as well. It is a balancing, centering process.

One of the striking characteristics of the acupuncture treatment setting is that patients seem comfortable in their own space and in their own thinking process. One patient explained, "I sat and thought about things in a slow way, as I did when I was 10 years old." Acupuncture treatment causes the perception of various relaxing bodily processes. Patients gradually gain confidence that their minds and bodies can function in a more balanced and autonomous manner. A hopeful process is developed on a private and personal basis, laying a foundation for the development of increasing self-awareness and self-responsibility.

The nature of recovery from alcohol addiction is that patients often have quickly changing needs for crisis relief and wellness treatment. Many persons in recovery have relatively high levels of "wellness" functioning. Even so, a crisis of craving or past association may reappear at any time. Conventional treatment settings are ill-equipped to cope with such intense and confusing behavioral swings. Often, merely the fear of a possible crisis can sabotage clinical progress. Acupuncture provides either crisis or wellness treatment using the same ear point formula. The nonverbal, present time aspects of the treatment facilitate response to a patient in any stage of crisis or denial.

Patients readily accept that it is possible to improve their acute addictive status. They seek external help to provide hospitalization and medication for withdrawal symptoms. The challenge develops when they encounter the necessity for internal change. Alcoholics perceive themselves as being unable to change from within. Their whole life revolves around powerful external change agents. Each alcoholic remembers countless examples of weakness, poor choices, and overwhelming circumstance, which lead them to the conclusion that they cannot help themselves become alcohol-free.

Acupuncture provides uniquely valuable assistance in coping with this challenge of internal redefinition. Patients often begin acupuncture treatment by seeking external escape and sedation as they do when they use drugs. When there is a rapid calming effect, they often assume there was some sort of chemical agent in the acupuncture needle. After a few treatments, they come to the astonishing conclusion that acupuncture works by revealing and employing their own capability. Regular participation in acupuncture helps patients use and revalue their internal resources much faster than is possible with conventional treatment processes. This effect contributes to the calm, cooperative atmosphere in most acupuncture settings. It reduces dropping out because of the fear of failure and low self-esteem that typify the early stage of treatment. Acupuncture creates a better atmosphere, enabling treatment staff to spend their energies on helping patients to make choices rather than be fatigued by trying to impose authority on a resistant clientele.

Acupuncture creates the foundation for psychosocial rehabilitation. At the beginning of treatment, building a proper foundation is very important. Once a foundation is established, the focus of treatment should shift away from acupuncture toward building a "house" of psychosocial recovery on that foundation.

Acupuncture is a nonverbal type of therapy. Words and verbal relationships are not necessary components of this treatment. Acupuncture is effective even when the patient lies to the therapist. With acupuncture, the verbal interaction that does take place can be quite flexible so that a patient who does not want to talk can be accommodated easily and naturally.

The most difficult-to-handle paradox in the field is the common reality that alcoholic persons usually deny that they need help. Such patients do not say anything that is helpful to the treatment process. Nevertheless, resistant patients often find themselves in a treatment setting because of referral or other pressures. Acupuncture treatment can bypass much of the verbal denial and resistance that otherwise limit retention of new and relapsed patients. Alcoholics are frequently ambivalent. Acupuncture helps therapists to reach the needy part of the psyche that wants help. Acupuncture can reduce stress and craving so that patients gradually become more ready to participate in the treatment process.

Alcoholic patients often cannot tolerate intense interpersonal relationships. Using a conventional one-to-one approach often creates a brittle therapeutic connection. It is easily broken by events or any stress. Patients have difficulty trusting a counselor's words when they can hardly trust themselves. Even after confiding to a counselor during an intake session, a patient may feel frightened and confused about expanding that relationship. Many concerns of these patients are so complex and troublesome that talking honestly about their lives can be difficult under the best circumstances. The ambivalence typical of alcoholics makes it easy to develop misunderstandings.

All of these factors support the usefulness of nonverbal technique during early and critical relapse phases of treatment and critical periods of relapse.

Acupuncture helps a program develop an underlying environment of acceptance, tolerance, and patience. There is ample space for ambivalence and temporary setbacks, which are a necessary part of any transformation. Patients can have a "quiet day" by attending the program and receiving acupuncture without having to discuss their status with a therapeutic authority figure. Since acupuncture reduces the agitated, defensive tone of the whole clinical environment, patients are able to interact with each other on a much more comfortable level. Their increased ability to listen to others and accept internal change has a profound effect on the quality and depth of communication in group therapy sessions and AA meetings. The primary community agenda can focus on the acceptance of each person and a tolerant encouragement of change rather than having to cope with defensive and antagonistic interactions.

NATIONAL ACUPUNCTURE DETOXIFICATION ASSOCIATION MODEL

The National Acupuncture Detoxification Association (NADA) was established in 1985 to promote auricular acupuncture for addiction while maintaining quality and responsibility in the field. Lincoln Recovery Center and NADA have trained more than 10,000 ADSes in the use of the Lincoln model.

Throughout the United States, NADA-inspired programs. in addiction and criminal justice settings number close to 1000. Independent NADA training and certification programs have been established in countries around the world. Acupuncture-based treatment has widespread roots in Eastern and Western European countries as well as Australia, Saudi Arabia, Nepal, India, Trinidad, Latin America, and Burma.

CONCLUSION

To really know the power of acupuncture in the treatment of alcoholism, listen to clients who have experienced it as part of their recovery transformation:

"Acupuncture has gotten me where I don't have a really manic life and I'm not depressed. I'm able to deal with everything that comes my direction because I have a lot of support also. I am energized, not miserable. I feel great about myself. I can smile today and the smile has feelings behind it. Acupuncture has hooked me up spiritually. I found my higher power—God—and He leads me each and every day."

"I was into prostitution and pornography—a violent woman . . . I behave differently today. I live with principles that I believe were ignited, sparked in me with acupuncture. As cumulative as acupuncture is, it has reached me on this level that I am able to change my beliefs more comfortably. I am given courage to take a look at my beliefs and empower myself, and now empower other women. I stand on the really strong truth that women can recover, and I know that acupuncture is the most valuable tool I know for recovery."

"Talking to [the counselor], getting acupuncture treatments—hate, anger jealousy, vengefulness, vindictiveness—all that changed into compassion and love. The acupuncture treatment just helped the thought process change and the detoxing and everything."

"It has a value that if you could share with them verbally you might be able to give it to them that way, and you can't give it to them that way. You can only give it to them through the acupuncture. It somehow helped me have a way to just be with myself long enough to see what it was I needed to work on—where I was wounded, how I could heal. And it's like a nonverbal way for one person to help to give treatment to another person. It's an experiential way to help sand the rough edges off what's going to be changed. It will give you a place to take all these other things into, to help create the change."

SUGGESTED READINGS

Brumbaugh A: Transformation and Recovery: A Guide for the Design and Development of Acupuncture-Based Chemical Dependency Treatment Programs.

Bullock ML, Culliton PD, Olander RT: Controlled trial of acupuncture for severe recidivist alcoholism. Lancet 1:1435–1439, 1989.

Guidepoints: Acupuncture in Recovery. The Professional's Newsletter on Innovative Treatment of Addictive and Mental Disorders.

Shwartz M, Saitz R, Mulvey K, Brannigan P: The value of acupuncture detoxification programs in a substance abuse treatment system. J Subst Abuse Treat 17:305–312, 1999.

Smith MO: Acupuncture for Addiction Treatment.

Voyles C: Some Lessons Learned.

Special Issues

FETAL ALCOHOL SYNDROME: ALCOHOL'S TERATOGENIC EFFECTS ON CENTRAL NERVOUS SYSTEM STRUCTURE AND FUNCTION

Sarah N. Mattson

Alcohol abuse during pregnancy can result in a spectrum of disorders in the offspring. This spectrum of effects includes, at one end, the fetal alcohol syndrome (FAS), which is characterized by a distinct pattern of malformation, growth deficiency, and central nervous system involvement. On the opposite end of the spectrum is normal development and offspring born without the physical or cognitive stigmata associated with FAS. Between these endpoints lies a broad array of effects, including physical, neurological, and neurocognitive changes that can have devastating effects on the children, their families and caregivers, and society.

FAS was first described in 1973 based on a small number of infants born to chronic alcoholic women. These authors noted a consistent pattern of facial features in these children, including short palpebral fissures, epicanthal folds, and a long, smooth philtrum. Based on their findings, they noted "an association between maternal alcoholism and aberrant morphogenesis in the offspring." Additional to this pattern of facial dysmorphology, the infants displayed prenatal or postnatal growth deficiency and evidence of central nervous system dysfunction. These three features are the diagnostic criteria for FAS. Since this pattern of malformation was first recognized in children of chronic alcoholic mothers, these diagnostic criteria have remained fairly constant. In 1996, the Institute of Medicine evaluated the status of the diagnosis of FAS and suggested a slightly modified diagnostic system. This system, which is detailed in Table 22.1, has received some support in the literature, although many researchers still use alternative labeling systems. For example, the term fetal alcohol effects (FAE) is still commonly used, although in many cases it could be substituted for partial FAS, as detailed in Table 22.1. Other research groups use more descriptive terminology that refers to the presence of prenatal alcohol exposure or facial dysmorphology. For example, the label *prenatal exposure to alcohol* (PEA) is used by our research group to describe children with histories of heavy prenatal alcohol exposure but without FAS. Most recently, the term *fetal alcohol spectrum disorder* has become more common, reflecting the belief that the effects of prenatal alcohol exposure occur on a continuum, as mentioned earlier.

Although the physical features (facial dysmorphology and growth retardation) comprise the primary features of FAS, it is the third

Table 22.1. Institute of Medicine Criteria for Fetal Alcohol Syndrome (FAS) and Related Disorders

FETAL ALCOHOL SYNDROME

1. FAS with confirmed maternal alcohol exposure

A. Confirmed maternal alcohol exposure
B. Evidence of a characteristic pattern of facial anomalies that includes features such as short palpebral fissures and abnormalities in the premaxillary zone (e.g., flat upper lip, flattened philtrum, and flat midface)
C. Evidence of growth retardation in at least one of the following:
  • Low birth weight for gestational age
  • Decelerating weight over time not due to malnutrition
  • Disproportionally low weight to height ratio
D. Evidence of CNS neurodevelopmental abnormalities in at least one of the following:
  • Decreased cranial size at birth
  • Structural brain abnormalities (e.g., microcephaly, partial or complete agenesis of the corpus callosum, cerebellar hypoplasia)
  • Neurological hard or soft signs (age appropriate), such as impaired fine motor skills, neurosensory hearing loss, poor tandem gait, poor eye-hand coordination

2. FAS without confirmed maternal alcohol exposure

B, C, and D as listed

3. Partial FAS with confirmed maternal alcohol exposure

A. Confirmed maternal alcohol exposure
B. Evidence of some components of the pattern of characteristic facial anomalies
Either C, D, or E:
C. Evidence of growth retardation in at least one of the following:
  • Low birth weight for gestational age
  • Decelerating weight over time not due to malnutrition
  • Disproportionally low weight to height ratio
D. Evidence of CNS neurodevelopmental abnormalities in:
  • Decreased cranial size at birth
  • Structural brain abnormalities (e.g., microcephaly, partial or complete agenesis of the corpus callosum, cerebellar hypoplasia)
  • Neurological hard or soft signs (age appropriate), such as impaired fine motor skills, neurosensory hearing loss, poor tandem gait, poor eye-hand coordination
E. Evidence of a complex pattern of behavioral or cognitive abnormalities that are inconsistent with developmental level and cannot be explained by familial background or environment alone, such as learning difficulties; deficits in school performance; poor impulse control; problems in social perception; deficits in higher level receptive and expressive language; poor capacity for abstraction or metacognition; specific deficits in mathematical skills; or problems in memory, attention, or judgment

(*continued*)

Table 22.1.   continued

ALCOHOL-RELATED EFFECTS

Clinical conditions in which there is a history of maternal alcohol exposure, and in which clinical or animal research has linked maternal alcohol ingestion to an observed outcome. There are two categories that may occur concurrently. If both diagnoses are present, both diagnoses should be rendered:

4. Alcohol-related birth defects (ARBD)

List of congenital anomalies, including malformations and dysplasias
- Cardiac
  - Atrial septal defects
  - Aberrant great vessels
  - Ventricular septal defects
  - Tetralogy of Fallot
- Skeletal
  - Hypoplastic nails
  - Clinodactyly
  - Shortened fifth digits
  - Pectus excavatum and carinatum
  - Radioulnar synostosis
  - Klippel-Feil syndrome
  - Flexion contractures
  - Hemivertebrae
  - Camptodactyly
  - Scoliosis
- Renal
  - Aplastic, dysplastic, hypoplastic kidneys
  - Ureteral duplications
  - Hydronephrosis
  - Horseshoe kidneys
- Ocular
  - Strabismus
  - Refractive problems secondary to small globes
  - Retinal vascular anomalies
- Auditory
  - Conductive hearing loss
  - Neurosensory hearing loss
- Other
  - Virtually every malformation has been described in some patient with FAS. The etiologic specificity of most of these anomalies to alcohol teratogenesis remains uncertain.

5. Alcohol-related neurodevelopmental disorder (ARND)

Presence of:
  A. Evidence of CNS neurodevelopmental abnormalities in any one of the following:
  - Decreased cranial size at birth
  - Structural brain abnormalities (e.g., microcephaly, partial or complete agenesis of the corpus callosum, cerebellar hypoplasia)

(*continued*)

Table 22.1.   continued

- Neurological hard or soft signs (age appropriate), such as impaired fine motor skills, neurosensory hearing loss, poor tandem gait, poor eye-hand coordination

and/or:

B. Evidence of a complex pattern of behavioral or cognitive abnormalities that are inconsistent with developmental level and cannot be explained by familial background or environment alone, such as learning difficulties; deficits in school performance; poor impulse control; problems in social perception; deficits in higher level receptive and expressive language; poor capacity for abstraction or metacognition; specific deficits in mathematical skills; or problems in memory, attention, or judgment

criterion, the effects on the central nervous system, that has the greatest impact on the child. The fact that heavy prenatal alcohol exposure affects brain development has been known for more than 30 years, and research for more than 10 years has identified a small number of brain areas that appear to be especially affected by this exposure. Additionally, a host of behavioral and neurocognitive features are common among children with FAS and heavy prenatal alcohol exposure. The following sections review the neuropsychological, behavioral, and neuroanatomical effects seen in children with heavy prenatal alcohol exposure, highlighting results from our research group. Although there exists a large body of literature describing studies of children with low to moderate levels of exposure, this chapter focuses on the effects of *heavy* prenatal alcohol exposure, with supporting evidence from prospective studies of lower levels of exposure if appropriate.

NEUROPSYCHOLOGICAL EFFECTS OF HEAVY PRENATAL ALCOHOL EXPOSURE

Although the neuropsychological features of heavy prenatal alcohol exposure are fairly broad, research over the past few years has focused on defining a profile of relative strengths and weaknesses in this population. Among the features commonly noted are lowered intelligence quotient (IQ) scores, academic difficulties, memory impairments, visual-spatial deficits, and executive function deficits. Each of these domains is reviewed herein.

Intellectual Functioning

FAS is one of the most common causes of mental retardation. Children with FAS typically have low IQ scores, although this is not a universal feature. A 1998 review of the literature revealed that of the cases of FAS that had been described at that point, the average IQ score was 72.26 with a range of 47.4 to 98.2. Our data suggest that alcohol-exposed children with the dysmorphic features of FAS and those without these features are impaired in their overall ability levels, although children with FAS tend to be slightly more impaired.

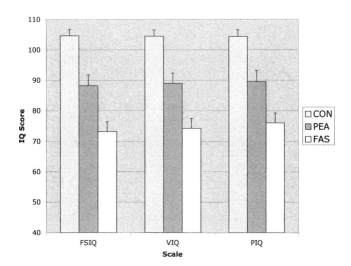

Fig. 22.1. Average IQ scores for children with fetal alcohol syndrome (FAS, $N = 32$), prenatal exposure to alcohol (PEA, $N = 24$), and non-exposed controls (CON, $N = 56$). Children were tested with WISC-III.

Figure 22.1 displays the average IQ scores for 56 children with FAS or PEA and 56 controls between the ages of 6 and 16 years. All children were tested with the Wechsler Intelligence Scale for Children, Third Edition (WISC-III). The average Full Scale IQ score for the combined alcohol-exposed group is 79.6, and both groups are impaired relative to controls (average Full Scale IQ = 104.6). These data are consistent with our previous report and indicate that even in the absence of facial dysmorphology, children with heavy prenatal alcohol exposure should be screened for intellectual impairments.

Academic Difficulties

Along with intellectual deficits, children with heavy prenatal alcohol exposure often experience academic failure. They are more likely to repeat grades and require special education services. Furthermore, despite being placed below their age-appropriate grade level, children with heavy prenatal alcohol exposure frequently work below their actual grade placement. Figure 22.2 illustrates the degree to which children in our sample are delayed academically. Both children with FAS and those with PEA are more likely to have achievement scores more than one grade behind their current grade placement.

Memory Impairments

Multiple studies have suggested that heavy prenatal alcohol exposure leads to deficits in learning and memory in both humans and animals. We have documented specific learning impairments in alcohol-exposed children. On the California Verbal Learning Test–Children's version (CVLT-C), children with FAS recalled fewer words

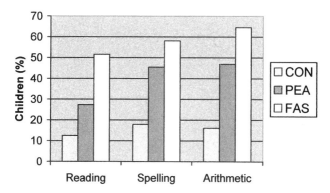

Fig. 22.2. Percentage of children with fetal alcohol syndrome (FAS, $N = 32$), prenatal exposure to alcohol (PEA, $N = 24$), and nonexposed controls (CON, $N = 56$) with academic achievement scores more than 1 grade below actual grade level.

than controls over five learning trials and after short (5-minute) and long (20-minute) delay intervals. In contrast, in comparison with controls, children with FAS retained a similar proportion of learned material after the 20-minute delay, suggesting that the deficit was at the level of encoding new information. We replicated these findings in children with heavy prenatal alcohol exposure but without FAS. Taken together, these studies suggest that the verbal memory deficits commonly reported in alcohol-exposed children might be secondary to encoding deficits present when new information is learned.

Less is known about learning and memory for nonverbal information. One study indicated that children with FAS recalled fewer objects after a 24-hour delay relative to controls, although immediate recall was similar between the groups and neither group appeared to forget a significant amount of information over time. In the same study, recall of spatial location by the FAS group was impaired in both immediate and delayed conditions, suggesting that loss of information over time (i.e., forgetting) was relatively unimpaired. A more recent study suggested that spatial memory deficits in children with FAS or FAE were secondary to deficits in perception or verbal memory and, therefore, not domain-specific. These studies are among very few to examine nonverbal recall in children with FAS and emphasize the importance of further examination of learning and memory in this domain.

We conducted a study that examined both verbal and nonverbal learning (i.e., acquisition) and memory (i.e., retention) in children with heavy prenatal alcohol exposure. Children with heavy prenatal alcohol exposure (both with and without FAS) displayed deficits in learning and recall of verbal and nonverbal information across all measures. On learning trials, they recalled fewer words and displayed a lower rate of acquisition. However, when delayed verbal recall data were analyzed after controlling for initial verbal learning, group differences were not apparent, indicating that verbal learning was more impaired than verbal memory. The same pattern did not occur for nonverbal information; children with prenatal alcohol exposure recalled less on delayed recall even when initial learning was taken into account. This study supported previous reports of immediate memory deficits but suggested that delayed memory for verbal and nonverbal information may be differentially affected. For verbal information, delayed recall deficits in this population are better accounted for by deficits in initial learning. In contrast, for nonverbal information, both learning and memory appear to be affected.

Visual-Spatial Deficits

In children with heavy prenatal alcohol exposure, the parietal lobe appears to be more affected than the temporal lobe. This pattern of damage may relate to specific aspects of visual-spatial functioning, namely the dorsal visual processing stream (the "where" system) and the ventral visual processing stream (the "what" system). In a pilot study, we demonstrated that children with heavy prenatal alcohol exposure had a relative weakness on measures of spatial location in comparison with object identification, supporting our hypothesis of a specific impairment on tasks sensitive to the where processing stream in comparison with tasks sensitive to the what processing stream.

Executive Function Deficits

One goal in the study of alcohol's teratogenicity is to define a profile of functioning, or core deficits, which best characterizes children with FAS and fetal alcohol spectrum disorders. This goal is still elusive; however, one characterization of deficits seen in this population is one of executive dysfunction. The domain of executive function encompasses abilities such as problem-solving, fluency, response inhibition, concept formation, and reasoning. These skills appear to be consistently affected in alcohol-exposed children. Three studies have addressed executive functioning and revealed specific deficits in planning and response inhibition, verbal and nonverbal fluency, and set-shifting and reversal learning.

BEHAVIORAL AND PSYCHOLOGICAL EFFECTS OF HEAVY PRENATAL ALCOHOL EXPOSURE

Disrupted behavioral development was among the cardinal features noted in the first descriptions of FAS. In the more than three decades since these first reports, both anecdotal and empirical evidence of behavioral alterations has been reported. One group of investigators noted that children born to alcoholic parents "are animated, agitated, turbulent, and quarrelsome in their play . . . they are also fearful and inhibited in the presence of an adult." Similarly, a description of 20 patients, including most of the original patients of the 1973 study mentioned earlier, noted that many of the children were hyperactive, distractible, and had attention disturbances.

General Behavior Disorders

Several studies have highlighted behavioral differences resulting from prenatal alcohol exposure. For example, the Child Behavior Checklist (CBCL) was used in a number of studies of children with prenatal alcohol exposure. In one retrospective study of children with fetal alcohol syndrome or effects (FAS/FAE), those with attention deficit disorder (ADD), and controls, parents rated both the FAS/FAE and ADD children as more hyperactive and inattentive using the CBCL and other behavioral rating scales. A similar study compared the CBCL profiles of children who had heavy prenatal alcohol exposure with those of a control group matched for age, sex, race, socioeconomic status, and IQ score. Significant differences were reported on five of the eight problem scales, including social problems, thought problems, attention problems, aggression, and delinquency. In contrast, no significant differences were found between the profiles of alcohol-exposed children with and without the features of FAS. These results emphasize that prenatal alcohol exposure results in significant and profound impairment in parent-rated behaviors and that these deficits are not explained entirely by facial dysmorphology, general intellectual level, or other demographic factors.

Other measures also reveal significant behavioral disturbance in children with prenatal alcohol exposure. Naturalistic observations of 4-year-old children with moderate prenatal alcohol exposure (mean = 0.45 ounces of absolute alcohol (AA)/day) revealed that prenatal alcohol exposure was related to decreased attention and compliance and increased fidgetiness. Similarly, in 6-year-old children with moderate to heavy prenatal alcohol exposure (mean = 0.89 AA/day), alcohol exposure was related to the impulsivity/hyperactivity scale of the Conners' Parent Rating Scale. The 11-year follow-up of a cohort of children exposed to varying amounts of alcohol also indicated alcohol-related behavioral differences on teacher ratings of classroom behavior. The most salient behaviors were those related to distractibility, restlessness, lack of persistence, and reluctance to meet challenges.

Psychological Disturbances

In addition to the behavioral problems described thus far, maladaptive behaviors such as poor judgment and difficulty perceiving social cues are often reported. These children also are reported to be at a higher risk for psychiatric or emotional problems. Two studies from a longitudinal cohort of alcohol-exposed children and their mothers indicated a relationship between prenatal alcohol exposure and attachment insecurity and child depressive features. One group of authors described the occurrence of secondary disabilities in individuals with FAS and FAE. Secondary disabilities, defined as "those that a person is not born with, and that could presumably be ameliorated through better understanding and appropriate interventions," were measured with the Life History Interview. The authors reported the following statistics from their sample of 473 people with FAS/FAE (age range, 3 years to 51 years): 94% of them had experienced "mental health problems"; 60% of those older than the age of 12 years had experienced "disrupted school experience"; 23% older than the age of 12 years had experienced inpatient mental health treatment; and 35% older than the age of 12 years had experienced "alcohol/drug problems."

Individuals with FAS often have disturbances of behavior that lead to psychiatric diagnoses. As mentioned earlier, in the secondary disabilities survey, an astounding 94% had a history of mental health problems. Attention deficits were the most frequently reported problems among children and adolescents (61%), whereas depression was the most frequent for adults (52%). In a later study, 25 adults (IQs greater than 70) with FAS or FAE were assessed by means of a structured psychiatric interview. Seventy-four percent had previous psychiatric treatment. The high rates of Axis I (clinical disorders such as depression or psychosis; 92%) and Axis II (developmental or personality disorders; 48%) diagnoses in this sample are alarming. Another study reported that the most common disorders in a sample of children with FAS were habits/stereotypes and emotional disorders, both occurring in nearly 50% of the group. Speech disorder (35%) and hyperkinetic disorder (32%) were the next most common diagnoses. Finally, in a study of 207 cases of FAS identified in Saskatchewan over a 20-year period, 45.9% had significant psychosocial problems. These included attention deficit (32.9%), "oppositional conduct" disorder (4.8%), depression (1.0%), psychotic features (3.9%), and autistic behavior (3.4%). Thus, prenatal alcohol exposure is related to high rates of psychiatric disturbances, which occur with and without mental retardation and persist into adulthood.

Hyperactivity and Attention Deficits

Hyperactivity and attention deficits are hallmark features of prenatal alcohol exposure. In fact, activity level may be a more sensitive indicator of alcohol's teratogenicity than physical features. Children with FAS have been described as tremulous, hyperactive, and irritable. Caretakers note that the children are "always on the go" and "never sit still." In a long-term follow-up of children with FAS, hyperkinetic disorders were among the most frequently diagnosed disorders and persisted throughout childhood. Additionally, hyperactivity may occur in the absence of intellectual impairment. One study of 15 alcohol-exposed children of average intelligence (IQ range = 82 to 113, mean = 98.2) reported all but one as being hyperactive. Even in the absence of the diagnosis of FAS, moderate levels of alcohol exposure (mean = 0.45 AA/day) are related to the offspring's being more "fidgety" and less compliant.

Additional to hyperactivity, attention deficits have long been associated with FAS and prenatal alcohol exposure. Early naturalistic observations of infants suggested that prenatal alcohol exposure was associated with an increased "nonalert state." That is, the infants spent more time with eyes open but not attentive. Such attention deficits appear to continue throughout childhood and may be similar to those of children with attention deficit disorder. Both adolescents and adults with FAS demonstrate deficits in tasks involved in the focusing (Talland Letter Cancellation Test), encoding (WISC-R Digit Span), and shifting (Wisconsin Card Sorting Test) of attention. Clearly, heavy prenatal alcohol exposure increases the risk for behavioral disturbance in childhood. Such behavioral disturbance is likely to lead to increased mental health treatment, decreased quality of life, and further increased risk for psychological problems as adults.

A recent study in San Diego examined the psychiatric diagnoses of children with FAS and prenatal exposure to alcohol (PEA) by means of a structured psychiatric interview. This study revealed that a high percentage of all children examined met criteria for an externalizing disorder. Of these, nearly all met DSM (Diagnostic and Statistic Manual [of Psychiatric Disorders])-IV criteria for attention deficit hyperactivity disorder (ADHD). Similarly, a recent case-control study of psychiatric inpatients revealed that patients with ADHD were 2.5 times more likely to have been exposed to alcohol than the controls. The authors suggested that prenatal alcohol exposure might have an association with ADHD in the offspring that is independent of other important risk factors for ADHD, such as smoking or familial factors.

Given the high rate of ADHD in children with heavy prenatal alcohol exposure, examination of attention in this population is critical. Multiple studies of lower levels of exposure have documented a relationship between prenatal alcohol exposure and deficits in attention, and three recent studies have specifically focused on visual and auditory attention deficits in children with heavy prenatal alcohol exposure and nonexposed controls. One group of investigators examined the sustained attention of children with prenatal alcohol exposure on a task that included both visual and auditory components. They showed that there was a specific deficit in visual sustained attention; that is, the processing of visual information was more affected than auditory sustained attention. In the second study, alcohol-exposed children and nonexposed control children were evaluated with use of a paradigm consisting of three conditions: visual focus, auditory focus, and auditory-visual shift of attention. For the visual condition, alcohol-exposed children responded with lower accuracy and slower reaction time for all intertrial intervals. In contrast, for the auditory condition, alcohol-exposed children were less accurate but displayed slower reaction time only on the longest intertrial interval. Finally, for the shift condition in which participants were required to alternate responses between visual targets and auditory targets, the alcohol-exposed (ALC) group had slower reaction time on the two longest intertrial intervals but had accuracy levels comparable with those of controls. These data suggest that children with heavy prenatal alcohol exposure have deficits in attention that are not global in nature. Rather, they appear to be able to shift attentional focus but have difficulty maintaining attention over extended intervals (i.e., at the long intertrial intervals). Additionally, deficits in visual attention were pervasive, whereas auditory attention deficits occurred only when intertrial intervals were long (greater than 10 seconds). Although these two studies provide convergent evidence of a selective deficit on visual attention, a third study of auditory and visual attention suggests conflicting results, with auditory deficits exceeding visual deficits.

Comparisons with ADHD

Previous research comparing children who had heavy prenatal alcohol exposure with children who had attention deficits but no prenatal alcohol exposure is limited, and the results are equivocal. Two separate studies compared children who had attention deficit disorder (based on DSM-IIIR) with children who had FAS/FAE on continuous performance tasks and parent ratings of behavior. One study's results showed that the two groups had similar task performance profiles. In contrast, the other study determined that the two groups did not have the same neurocognitive or behavioral profile and that the children with primary ADHD performed more poorly on conventional tests of attention.

Thus, distinguishing children with heavy prenatal alcohol from children with ADHD is still an important research question. In recent studies, we addressed the issue of attention in our sample of children with FAS and PEA. In the first study, we compared three groups of children: those with heavy prenatal alcohol exposure, those with ADHD but no prenatal alcohol exposure, and nonexposed, non-ADHD controls. Our results suggested a different pattern of performance on a standard continuous performance task in the two clinical groups. Inattention was representative of children with ADHD with or without heavy prenatal alcohol exposure, but impulsivity was specific to nonexposed ADHD children. Thus, these types of errors may be useful for distinguishing children with heavy prenatal alcohol exposure from nonexposed children with ADHD. In the second study, we attempted to distinguish children with heavy prenatal alcohol exposure from nonexposed controls using logistic regression. A model including the Freedom from Distractibility index from the Wechsler Intelligence Scale for Children, Third Edition, and the Attention Problems scale from the Child Behavior Checklist correctly classified more than 90% of the overall sample. These data indicate that children with heavy prenatal alcohol exposure can be distinguished from nonexposed controls with a high degree of accuracy using two commonly used measures.

Pharmacological Treatment

Children with behavioral disorders often require pharmacological treatment. Children with heavy prenatal alcohol exposure are not an exception. The high rate of behavioral disorders is paralleled by a high rate of medication use in this population. Preliminary data from our laboratory indicate that of 64 individuals with heavy prenatal alcohol exposure surveyed by questionnaire, 57.8% had taken psychoactive medications at some point and 39.1% had taken more than one medication. These drugs included stimulants (54.7%), antidepressants (50%), neuroleptics (15.6%), mood stabilizers (10.9%), and alpha-adrenergic agonists (e.g., clonidine), which are used in the treatment of ADHD (21.9%). In a separate investigation, information gathered at the time of testing at the Center for Behavioral Teratology indicates that 39% of our sample of children with heavy prenatal alcohol exposure currently take medication (as opposed to 2% of controls). As in the aforementioned survey, many (25.4% of total sample) were taking more than one medication. Additionally, several classes of drugs were being used, including: stimulants (15.3%), antidepressants (23.7%), neuroleptics (6.8%), mood stabilizers (6.8%), and clonidine (11.9%). Thus, children with heavy prenatal alcohol exposure are commonly prescribed psychoactive medications, despite the lack of empirical data on the efficacy of these treatments in this population.

NEUROANATOMICAL EFFECTS IN CHILDREN WITH HEAVY PRENATAL ALCOHOL EXPOSURE

Additional to its effects on cognitive functioning and behavior, heavy prenatal alcohol exposure can have devastating effects on the structure of the developing brain. The earliest descriptions of FAS included an autopsy of a 5-day-old infant with FAS. The brain of this infant was grossly abnormal and was characterized by microcephaly, neuroglial heterotopias, agenesis of the corpus callosum, and cerebellar hypoplasia. Since that time, only a small number of autopsies have been reported. Descriptions of these autopsies indicated a wide array of brain damage that did not lend itself to a clear picture of the effect of heavy alcohol exposure. In fact, some interpreted these autopsies as suggesting only diffuse damage and speculated that no consistent pattern of structure or function would be found. However, as detailed in the following section, there does appear to be a pattern of brain changes seen in children with heavy prenatal alcohol exposure. The importance of such a pattern, if it does exist, is the suggestion that the collective changes seen after heavy prenatal alcohol exposure may be specific to this exposure. Furthermore, such specificity provides the basis for understanding the mechanisms of alcohol's effects and the development of treatment and intervention strategies.

Although the autopsy studies provided critical early information on the effect of alcohol on the brain, providing clear evidence of the damaging effects of alcohol consumption in pregnancy, the cases represented the most severely affected children. This truncated sample makes generalities to those living with FAS problematic. For more than 10 years, the use of magnetic resonance imaging (MRI) has provided a more detailed and systematic examination of children with FAS and heavy prenatal alcohol exposure. Most recently, functional brain imaging and novel analysis techniques have provided even greater detail on the effects of heavy prenatal alcohol exposure on the brain.

Structural Brain Imaging

MRI studies of the brain have suggested that, in contrast to previous speculation, certain structures in the brain are more affected than other structures. These studies rely on highly technical image analysis techniques that compare the volume of specific brain structures or regions with those of nonexposed controls. Importantly, these volumetric studies reveal brain differences where clinical studies (e.g., radiological reports) suggest relatively normal brain development (i.e., no gross abnormalities). Additional to the volumetric experiments, other studies of the brain in individuals have focused on brain morphology, including the shape and structure of specific brain regions. Both volumetric and morphologic studies are reviewed later. These studies suggest that in addition to reductions in the overall brain volume, there are three main areas affected by heavy prenatal alcohol exposure: the corpus callosum, the basal ganglia, and the cerebellum.

Corpus Callosum

As mentioned previously, the first autopsy study revealed agenesis of the corpus callosum along with diffuse damage throughout the brain. The first study reporting MRI findings in living children with FAS also described a child with agenesis of the corpus callosum and a second patient with hypoplasia of the corpus callosum. After this first study, additional cases of callosal agenesis in children with FAS were documented. In the San Diego sample, we suggested an approximate rate of this abnormality of 6%, and others have suggested that prenatal alcohol exposure might be the most common cause of agenesis of the corpus callosum. Fig. 22.3 illustrates callosal agenesis in a child with FAS. In addition to callosal agenesis, the size of the corpus callosum is reduced, particularly in the anterior and posterior regions. Interestingly, the anterior corpus callosum is significantly

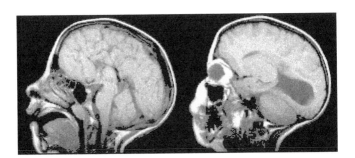

Fig. 22.3. Magnetic resonance images of a 9-year-old girl with fetal alcohol syndrome. These sagittal images illustrate agenesis of the corpus callosum (left) and colpocephaly (right) present in this child. (Mattson & Riley, 1995)

reduced in children with attention deficit hyperactivity disorder (ADHD), and there is some evidence that reductions in the posterior corpus callosum also are seen in children with ADHD who have secondary learning disabilities. Morphometric studies of the corpus callosum in individuals with heavy prenatal alcohol exposure suggest that in addition to reductions in size, the corpus callosum also is spatially displaced in comparison with controls. Specifically, the posterior corpus callosum in the alcohol-exposed individuals was located more anteriorly and inferiorly than in the control participants. This displacement was apparent in individuals with either FAS or PEA, although it was less severe in the latter group. Finally, the shape of the corpus callosum was examined in a subsequent study, which corroborated the first study's findings, suggesting that callosal shape is strongly related to prenatal alcohol exposure.

Basal Ganglia

The basal ganglia are a group of subcortical structures composed of the caudate and lenticular nuclei (the globus pallidus and the putamen). This group of gray matter structures has traditionally been thought to have primary motor functions; however, certain studies have suggested possible roles for the basal ganglia in cognitive function. Importantly, the motor functions of the basal ganglia are associated with the putamen, whereas the cognitive functions are associated with the caudate. MRI studies indicate that the basal ganglia and, in particular, the caudate nucleus are reduced in size in children with heavy prenatal alcohol exposure. Of note is that the reduction seen in the caudate persists even when overall brain size is controlled, suggesting that this brain region is disproportionately affected by prenatal alcohol exposure.

Cerebellum

The third brain region that appears to be affected is the cerebellum. Like the basal ganglia, the cerebellum has traditionally been thought of as having a primarily motor function but now is understood also to have cognitive functions. In addition to the reductions in overall brain size, the volume of the cerebellum is reduced in children with heavy prenatal alcohol exposure. In addition to these overall volume reductions, the area of the anterior vermis is reduced, although the posterior and remaining regions are not. Hypoplasia of both the vermis and the overall cerebellum was noted in one description, confirming the effect of heavy prenatal alcohol exposure on this brain region.

Additional Brain Areas Affected by Prenatal Alcohol Exposure

Besides the corpus callosum, the basal ganglia, and the cerebellum, heavy prenatal alcohol exposure may affect other brain regions. One structure previously hypothesized to be affected is the hippocampus. MRI studies of this structure have yielded equivocal findings, with some studies suggesting reductions and others suggesting relative sparing of this structure when overall brain size was adjusted for statistically.

Some studies have suggested that in addition to overall brain volume changes (i.e., microcephaly), specific regions of the cortex might be particularly affected by heavy prenatal alcohol exposure. Specifically, an analysis of the overall shape of the brain indicated narrowing in the inferior parietal/perisylvian region as well as reduced growth in the inferior frontal region. Mapping of the density of the gray and white matter in the brain also supported abnormalities in the temporal-parietal regions of the brain, particularly in the left hemisphere. Increased gray matter and decreased white matter were apparent in individuals with heavy prenatal alcohol exposure. These results are consistent with those of another research team that suggested decreased overall parietal volume and decreased white matter volume in this region. Thus, it appears that the parietal region of the brain may be an additional target of heavy prenatal alcohol exposure.

Functional Brain Imaging

Only a small number of published studies have used functional imaging techniques in children with heavy prenatal alcohol exposure. Several early studies have reported electrophysiological changes in the brains of infants and young children with heavy prenatal alcohol exposure with or without fetal alcohol syndrome. These studies have shown that the observed changes were a sensitive indicator of alcohol's teratogenic effects. More recent studies have found clinically suspect electroencephalograms in about 50% of individuals tested, with specific changes seen in the left hemisphere.

Two studies have described the results of single photon emission computerized tomography (SPECT) in individuals with FAS, although both had relatively small samples. One study of 11 patients with FAS demonstrated mild hypoperfusion of the left hemisphere in all patients, especially in the parietal-occipital region, which is consistent with the left-sided changes noted in gray/white distribution and the shape changes in this region. The second study included only 3 patients but noted blood flow reductions in the temporal region.

Only one published study has described positron emission tomography (PET) results from individuals with FAS. This study included 19 young adults and adults (aged 16 to 30 years) who were relatively high functioning (IQ range = 66 to 92) and had received structural brain imaging studies that were normal in all but one case (callosal hypoplasia in one case). PET results revealed bilateral reductions in activity in the thalamus and the basal ganglia. Thus, additional to volumetric reductions in the subcortical regions as described earlier, metabolic activity also appears disrupted, again suggesting that these regions may be especially sensitive to the teratogenic effects of alcohol.

CONCLUSIONS

The effects of heavy prenatal alcohol exposure are devastating and lifelong, particularly the effects on the central nervous system. Children with FAS have a characteristic triad of features and often exhibit significant learning and behavior difficulties. These difficulties present the greatest impediment to the children and their families, and the effects of these impairments are felt throughout the community and society. Future research should focus on further understanding of alcohol's effects on the brain, the mechanisms by which these occur, and the development of strategies to prevent these devastating effects.

ACKNOWLEDGMENTS

The author acknowledges the support of the Center for Behavioral Teratology, especially its director, Dr. Edward P. Riley, the families who have graciously participated in our research, and the continued support of National Institute on Alcohol Abuse and Alcoholism (Grants AA10820, 12596, and 10417).

SUGGESTED READINGS

Archibald SL, Fennema-Notestine C, Gamst A, Riley EP, Mattson SN, Jernigan TL: Brain dysmorphology in individuals with severe prenatal alcohol exposure. Dev Med Child Neurol 43:148–154, 2001.

Autti-Rämö I, Autti T, Korkman M, Kettunen S, Salonen O, Valanne L: MRI findings in children with school problems who had been exposed prenatally to alcohol. Dev Med Child Neurol 44:98–106, 2002.

Coles CD, Platzman KA, Lynch ME, Freides D: Auditory and visual sustained attention in adolescents prenatally exposed to alcohol. Alcohol Clin Exp Res 26:263–271, 2002.

Coles CD, Platzman KA, Raskind-Hood CL, Brown RT, Falek A., Smith IE: A comparison of children affected by prenatal alcohol exposure and attention deficit, hyperactivity disorder. Alcohol Clin Exp Res 21: 150–161, 1997.

Mattson SN, Riley EP: Prenatal exposure to alcohol: what the images reveal. Alcohol Health Res World 19:273–278, 1995.

Mattson SN, Roebuck TM: Acquisition and retention of verbal and nonverbal information in children with heavy prenatal alcohol exposure. Alcohol Clin Exp Res 26:875–882, 2002.

Roebuck TM, Mattson SN, Riley EP: A review of the neuroanatomical findings in children with fetal alcohol syndrome or prenatal exposure to alcohol. Alcohol Clin Exp Res 22:339–344, 1998.

Sowell ER, Thompson PM, Mattson SN, Tessner KD, Jernigan TL, Riley EP, et al: Regional brain shape abnormalities persist into adolescence after heavy prenatal alcohol exposure. Cereb Cortex 12:856–865, 2002.

Stratton K, Howe C, Battaglia F: Fetal Alcohol Syndrome: Diagnosis, Epidemiology, Prevention, and Treatment. Washington, D.C.: National Academy Press, 1996.

ALCOHOL AND COMORBID PSYCHIATRIC CONDITIONS: TREATING THE DUALLY DIAGNOSED PATIENT

Sylvia J. Dennison

Alcohol use disorders commonly occur concomitantly with other psychiatric conditions. Largely unknown approximately a decade ago, this fact is increasingly well recognized today. The two largest studies conducted to evaluate the prevalence of mental illness in the United States found that nearly half of all individuals with alcohol use disorders suffer from other psychiatric problems as well. Such comorbidity, or "dual diagnoses," renders the treatment of either condition more than doubly difficult; each complicates, magnifies, and interferes with the other.

Care of dually diagnosed patients claims a disproportionately high percentage of the health care dollar. Comorbidity is associated with an increased risk of being the victim or perpetrator of violent crime, of being homeless, of being incarcerated, of being poorly compliant with medication, and of having an overall poorer prognosis. These facts make it clear that it is imperative to develop approaches targeting the specific needs of the dually diagnosed both to improve quality of life and to reduce the cost of care.

Despite the frequency with which comorbidity occurs, treatment providers have been slow to develop effective interventions for dealing with the unique needs of dually diagnosed clients. Instead, for many years, such patients have been placed in alcohol treatment programs that are ill equipped to meet their needs, and often to the patients' detriment. It was an accepted practice to insist that the patient be "dry" for a minimum of 6 months before offering medication for a condition such as major depression or anxiety disorder or to withhold medication from psychotic individuals who were actively drinking. The intention in the former situation was to ensure that the symptoms observed were not simply the result of the alcohol or its residual effects. In the latter case, fear of alcohol-medication interactions was a concern of the treatment provider. Unfortunately, the result of such an approach was that those with the untreated comorbid condition tended to be among the earliest relapsers. Studies show that treating such conditions helps decrease the relapse rate and improves the patient's overall outcome. In the latter case, the untreated psychotic individual was guaranteed a worsening of psychosis.

APPROACHING THE DUALLY DIAGNOSED PATIENT

Various models have been proposed for treating the dually diagnosed. Three in particular summarize the approaches that have been used. The first, the sequential model of treatment, proposes that first one and then the other condition be treated. The idea is that one condition must be controlled before the second can be adequately addressed. A problem, of course, is which condition should be addressed first? Can an alcoholic individual with schizophrenia truly benefit from alcohol treatment if voices convince the individual that they are a Higher Power, and that this Higher Power is telling the individual to drink? On the other hand, the patient who is drinking a fifth of whiskey per night can hardly be expected to receive maximal benefit from taking haloperidol, and needs to have the use of alcohol addressed—vigorously. The conditions are inextricably linked.

Next is the parallel model in which both conditions are addressed simultaneously, but in different programs with different staff. A problem here, however, is that the patient often receives conflicting messages from treatment providers with different goals and lack of knowledge about the condition they are not directly addressing. In the alcohol treatment program, for example, total abstinence from all psychoactive substances, prescription or otherwise, might be a stated goal. The mental health provider, on the other hand, might be striving for rigid adherence to a medication regimen. Thus, a patient with bipolar illness might be told in one program that "everybody gets depressed sometimes" and encouraged to stop taking a mood stabilizer. At the same time, the mental health care provider might jump to treat the same patient's anxiety symptoms with a benzodiazepine, without thinking of the possibility that the patient's early recovery from alcohol might be endangered by this approach.

Finally, the integrated model is one in which both conditions are treated simultaneously by providers who are knowledgeable about both conditions. Clearly the ideal, widespread use of this approach is made difficult by the fact that there are insufficient numbers of skilled individuals available to treat the large quantity of patients who need such help.

Regardless of the model used, helping the dually diagnosed patient into recovery is a process that occurs over time. The more severe the psychiatric illness of the individual, the more protracted the treatment required. It may seem obvious to the point of being unnecessary to say it, but no two dually diagnosed patients are alike. It is emphatically *not* true that "an alcoholic is an alcoholic." An "alcoholic" is an individual who has a physiological dependence on alcohol in addition to having other human traits and needs. It is also not true that any one approach can be used for treating all dually diagnosed patients. The approach taken with each must be customized to meet the person's particular needs.

Those who adhere to Alcoholics Anonymous have typically offered a very simple prescription for recovery: "Go to meetings. Read the Big Book. Do what it says." Although this has worked well for many people without comorbid conditions, individuals with dual diagnoses have often done very poorly in traditional AA groups and in traditional alcohol treatment programs. Because of the complex interplay of one condition with the other, simply focusing on the alcohol use may not be sufficient to help the dually diagnosed patient. Instead, treatment providers must help patients gain an understanding of both their alcohol dependence and their mental illness, and of the impact one has on the other. It is then necessary to develop strategies for recognizing and dealing with each. Strategies often include medication, especially for individuals with psychotic disorders.

TREATMENT ISSUES

It is helpful to learn whether the patient's psychiatric condition improves or disappears when drinking is discontinued. It is also helpful to find out if the psychiatric symptoms predate the onset of alcohol use. Often, it is impossible to determine the onset of either of the aforementioned conditions. If the patient drinks daily and has no substantial periods of clean time, clearly it is not possible to know whether symptoms improve with alcohol cessation. Likewise, if the patient has been drinking for many years, memory may not prove accurate as to whether the drinking or the symptoms came first.

There is a school of thought that suggests withholding treatment of psychiatric disorders unless the patient is abstinent. There is much evidence to show, however, that working with patients and helping to treat their other symptoms can improve the chances of engaging them in alcohol treatment, increase the likelihood of decreasing their alcohol consumption, and reduce symptoms even if they continue to drink. As long as patients can be treated safely, doing so can be justified. Sometimes the decision of whether or not to medicate comes down to the clinician's level of comfort and best judgment based on knowledge of the patient and of the mental illness. Therefore, it is helpful to know a few basic facts about the relationship of alcohol and psychiatric symptoms and conditions.

It comes as no surprise to find that heavy alcohol consumption worsens symptoms of psychosis. Untreated, individuals with primary psychotic disorders who continue to drink heavily can be expected to get worse. Data are lacking regarding the effect of mild alcohol consumption on psychotic symptoms. Therefore, withholding medication from individuals with psychoses because they consume alcohol—a common practice—ensures rapid deterioration of their condition not simply because they have been drinking but because they are unmedicated as well. Reviews of the literature do not demonstrate a significant problem with interactions between alcohol and antipsychotics alone. The problem, however, is that a large percentage of individuals with psychotic disorders take multiple medications, thereby increasing the risk of interactions. For this reason, it is probably best for clinicians to limit supplies of medication available to patients so as not to risk accidental overdose. Patients should then be encouraged to continue taking their customary medications, even if a drinking binge should occur.

More women than men with alcohol dependence have a primary depression, just as is the case in the non–alcohol-dependent population, although depression is substantially increased among alcohol-dependent men as well. The majority of men and women who meet the diagnostic criteria for major depression when they are actively drinking improve within 2 weeks of abstinence without additional treatment. Those who do not improve, however, continue to meet those criteria and are likely to require further treatment for affective disorder. Untreated, such patients are prone to earlier relapse than their nondepressed counterparts. Major depression can be treated even if the patient continues to drink. Furthermore, treating the condition may be associated with a decrease in alcohol consumption.

The problem is the large number of patients in the middle who achieve either intermittent or no abstinence and meet the criteria for depression. In such cases, it is best to err on the side of continuing treatment. If the patient can be engaged by receiving medication in very limited supplies, it may be best to do so. Reiterating the aforementioned: Major depression can be treated effectively in actively drinking patients and this treatment may help them decrease alcohol consumption.

Anxiety disorders too are frequently associated with alcohol use disorders. Some anxiety disorder sufferers (e.g., those with panic disorder) may find temporary symptomatic relief when they use alcohol. This furthers the likelihood of continued drinking if the anxiety is left untreated. Flashbacks associated with post-traumatic stress disorder (PTSD) are a strong and common relapse cue for resumption of drinking.

Since there is a strong anxiety component to alcohol withdrawal due to the autonomic hyperarousal that characterizes it, treatment providers have been particularly resistant to treat anxiety disorders in actively drinking patients. The anxiety disorders, however, are a constellation of nine conditions joined together by the common bond of anxiety. Unlike the case of the patient with depression, it is often easy to determine that the anxious patient with comorbid alcohol use disorders has a primary psychiatric condition. Onset of these conditions typically occurs when patients are in their teens and twenties. A precipitating event must occur to account for PTSD. A patient with anxiety disorders can often give a lucid history of onset of anxiety symptoms well in advance of onset of drinking. As in the case of the depressed patient, treating the anxiety may help the patient decrease alcohol use as well

Medication alone is not sufficient to control the depressed, psychotic, or anxious patient's drinking. In each case, however, medication may provide symptomatic relief, enable the patient to engage in treatment, and, concomitantly, help to decrease alcohol consumption.

TREATING SPECIFIC CONDITIONS

Joe M had always had a few beers in the evenings. They helped him unwind, made him more sociable, helped him sleep, and so forth. When he was laid off at the plant, he had time on his hands, and he found himself occasionally drinking during the day. Things had been bad between him and his wife for quite a while, but the added financial strain pushed things over the edge. She left and took the children with her. After that, he did not sleep at all without a drink. He cried all the time, but the pain was less when he was drunk. Joe knew he was in trouble. He was depressed, ashamed of his drinking and ashamed of himself, and he thought about suicide. He did not want to take his life because of the impact his death would have on his children. When he was sober, however, he was afraid he would find the courage to kill himself during one of his drinking episodes.

In the traditional approach to recovery, Joe would be told to go to AA, obtain and maintain sobriety, and be assured that things would get better. Unfortunately, for a significant number of the Joes of the world, life does not work that way. Ignoring oe's depression places him at higher risk of relapse, and thereby increases his feelings of failure.

It can be assumed that Joe does not require hospitalization for detoxification from alcohol. Encouraging participation in AA or a similar recovery group might be advisable if Joe could find a group whose members would not feel a need to ascribe all his feelings to alcohol. There is danger of trivializing Joe's emotions and furthering self-loathing. Many members of self-help groups recognize that for medical and psychiatric issues, the member should talk to a physician. For help with sobriety, Joe should talk with the members of a group. If Joe could find such a group, he would benefit greatly. He is isolated, a fact that must be countered, and participation in an organization that additionally encourages abstinence would only work to his advantage.

If, however, he finds himself in a group whose members insist that he does not need medication and that he should merely turn himself over to a Higher Power, he should be encouraged to look for another group. Many truly supportive groups exist, and Joe should be supported in his search for one. Joe has suffered multiple losses: job, income, family, self-esteem. He is depressed. With his heavy drinking, despite his having a strong motivation for living, he recognizes that with the disinhibiting effect of alcohol, he is capable of suicide. He needs professional help rather than pressure.

If Joe drinks throughout the day because he has no structure and has time on his hands, he should be encouraged to spend that time in specific activities. He could go to self-help meetings. He could volunteer at a school or a hospital or help out at a church, mosque, or synagogue. He could be paired with nondrinking friends, family members, or group members, each of whom would spend time with him each day—providing anything to reduce his isolation and decrease his time in an environment conducive to drinking.

Next, Joe requires medication. It is generally accepted that psychotherapy has an efficacy equal to that of medication for the treatment of mild to moderate depression. Joe, however, appears to be severely and suicidally depressed. Medication is going to be an essential part of his recovery from depression and may help decrease his drinking as well. The questions are which medication and whether it will work if he continues to drink?

Although it would obviously be best to wait for Joe to be completely abstinent for a couple of weeks, it might be impractical to think he could accomplish this consistently for some time. Refusal to address his depression may further contribute to his discouragement. Besides, Joe is seriously considering ending his life. Therefore, the treating clinician must work with Joe to encourage him to decrease and eventually stop his alcohol use while his depression is treated in the safest, most effective way available.

A number of studies have demonstrated that depression can be treated effectively in actively drinking alcohol dependent individuals. Some of those studies, however, used medications that raise safety issues. Tricyclic antidepressants, for example, have been shown to be beneficial in this regard. Although in a tightly controlled experimental situation this might be successful, the potential for lethal interaction between the medication and alcohol makes this inadvisable.

Instead, the selective serotonin reuptake inhibitors (SSRIs) have to date had the best track record of safety and efficacy and they could safely be prescribed for Joe. It would be advisable while Joe is feeling very bad to limit the amount of medication he has on hand. As single agents, the SSRIs have been found to be generally safe, even in large quantities, although some patients have developed complications such as serotonin syndrome. It is in combination with alcohol and other drugs that problems have arisen. Therefore, keeping Joe's supply of medication limited and making frequent visits to him would be the safest approach while he is trying to address his drinking.

Neither bupropion nor nefazodone can be recommended for an actively drinking individual with an alcohol use disorder. The former is well known for lowering the seizure threshold and the latter has been described as being associated with hepatotoxicity, even in individuals with normal liver function. Therefore, these agents should be avoided. Likewise, venlafaxine is metabolized in the liver. In an individual with normal hepatic function, it might be safe to use this drug. To date, however, there is simply not sufficient evidence with actively drinking patients to know whether mirtazapine and venlafaxine will prove safe and effective. There are no known absolute contraindications; there is simply not enough known at this point. Thus, the SSRIs remain the treatment of choice.

Every time Sarah tried to become sober, the same thing happened: She felt the man's hand over her mouth, felt the knife at her throat, relived the rape, thought she was going to die. Her hands would shake. She felt tightness in the pit of her stomach and could hardly breathe. Sometimes, she thought she would pass out. It was hard to keep from drinking when she knew that just a few shots of whiskey would be enough to calm her nerves and push the memories back into some dark corner of her mind where they would not hurt and terrify her.

Sarah's scenario is all too common: PTSD hand in hand with alcohol. The two work together like a child's teeter-totter: push one down and the other one pops up. This is indeed what happens. As the sufferer tries to become dry, painful memories erupt, which the patient can subdue only by diving back into alcohol. The reemergence of these traumatic memories often acts as a powerful relapse cue.

In general, addiction treatment providers have discouraged patients from confronting the trauma until they have established some sobriety and some relapse prevention skills. Having these skills in place is very important. The patient must develop and practice alternatives to drinking as a means of coping with the intensity of emotions the traumatic memories evoke in order to deal effectively with them without relapse. Such techniques as guided visualization may be quite helpful. In a session during which a patient such as Sarah would feel safe, she would be encouraged to create a calm scenario and practice being a part of it. For example: a woman in a long, flowing dress walks through a field of aromatic deep orange flowers. The wind blows her dress and hair. The sun is warm and comfortable on her skin. The scent of the earth and blossoms pleasantly caresses her nostrils, etc. Sarah produces the scene, adding comfortable images, aromas, other sensations. When distressing memories leap into consciousness, she is instructed to force herself to return to this quiet, safe, practiced place to calm and comfort herself instead of reaching for a drink.

It is important that the patient develop or help produce the scene so that no material with negative connotations is introduced into the imagery. In the aforementioned example, for instance, a woman with a deathly allergy to bees might find her heart racing as the image of flowers makes her think of these insects and of anaphylactic shock rather than of comfort and serenity.

Again, medication may also be of great benefit. The benzodiazepines are a class of drugs that often come quickly to mind when one thinks of dealing with anxiety and may provide rapid, temporary, symptomatic relief for some PTSD sufferers. In the world of addiction medicine, however, their use is highly controversial. There are studies indicating that some individuals with a history of addictive disorders can and do use such agents responsibly. Treatment providers working with this population, however, do not generally see the study group. Instead, they see that a high incidence of misuse of these drugs seems to be the norm, and therefore avoid their use if possible. Furthermore, if the PTSD sufferer relapses to alcohol use, the combination of alcohol and benzodiazepines is a potentially lethal one, further supporting avoidance of their use. If medication is used, much evidence again shows that an SSRI is the medication of choice.

David was diagnosed with schizophrenia at the age of 19 years. During his initial hospitalization, his condition was dubbed a "substance-induced psychosis" because there was a prominent odor of alcohol about him, and his toxicity screen showed that he had been using marijuana. Now, 8 years later, he is a "revolving-door patient"—in the hospital nearly as much of the time as he is out, poorly compliant with his medications, drinking often, and continuing to dabble with marijuana.

David is typical of many individuals burdened with schizophrenia. It is frustrating for providers to work with him, but his refusal to accept his lot is understandable. He is young, has an illness that can have devastating consequences, and wants to try to be normal without medication and hospitalizations. The Davids of the world are best helped over time, by gradually developing a relationship with a provider whom he trusts, typically after a protracted period of engagement.

A common reaction in the past was for the provider to refuse to medicate someone like David. There are a variety of rationales for such an approach. Some have worried about a potentially lethal interaction between antipsychotic medications and ethanol. In other cases, there may have been a more punitive intent behind the refusal to treat—if patients would not do as they were told, treating clinicians would not be bothered.

Regardless of the reason, withhholding treatment has one inevitable result: the worsening of the patient's psychosis. To minimize the severity of the psychosis and increase the likelihood that a patient such as David can continue to function in an out-of-hospital environment, he should be encouraged to remain on his antipsychotic medication, even if he is drinking. Once again, the clinician should do what feels comfortable. Thus, limiting the supply of medication available to the patient on multiple medications to decrease the risk of accidental overdose is reasonable. It would not be unthinkable for intoxicated patients taking several medications to forget whether or not they had taken their medications and to take their "normal" doses repeatedly over a brief period of time.

Considering how long they have been in use, there is surprisingly little in the literature about low-potency antipsychotics and alcohol. As they have fallen out of favor, however, how these agents could interact with alcohol might not be so important to clinicians as they might have been in the past. The high-potency medications, on the other hand, have been proved generally safe when combined as single agents with alcohol. The addition of an anticholinergic agent such as benztropine or trihexyphenidyl, however, is not advisable in the actively drinking patient because of the chance of furthering sedation. Again, reports of significant problems of antipsychotics combined with alcohol have occurred with patients only when they have been on other medications as well. In addition, it should be noted that the anticholinergics themselves are known to have abuse potential in their own right. Thus, if David is placed on a typical antipsychotic, he should have a high-potency agent, be given limited amounts of the drug, and should avoid anticholinergic agents.

Among the newer agents, clozapine is unique in that patients who take this medication have been found to decrease the use of alcohol and other drugs. Although this might theoretically appear to make it the ideal agent for treating the individual with both schizophrenia and alcohol dependence, there are actually some very significant

**Table 23.1.   Summary: Alcohol and Selected
Psychiatric Conditions**

Condition	Treatment Issues	Medication
Depression	↑ incidence of depression with alcohol use disorders Untreated depression → ↑ risk of relapse	SSRI preferred TCA effective → risk of interaction with alcohol MAOI → risk of interaction Venlafaxine/mirtazapine → insufficient data Nefazadone/venlafaxine → extensive hepatic metabolism Bupropion → ↓ seizure threshold
Anxiety disorders	↑ incidence of most anxiety disorders with alcohol use disorders Flashbacks in PTSD strong relapse cue Alcohol → temporary relief of some symptoms	SSRI preferred Benzodiazepines → ↑ risk of dependency with history of alcohol dependency Buspirone: relatively ineffective with some anxiety disorders
Schizophrenia	High incidence of comorbidity Alcohol use disorders → overall worse prognosis	High potency typical antipsychotic, most data available

MAOI = Monoamine oxidase inhibitor; PTSD = post-traumatic stress disorder; SSRI = selective serotonin reuptake inhibitor; TCA = tricyclic antidepressant.

drawbacks. Clozapine decreases the seizure threshold. Furthermore, it can cause blood cell abnormalities. Both of these problems are also potential complications of alcohol use. In addition, patients with alcohol use disorders tend to be more poorly compliant with medications than other patients. To obtain clozapine, a patient must submit to weekly blood tests. Failure to do so results in the pharmacy's withholding the medication. Thus, clozapine is less than an ideal drug for a patient such as David. Perhaps if David were in a controlled environment for a period of time, during which clozapine could be initiated and its positive effects appreciated so that David had some insight into the need to take this agent, it might be a good choice. In an outpatient venue, however, the wisdom of its use is highly questionable.

Other atypical drugs may also be quite good choices. Data are accumulating with risperidone to support its safety and efficacy in actively drinking, alcohol-dependent individuals. Less information is available at this time, however, to ensure the safety of other, newer agents.

SUGGESTED READINGS

Dennison S: Treating the Dually Diagnosed: Psychiatric and Substance Use Disorders. Baltimore: Lippincott Williams and Wilkins, 2003.

Miller WR, Rollnick S: Motivational Interviewing: Preparing People to Change Addictive Behavior. New York: Guilford Press, 1991.

Weiss RD, Najavits LM: Overview of treatment modalities for dual diagnosis patients. In: Kranzler HR, Rounsaville BJ (eds.), Dual Diagnosis and Treatment: Substance Abuse and Comorbid Medical and Psychiatric Disorders. New York: Marcel Dekker, 1998, pp. 87–105.

PREVENTION

Stuart Gitlow

When we speak of prevention of alcoholism, we must define our terms. Are we talking about preventing alcoholism, the disease defined as a complex relationship between specific behaviors and typical consequences? Or are we talking about preventing the use of alcohol among those diagnosed with the disease? Or perhaps we are trying to prevent alcohol use among our youth, or in those likely to develop symptoms of alcoholism based on their genes or on their environment during their upbringing. We know that alcoholism itself is a disease based not on quantity of alcohol used, nor upon frequency with which alcohol is imbibed, but on a certain inherent response to the drug leading to a collection of behaviors and resulting sequelae. As for origin, we know that alcoholism has both genetic and environmental predetermining factors, and that, to some extent, both need to be present for development of the illness. From a psychological perspective, in our culture, the use of alcohol is not only socially accepted but encouraged and expected as well. Thus it is that peer pressure generally is perceived as a factor leading to use rather than nonuse of alcohol, although such pressure could hypothetically be present in either direction. Prevention of alcoholism may be viewed as having multiple potential sites of action.

PRIMARY PREVENTION

The primary form of prevention focuses on preventing the disease from ever occurring and thus reducing the incidence of disease. Successfully targeting of the root cause of a disease causes the incidence to drop, leading to a resultant decrease in prevalence for chronic illnesses. The currently accepted definition of alcoholism indicates in part that the illness is a chronic disease state that starts when a certain set of criteria is met. It is essentially impossible for someone to meet the criteria set until use of alcohol has begun. Therefore, each patient has a period of time free of the illness followed by a period of time with the illness. This is equivalent to hypertension, a chronic illness that starts only when blood pressure initially rises above a certain level on an ongoing basis. The hypertensive 40-year-old rarely had hypertension when he was 20. There may be steps this 20-year-old individual can take to prevent or delay the development of hypertension. Is that true in the alcoholic? More specifically, looking at the issue of primary alcoholism prevention, let us look at two individuals at age 20 years. Young Mr. A will one day meet the criteria for alcoholism, but as of this moment, he has never tried alcohol. He grew up in a strict family setting and has just moved out of his parents' home for the first time. Young Mr. B is also 20 years old. He plans to celebrate his 21st birthday by drinking with his friends. He too grew up in a strict environment and has never tried alcohol. But with the knowledge of the future that we have, we know that Mr. B will not have alcoholism. Let us add one additional factor. Many studies have indicated that there are genetic and behavioral markers in adolescents who later go on to develop alcoholism. We must, therefore, address the question as to whether Mr. A has alcoholism right now, despite the fact that he has not picked up his first drink. More fundamentally, is there something wrong with the 10% to 15% of the population for whom alcohol use becomes a form of self-treatment rather than a social activity? Is that "something" at the heart of what the disease truly is, and, therefore, should primary prevention be directed at *that* thing rather than at alcoholism as defined? We know that this premorbid state is likely to have several genetic factors that we will one day be able to identify. There also appear to be perceptual differences that have yet to be fully described and researched in the literature. These issues require further exploration.

There are several possible sites of action for a primary prevention campaign on alcoholism. If we look solely at the definition of alcoholism, we may target alcohol itself because it appears to be a virtual requirement for the disease to be present. This was attempted in a broad cultural experiment called Prohibition, and there have been many resulting papers studying both the successes and failures of that effort. If we look at the psychology of the disease, we may target peer pressure and behavioral norms, as in the "Just Say No" and "This is your brain on drugs" campaigns. We can curtail marketing of alcohol, discontinue promotions targeting young people, and place public information programs where necessary. Price controls have proved useful as an economic incentive to decrease alcohol intake. If we look at the origin of the disease, we will encourage research determining the identification of markers so as to determine which adolescents are most likely to have alcoholism before the first drink. We would then look to prevent development of the illness through education of the identified individuals, their teachers, and their families.

As an anecdotal point, an alcoholic patient in recovery told me of his early childhood. "My mother was very direct with me. From the time I was 7 years old, she told me that alcoholism runs in my family and that I should stay away from alcohol. She repeated it again and again before I ever picked up a drink." I asked him if this temporarily stopped him from drinking or if he felt that it simply encouraged him to drink. "Neither," he responded, "I just ignored it entirely. I knew in the back of my mind that I might get into trouble with it, but I really didn't think it would happen to me." I asked him what differentiated him now in recovery from him before he had ever picked up a drink. "The lack of doubt," he replied. He went on to indicate that he no longer had any doubt that alcohol would hurt him. Every time he picked up alcohol in the past, it was always because at that time he felt that just maybe there was a chance he would not get hurt. In alcoholism, it is important that all doubt as to the danger of alcohol be removed from patients at risk. If that is the difference between the alcoholic before picking up and the alcoholic in recovery, that is what we must teach. The catch, however, is that we do not yet know how to identify the premorbid alcoholic. We, therefore, have as much doubt as the patient-to-be.

SECONDARY PREVENTION

The process gets simpler with the secondary form of prevention because the disease is now present and easily diagnosed. Find and treat disease within the early stages. Such is the model of secondary prevention. The disease process has already begun, but there is yet to be any significant rise in resulting morbidity. Secondary prevention does not alter incidence, but its goal is to decrease prevalence. This is possible with alcoholism if we define prevalence as *not* including individuals in recovery. Within our analogy with hypertension, our patient is from a family with a high incidence of high blood pressure. He therefore comes in for frequent checkups and follows an exercise and dietary regimen he thinks will be less likely to lead to hypertension. Despite these primary prevention techniques, one day he is noted to have a significant rise in his baseline blood pressure. He is started on an antihypertensive and lives the rest of his life without further blood pressure-related difficulties. Starting the antihypertensive at that point in the development of the illness was a form of secondary prevention. For alcoholism, we might look at this patient:

Mimi is a 29-year-old patient who drinks a quart of vodka each weekend. She began drinking 2 months ago after a 6-year period of sobriety, which was self-imposed after her own recognition that alcoholism ran in her family and that her own use of alcohol was dissimilar to the patterns of her friends. After the 6 years of sobriety, she re-thought the situation and hoped that she could now drink responsibly, as many of her friends did. Within a month, she noticed that when she went out with friends for dinner, she and they would have a glass or two of wine with the meal, but that she would stop at the liquor store on her way home to buy another bottle of wine. She would then finish that bottle on her own. A few weeks later, she was buying vodka instead of wine. Although she had no medical complications, was still doing well at work, and was having no subjective difficulties relating to others, she made an appointment with her doctor because of her own concern that things would get worse. Shortly after her doctor recommended that she attend Alcoholics Anonymous (AA) meetings, she returned and said, "The stories other people tell at these meetings are horrendous. Lost marriages, liver replacements, kids never talking to their parents again—I don't have any of that." She was told that each of those people once passed through a period of time like the one she was currently experiencing. They passed there on their way to the bottom that they described at the meetings. "Do I need to get worse before I can stop drinking this way," she asked.

Mimi's question is key to the issue of secondary prevention. Do patients need to "hit bottom" before they can be receptive to treatment? Can they attain a lasting recovery and sobriety without experiencing any significant alcoholism-related morbidity? Presuming that secondary prevention is useful, early detection is critical. As noted earlier, diagnosis is straightforward, but only if the clinician is actually looking for a substance use disorder. The CAGE (*C*ut down, *A*nnoyed, *G*uilty, *E*ye-opener [test for problem drinking]) questionnaire represents one quick form of screening test. Some have noted that the traditional placement of addictive substance use in the patient's social history rather than in the medical history makes it more likely to be overlooked. In fact, interventions at the early stages of the disease are often effective, but clinicians often feel pessimistic regarding their chances of helping the patient effectively. There is a general lack of appreciation in the medical field as to how to best treat patients in the early stages of alcoholism. Training and educating medical professionals is likely, therefore, to be a significant and useful approach to addressing secondary prevention.

TERTIARY PREVENTION

Tertiary forms of prevention apply to those individuals who demonstrate characteristics consistent with a generalized disease state, complete with sequelae and related morbidity. Tertiary prevention often involves taking individuals away from their environment. Halfway-house placement, extended periods of rehabilitation, treatment of concurrent psychiatric illness if present, and initiation of self-help participation are all forms of tertiary prevention. The initial steps toward rehabilitation after significant injury, as part of an overall prevention plan, should lead to a lower incidence of relapse. A hypertensive patient who receives medication resulting in normal blood pressure is essentially identical to the nonhypertensive, with the exception of an increase in expected morbidity based on the duration for which the patient experienced elevation of blood pressure. Is that true for the alcoholic as well? Can we say that an alcoholic who has been in recovery for 5 years, attending AA meetings regularly, with no relapses during that time period, is identical to a nonalcoholic, with the exception of any morbidity related to the use of alcohol experienced by the patient before entering sobriety? Do we define recovery as sobriety, or is there more to it than that? Perhaps sobriety is all that is necessary to reduce medical morbidity, but more is necessary to achieve recovery of both medical and psychological status. If tertiary prevention is what we apply to individuals with chronic disease states so that they can achieve the equivalent of a disease-free state, what term applies to the ongoing preventive measures that we hope will reduce the risk of relapse in those already in long-term recovery? We should return to the primary prevention model again for this group because, medically, there is little to differentiate the premorbid group from the recovery group. However, to distinguish the two, because additional preventive measures can be taken with the recovery group, we use the term "relapse prevention" for the latter group.

RELAPSE PREVENTION

Some clinicians distinguish between a "slip" and "relapse." For ease of communication with patients, I use the term "relapse" to refer to all use of addictive agents other than nicotine after a period of sobriety. To study the area of relapse prevention, let us look at measures that are likely to lead to relapse:

(1)   After detoxification, sending patients back to their original home environment without implementing any protective measures.

(2)   Attempting rehabilitation while patients continue to live in their original home environment.

Triggers for patients to return to use of alcohol include exposure to certain people and places. The bar on the corner where everybody knows your patient's name is far more likely to call out to your patient than an unfamiliar setting. The "friends" that the patient had while drinking often encourage a return to drinking for your patient, to better meet their own needs. Although geographic cures do not generally work, a temporary move can be quite useful in the early stages of recovery.

(3) After successful rehabilitation, failing to arrange for ongoing outpatient visits.

(4) Having the patient followed by a string of frequently changing healthcare professionals.

(5) Providing only the care allowed by the patient's insurance after the patient's attainment of sobriety, ending outpatient visits after 5 to 10 sessions.

Figure 24.1, which demonstrates the life cycle of alcoholism, indicates that before general exposure to society, there is exposure to interpersonal relationships and education regarding emotional expression. Will feelings be expressed or stifled? Will children be cared for, or will they be only the caretakers? This education, which takes place quite early, needs to be repeated in sobriety, this time with the patient taught how to properly interact with others and how to properly express feelings. Self-help groups such as AA are one environment where this takes place. The clinical setting represents another such environment. If patients consider their physicians to be mentors, the parents they never had, or simply individuals they hold in high esteem, it does not do for those clinicians to discontinue

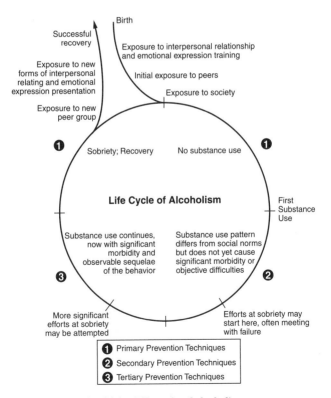

Fig. 24.1. Life cycle of alcoholism.

care shortly after initiating it. Such an action is seen as the type of treatment these patients received earlier in life from other such figures, and the information the clinicians provided will be discounted as being as worthless as the information the patients received from those others. Similarly, the usual psychiatric wall between clinician and patient should not apply here. The relationship is what will lead to improvement and solidity of recovery. Development of that relationship requires participation on both sides.

(6)   Treating the patient's insomnia or anxiety with potentially addictive medications, including benzodiazepines such as imidazopyridine with zolpidem tartrate (Ambien), and zaleplon (Sonata).
(7)   Treating the patient's concurrent muscular difficulties with potentially addictive medication, such as carisoprodol (Soma), which is metabolized to meprobamate, an addictive sedative agent.

Patients need to be educated regarding the many medications that are inappropriate for them, but which, nevertheless, may be offered to them by other physicians. There are patients for whom narcotic agents may be necessary to treat ongoing pain, and there are rare patients for whom methylphenidate (Ritalin) or similar medications are necessary for control of primary psychiatric disorders. Although some may choose to argue, I do not believe there are any patients with addictive disease for whom benzodiazepines or other sedative agents are ever appropriate. Proper detoxification and rehabilitation of patients with alcoholism includes discontinuation of all such agents before discharge.

(8)   Accepting the patient's statement, "I tried going to AA, but I didn't find it useful," as a reason not to encourage participation in 12-step program activities.

Patients in early recovery do not want to go to AA. They feel they do not fit in, do not belong, and will not be accepted. They do not want to speak in front of a group. They do not want to meet any of the strange people they see at these meetings. If they go at all, they arrive late, sit in the back quietly, and slip out before the meeting ends. I tell my patients that if they attend regularly on my terms, including their obtaining of a sponsor with whom they speak daily, for a certain amount of time, usually 6 months, that I will accept their decision regarding its effectiveness for them. But until that time, their attendance is a requirement.

(9)   Scheduling regular toxicology screens as a preventive measure rather than establishing a significant rapport with the patient.
(10)   Discharging the patient after a period of relapse, or after an attempt at gamesmanship by the patient regarding substance use.

As the issue of importance is the relationship, and because patients have been let down by so many other relationships in their lives, the therapist will be tested. Patients will lie to the therapist about their use. Almost without fail, each patient will at least once be intoxicated during an early visit, will lie about it, and will be focused closely upon your response as the clinician when the truth eventually comes out, either from a relative, from a toxicity screen, or from the patient. Discharging the patient at that point is the equivalent of an internist discharging a hypertensive patient who is noncompliant with medication. The illness is worse and care should be stepped up, not down. A reasonable response to relapse is, "These weekly sessions don't seem to be enough for your illness. Let's go to twice a week to see if that would be more helpful for you."

(11)   Focusing on other issues, such as a primary mood disorder, at the expense of the substance-use disorder.

Concurrent depressive disease is comparatively easy to treat. Give a medication and follow the symptom severity over time. We can raise medication dosages, add adjunctive therapy, focus on side effects, and change to any of several dozen medications. That is often easier than focusing on the relationship and the patient's overall sense of well-being, which are at the heart of a solid recovery.

SUGGESTED READINGS

American Society of Addiction Medicine: Public Policy on Prevention. http://www.asam.org/ppol/Prevention.htm.

Gitlow S: Substance Use Disorders: A Practical Guide. Philadelphia: Lippincott Williams & Wilkins, 2001.

Substance Abuse and Mental Health Services Administration (SAMHSA): Prevline, Prevention Online is an extensive series of related material available at http://www.health.org/.

Wallace RB: Public Health and Preventive Medicine, 14th Edition. New York: Appleton & Lange, 1998 (Chapters 45–46 are of interest).

ALCOHOL AND HIV/AIDS

Harold W. Goforth
Margaret Primeau
Francisco Fernandez

Human immunodeficiency virus (HIV) is a retrovirus discovered first in the 1980s and soon thereafter associated with men who have sex with men in the United States. The continued spread of HIV and its rapidly increasing presence among children, intravenous drug abusers, heterosexual couples, and chronically mentally ill persons has helped to change the belief that HIV is a disease of gay men only and has spurred a new urgency toward a more complete understanding of HIV. Although intravenous drug use (IVDU) is most prevalent in the United States and Europe, emerging nations also identify it as an increasing risk factor among their populations, especially in Southeast Asia.

Transmission of HIV occurs primarily during microtransfusions of infected blood during IVDU and arises primarily through the sharing of needles among addicts. Theoretically, it would be possible to arrest the spread of HIV from IVDU by teaching proper injection techniques such as cleaning needles with a bleach solution after each injection or a needle exchange program. These questions have encouraged much policy debate in the field over the most efficient and moral way by which to accomplish the objective of ending the further spread of HIV. This imperative is made even clearer when one examines the statistics surrounding perinatal HIV transmission. In urban areas, IVDU has become the primary means for perinatal transmission. The New York City Department of Health in 1990 estimated that approximately 90% of perinatal cases involved transmission from an IV drug-abusing mother or from a mother who had a sexual relationship with an IV drug abuser.

In addition to the public health concerns, HIV associated with IVDU has transformed itself into a variant of the original disease identified in homosexual males. IV drug users with HIV are less likely to develop Kaposi's sarcoma and have shorter life expectancies after developing AIDS. In addition, patients with IVDU-associated HIV die of a variety of infections, usually before developing the opportunistic infections associated with AIDS, leading to a possible underestimation of the prevalence of the disease.

In spite of the challenges confronting the study of HIV in drug-abusing populations, several risk factors for contracting HIV have emerged from the gathered data. Frequency of IV drug injection and the number of partners sharing needles are both proportionate to the risk for contracting HIV infection and subsequent disease. Additionally, certain drugs seem to make one more predisposed to contract HIV, such as heroin and cocaine injection, as opposed to amphetamine injection, which carries a smaller risk. There is as yet no explanation for this pattern.

PATHOGENESIS

HIV types I and II are now deemed the causative viruses of acquired immune deficiency syndrome (AIDS). Currently, the standard diagnostic procedure used to diagnose infection with HIV is testing for the presence of antibody to the virus, but this test is complicated by the relatively long latency period for HIV antibodies to appear after exposure (up to 6 months). After exposure to HIV through sexual or other blood-borne contact, a person typically develops an immune response that is detectable after 6 months by currently available assays in 99% of cases. Currently available methods to screen for the presence of HIV antibodies involve a two-step process. First, a screening is performed by ELISA (enzyme linked immunosorbent assay) techniques that have a high sensitivity (greater than 99%) but lower specificity and may cross-react with other common viruses, including influenza A . If the ELISA screen is confirmed as positive on repeat testing, the sample is submitted to additional, more rigorous testing using Western blot or immunofluoresence assay (IFA), both of which have high degrees of specificity for the virus. Both the ELISA and the Western blot or IFA must be positive for antibody diagnosis. Since approximately 1998, the nation's blood supply has been additionally subjected to HIV serum antigen (p24) testing as well.

Once an individual is infected, HIV systematically destroys the immune system, resulting in opportunistic infections and malignancies. Virtually all people who contract the HIV virus will eventually develop AIDS, with an average latency period of 8 to 10 years. The manifestation of AIDS has been consistently noted to vary across geographic areas as well as at-risk subgroups with the disease. For example, Kaposi's sarcoma appears more commonly in male homosexual subgroups than in IVDU subgroups. Mortality for all groups with fully developed AIDS is nearly 90% at 5 years of diagnosis.

AT-RISK POPULATIONS

Intravenous drug abusers are one of the most highly at-risk populations for contracting HIV. They currently comprise the most rapidly rising segment of the HIV population and contribute disproportionately to the new cases of HIV in the United States. A study by Rees and colleagues in 2001, which examined the role of alcohol in mediating risk-taking behavior among subjects with IVDU, found that sexual risk-taking was significantly associated with alcohol abuse among women with IVDU, and that women had more risky sexual behavior than men in this subgroup. Surprisingly, however, alcohol use did not predict that users take an increased risk in injection behavior, which suggests that alcohol mediates HIV transmission primarily though an influence on sexual behavior instead of increasing at-risk behavior at large.

A 2001 study by Purcell and associates, which was associated with the Centers for Disease Control (CDC), examined more closely the role of alcohol in mediating transmission risk behavior and unsafe sexual practices in HIV-infected men and their HIV-negative or status-unknown partners. Not surprisingly, it was found that men who engaged in high-risk transmission behaviors had increased likelihood to abuse various substances, including alcohol. Of the groups of HIV-infected subjects who used alcohol, those who consumed it around the time of or during sexual intercourse were found to be more likely to engage in unprotected insertive anal intercourse with casual partners. Conversely, those men who consumed drugs other than alcohol during these seemingly key times were more likely to engage in unprotected receptive anal intercourse. Given that a high degree of both alcohol abuse and illicit drug abuse has been demonstrated to be quite extensive in the HIV community, the use of alcohol and other illicit drugs seems to aid in the further transmission and perpetuation of this disease.

A similar study by Bagnall and coworkers (1990) examined the relationship between AIDS-related risks in a cohort of young adults and their corresponding alcohol, tobacco, and illicit drug use. A minority reported consistent use of barrier protection (condoms) during sexual activity, but over one half of respondents reported having only a single sexual partner in the previous year. Respondents who often combined alcohol and sex were estimated to be seven times less likely than others to always use condoms for vaginal intercourse. The numbers of respondents in the study who reported illicit drug use and sexual behavior were few, so conclusions are limited. However, four of six reporting males and three of four reporting females stated that they had seldom used condoms in the previous year. Available conclusions lend some support to the notion that use of alcohol and illicit drugs of abuse increase the likelihood of risky sex.

Although HIV disease is a growing concern among developed Western nations, it has reached epidemic proportions in sub-Saharan African nations, where an estimated 30% of the population carry HIV, particularly in countries such as South Africa and Zimbabwe. A study that investigated the association between alcohol consumption and HIV seropositivity in rural Uganda found a significant role for alcohol in encouraging transmission of the disease. By means of epidemiological surveillance for HIV infection coupled with a questionnaire survey, it was found that the overall rate of HIV infection for 15 surrounding villages was 8%. However, among those subjects who lived in households where alcohol was sold, the infection rate rose to fifteen percent of the population. In fact, only age, marital status, and the independent consumption of alcohol predicted HIV seropositivity in this rural population. These authors also note that the role of alcohol in promoting the transmission of HIV disease and risk-taking behavior may help to explain the lower incidence of HIV among Muslims, whose religious tenets forbid the consumption of alcohol.

Although it seems that alcohol and illicit drug use can contribute to increased risky sexual behavior as noted in other subgroups, the actual means by which consumption of these substances works to increase this behavior remains unclear. McKirnan and colleagues, in 2001, tested the hypothesis that sexual risk-taking is related to the combination of alcohol and drugs with sexual practices, which allows a cognitive escape from the awareness of HIV risk during social and sexual settings. A stratification of sexual risk-taking was identified during this study. The patients who used illicit drugs of abuse during sexual practice reported higher rates of sexual risk-taking and hepatitis B infection than all other groups. Subjects that used alcohol alone were less likely to have increased sexual risk-taking behavior, and subjects who only occasionally combined substances with sex were least likely to demonstrate high-risk sexual behavior. The authors concluded that men who used drugs of abuse and alcohol during sexual encounters had a significantly diminished capacity to avoid high-risk sexual practices or use preventive methods such as condoms.

Special Populations

Given the high rates of alcoholism found in the Native American subculture, the interplay between alcohol and HIV has been better characterized by examining this high-risk population. In 2000, a study by Baldwin and associates that examined the patterns and behaviors of Native Americans and Alaskan Natives found that there was a disproportionately high rate of alcohol abuse among active crack and injection drug users of this culture. IVDU showed the highest frequency and quantity of alcohol use within the preceding 30 days, and a significant association was identified between crack and alcohol use within 48 hours. Importantly, those individuals who identified increased episodes of either drug or alcohol use before or during sexual intercourse also reported significantly more episodes of unprotected sexual intercourse. Also of special concern is the fact that that many participants in this group reported blackout episodes. When they awakened, they discovered that they had had sexual intercourse with either an unknown or unsatisfactory partner. Given these scenarios, the implications for increased risk of HIV transmission are obvious. Especially of concern among this population is that members of minority groups often have limited access to health care and preventive medicine. Thus, when these individuals do contract HIV disease, the diagnosis is often delayed until later and less treatable stages in the illness.

Data emerging from the CDC indicate an increased rate of transmission of HIV among adolescents, who are too young to have been influenced by the initial scare of HIV disease in the 1980s and 1990s. Attitudes among young adolescents have reflected a growing nihilism, as evidenced by such as the idea that a homosexual lifestyle is necessarily linked with HIV, which minimizes the need for safe sexual practices. The lack of protective sexual practices, combined with a relatively high rate of alcohol and drug abuse leading to increases in impulsive behavior in this population, reinforces the groundwork for a possible explosion of HIV cases in the very young unless this subgroup undergoes extensive education regarding the disease.

However, the relationship between active substance use and disease progression continues to be a controversial one. In the Multicenter Cohort Study of Homosexual Men, the authors found no statistically significant difference in the rates of progression to AIDS over 18 months among users of alcohol and illicit drugs compared with a non–substance-abuse, HIV-infected population. Furthermore, no other manifestations of immunodeficiency were positively associated with substance use before enrollment; therefore, drug or alcohol use in this study was not associated with greater subsequent decline in CD4 counts.

HIV-ASSOCIATED CNS DISORDERS

Similar to syphilis, HIV virus has often been called a "great mimicker" and can appear as many different psychiatric illnesses, of which the most common are the organic mental disorders including delirium, dementia, and mood disturbances. Psychotic features may or may not be present. Individuals with comorbid substance abuse further complicate the diagnostic dilemma because these substances can independently cause psychiatric disturbances indistinguishable from those associated with HIV illness or general psychiatric disorders.

Delirium

Delirium is the most frequent mental disorder associated with HIV disease, with an incidence noted by some studies approximating 30%. It is imperative to diagnose these disorders because etiologies may be life threatening, and a failure to diagnose may lead to poor treatment and outcome. However, delirium is also one of the most underdiagnosed conditions in medicine.

Delirium can be ascribed to a global cerebral process characterized by metabolic dysfunction, as evidenced by generalized slowing on electroencephalography. A prodromal phase of delirium has been described, which includes difficulty in thought processing, restlessness, irritability, and fragmented sleep with vivid nightmares. Other nonspecific neurological findings include asterixis, tremor, and multifocal myoclonus. Often, the patient becomes severely disoriented and agitated, requiring chemical and physical restraints to protect the integrity of dressings, IV lines, and other medical equipment. When confronted with the early prodromal phase of delirium, the patient should undergo an extensive evaluation to determine the precise etiology with the focus in HIV disease on infectious, metabolic, and central nervous system (CNS) processes. In addition, HIV patients are more predisposed to opportunistic infections, including herpes, *Toxoplasma gondii* encephalitis, cryptococcal meningitis, tumors, multifocal leukoencephalopathy, and antiviral neurotoxic effects.

Patients who are agitated may require chemical restraints as a result of the delirious process. Oral and parenteral high-potency neuroleptics, preferably haloperidol, have been used. As with all patients with significant cerebral pathology, HIV patients are more sensitive to the neuroleptics and more prone to develop significant extrapyramidal symptoms, which necessitates a lower dose. However, extrapyramidal side effects have long been noted to be less frequent if the neuroleptic is given by an IV route. IV haloperidol is generally safe from a cardiovascular standpoint if the patients do not have hypovolemia, hypomagnessemia, or an underlying electrolyte disturbance. Data also suggest a role in treating delirium with the atypical antipsychotics, including risperidone, olanzapine, quetiapine, and ziprasidone. The use of ziprasidone or olanzapine has not yet been reported in patients with HIV/AIDS.

Dementia

Another common manifestation of HIV-linked CNS pathology is the HIV-associated dementia complex (HADC). Although there has been a clear link between illicit drug and alcohol abuse and contraction of HIV disease, the direct effects of such substances upon the neural substrate have not been clearly linked.

HADC is most often identified in patients with significant immunocompromise due to AIDS. Although various neurological symptoms have been identified in conjunction with HADC, early motor slowing is a common and predominant one, as evidenced by neuropsychological testing that demonstrates frontal and subcortical deficits superimposed on memory impairment. Imaging of the HADC brain usually reveals generalized atrophy consisting of enlarged ventricles and widened sulci. Average life span after the diagnosis of HADC is approximately 7 months. On autopsy, pathological features include a reduction in the number of neurons, abnormal dendritic arborization, and neuronal apoptosis.

Toxins implicated in this process include quinolinic acid, arachidonic acid metabolites, and others. Quinolinic acid has been of special interest, for it and the gp120 HIV protein interact with the *N*-methyl-d-aspartate receptor, with resultant excitatory receptor neurotoxicity. While HIV *tat* and *rev* have also been identified as neurotoxic in vitro, actual studies linking HIV viral load to HADC are lacking.

TNF-alpha may play a pivotal role in the production of neurotoxic metabolites because TNF-alpha has been shown to stimulate gliosis as well as independent altering of neuronal function by direct toxicity to oligodendrocytes in vitro. In addition, it stimulates mononuclear phagocytes and astrocytes to produce several neurotoxins, including quinolinic acid and nitric oxide. It also potentially increases the HIV viral load, which indirectly compromises further the remaining CNS function. The effects of alcohol and illicit substances are of great interest, because they likely affect these cytokines indirectly and directly, thereby modifying the disease process.

Inflammatory cytokines linked either directly or indirectly to neurotoxicity include TNF-alpha, IL-1, IFN-gamma, and IL-6. These cytokines act to stimulate predominantly mononuclear phagocytes and astrocytes as well as to generate other cytokines and inflammatory precursors such as eicosanoids, nitric oxide, quinolinic acid, and superoxides. TNF-alpha, IL-1, and IL-6 potentiate HIV replication, while HIV stimulates the production of these cytokines in an autocrine loop.

When alcohol or illicit drug abuse is present along with features of HADC, neuropsychological testing has given support to the theory that drugs of abuse may hasten or worsen the HIV-related disease process, the immune decline, and the cognitive dysfunction. However, clinical studies have failed to validate these findings, inclusive of the laboratory findings in alcohol-related immune effects. Of interest is the fact that many of the described pathological abnormalities associated with HADC are also associated with chronic ethanol abuse. Dementia is a feature common to both HIV and chronic alcohol disease. Similarly, neuropsychological testing indicates that both cognitive deficits and frontal lobe dysfunction are present in both sets of patients. Comparative imaging reveals similar degrees of generalized atrophy predominantly in the frontal lobes, and cerebral functional imaging reveals gray matter abnormalities in the frontal regions. Finally, anatomic pathology studies indicate a similar pattern of neuronal loss, dendritic arborization abnormalities, and frontal cortex neuronal dropout. The two conditions are so similar that chronic alcohol abuse has been offered as a possible etiologic link in HADC.

Although cytokines have been implicated in the pathogenesis of CNS dysfunction related to both alcohol and HIV, relatively little work has been done regarding the direct effect alcohol plays on the immune system of the CNS. Evidence that ethanol dysregulates the immune system is quite convincing, however. Chronic alcoholics have alterations in their native cytokine levels, presumably making them more susceptible to infectious agents, including intracellular retroviruses. Similarly, the growth of *Mycobacterium avium* has been reported to be greater in cultured human macrophages exposed to ethanol than in those that had not been exposed to alcohol. Evidence is also available that the HIV *tat* protein responsible for oxidative damage, bone marrow toxicity, and polymorphonuclear neutrophil defects is enhanced by the chronic presence of alcohol.

The treatment of HIV-associated dementia complex is one of the most challenging aspects of HIV/AIDS care. At present, no definitive treatment exists and chronic decline of cognitive function is the rule. Cognitive decline appears to occur independently of CD4 counts and serum viral load. Also, a higher number of HADC cases are being identified as HIV patients are living longer. The blood-brain barrier is presumed to share a significant role in HADC because it is responsible for sequestering the brain from the antiviral effects of HIV medications. HIV, therefore, is protected in the CNS and progresses somewhat independently of the systemic illness, leading to cognitive decline even in some otherwise healthy individuals with low viral loads. Symptomatic management of behavioral difficulties can be accomplished with typical neuroleptic agents in a manner similar to that used in the treatment of delirium. However, HADC patients are often exquisitely sensitive to high-potency agents and develop extrapyramidal effects even at low doses. Similarly, use of the low-potency agents are not recommended owing to their significant anticholinergic component, which may further impair remaining cognitive ability. If neuroleptics are required in these patients, one must be cautious and begin use with low doses of the high-potency or medium-potency agents such as molindone. Alternatively, the atypical neuroleptics are gradually becoming more widely used, including low-dose risperidone and quetiapine.

In summary, both alcohol and HIV have been demonstrated to cause similar central nervous system pathology characterized by neuronal loss and abnormal microscopic structure, likely mediated both directly and indirectly by numerous cytokines and the HIV virus itself. Although large studies are lacking to examine specifically the effect of alcohol on current HIV illness, it can logically be presumed that when the two agents are placed together, a synergistic effect may occur characterized by more rapid progression of HIV disease, including CNS pathology.

ALCOHOL-ASSOCIATED CNS DISORDERS

Delirium

Alcohol-induced CNS disorders include a withdrawal syndrome that may progress to delirium, Wernicke's syndrome, Korsakoff's psychosis, and seizures. Alcohol withdrawal syndrome is a cluster of symptoms involving tremulousness, transitory hallucinations, tachycardia, tachypnea, hypertension, diaphoresis, and tonic-clonic seizures. Delirium tremens occurs infrequently and is often associated with an underlying medical illness. Common medical illnesses include hepatic insufficiency, pneumonia, subdural hematomas, pancreatitis, and major bone fractures. A diagnosis consists of gross memory deficits in addition to agitation and hallucinations; it usually begins approximately 2 to 3 days after the cessation of alcohol intake and lasts between 1 and 5 days. Mortality associated with delirium tremens has been estimated at 20% in some studies and is a true medical emergency. Treatment involves supportive measures along with rapid benzodiazepine sedation followed by a slow wean over a 3-day to 5-day period. In some severe cases, an even slower taper may be required.

Dementia

Alcoholism is associated with disease of the nervous system primarily through its link with B-vitamin deficiencies and malnutrition. Wernicke's syndrome resulting from thiamine deficiency consists classically of ocular disturbances that involve nystagmus or sixth nerve paresis, ataxia, and confusion. However, it is important to note that all three signs of Wernicke's syndrome have been estimated to occur in only approximately 30% of the population that has true Wernicke's syndrome. In the remainder, only one or two of the signs may be initially present; therefore, a high degree of clinical suspicion is warranted in diagnosing this entity. With prompt treatment consisting of relatively large doses of thiamine, the deficiencies usually clear rapidly but may persist and develop into Korsakoff's psychosis. The typical dose recommended for the acute treatment of Wernicke's syndrome consists of thiamine, 300 mg per day for 3 days, administered either intravenously or intramuscularly, and followed by conversion to an oral formulation if gastric absorption is not compromised. Thiamine and the remainder of the B-vitamins are water-soluble and safe if given in large doses.

Short-term memory loss is the most characteristic feature of Korsakoff's psychosis and is classically accompanied by "confabulation." The Wernicke-Korsakoff syndrome is related to hemorrhagic necrosis of the mammillary bodies, thalamus, and brainstem. Although thiamine is useful in the treatment of early Wernicke's syndrome, it appears that Korsakoff's syndrome is typically unresponsive to thiamine replacement and tends to be a chronic condition. However, there are case reports in the literature that point to gradual and sustained improvement in memory deficits related to Korsakoff's syndrome if treatment with thiamine is extended to several months at high doses.

SUMMARY

In summary, the subset of patients who abuse alcohol and are HIV-infected is challenging from both a clinical and a public health standpoint. This group of patients appears more likely to engage in high-risk behavior and expose others to the disease as well as to suffer from a higher number of comorbid conditions. Education and prevention interventions remain the key to treating this subgroup. Treatment must center on both alcoholism and HIV-related issues. Medical treatment of these patients is complicated and must involve collaborative care among a general medicine practitioner, an infectious disease specialist, and a psychiatrist experienced in using the specific group of medications that these patients will likely receive and in treating patients with addictions. As researchers further clarify the role of alcohol and its interaction with primary HIV disease, additional treatment options should become more available.

SUGGESTED READINGS

Bagnall G, Plant M, Warwick W: Alcohol Drugs, and AIDS-Related Risks: Results from a Prospective Study. AIDS Care 2:309–317, 1990.

Baldwin JA, Maxwell CJ, Fenaughty AM, Trotter RT, Stevens SJ: Alcohol as a risk factor for HIV transmission among American Indian and Alaska Native drug users. Am Ind Alaska Native Ment Health Res 9: 1–16, 2000.

Cournos F, McKinnon K: Substance use and HIV-risk among people with severe mental illness. NIDA Res Monogr 172:110–129, 1997.

Fernandez F, Ringholz GM, Levy JK: Neuropsychiatric aspects of human immunodeficiency virus on the central nervous system. In: Yudofsky SC, Hales R (eds.), The American Psychiatric Textbook of Neuropsychiatry and Clinical Neurosciences. Washington, D.C.: American Psychiatric Press, 2002, pp. 783–812.

Kaslow RA, Blackwelder WC, Ostrow DG, Yerg D, Palenicek J, Coulson AH, et al: No evidence for a role of alcohol or other psychoactive drugs in accelerating immunodeficiency in HIV-1-positive individuals. A report from the Multicenter AIDS Cohort Study. JAMA 261:3424–3429, 1989.

McKirnan DJ, Vanable PA, Ostrow DG, Hope B: Expectancies of sexual "escape" and sexual risk among drug and alcohol-involved gay and bisexual men. J Subst Abuse 13:137–154, 2001.

Purcell DW, Parsons JT, Halkitis PN, Mizuno Y, Woods WJ: Substance use and sexual transmission risk behavior of HIV-positive men who have sex with men. J Subst Abuse 13:185–200, 2001.

Rees V, Saitz R, Horton NJ, Samet J: Association of alcohol consumption with HIV sex- and drug-risk behaviors among drug users. J Subst Abuse Treat 21:129–134, 2001.

ALCOHOLISM AND THE ELDERLY

Roland M. Atkinson

For more than 20 years, studies have indicated that alcohol use disorders (AUDs—alcohol dependence and abuse) are common among aging individuals. The elderly are a highly heterogeneous population with substantial variability in physical and functional status. As such, the clinical presentations, consequences, and complications of alcohol-related illness among aging persons are wide ranging. Major psychiatric, physical, and social disabilities occur in this age group, either related or coincident to AUDs. In this chapter, I summarize current knowledge about the use and abuse of alcohol by older adults, emphasizing special treatment issues in this age group and associated health and social problems.

EPIDEMIOLOGY OF ALCOHOL USE AND ABUSE

Prevalence

Alcohol use and alcohol problems decline with age but still constitute a significant public health problem. Community surveys show that *alcohol use* in the United States is most prevalent in the group aged 25 to 45 years, declining stepwise in older age cohorts to 12-month prevalence levels, in persons aged 55 years and older, of about 50% who report any alcohol use and 30% who report having consumed at least 12 drinks in the past 12 months. Rates of any recent alcohol use continue to decline after age 55 years to 25% of persons aged 85 years and older. Rates for *"risky" drinking* (defined as heavy nonproblem drinking) and *problem drinking* (which may or may not meet DSM [Diagnostic and Statistical Manual of Mental Disorders]-IV criteria for an AUD) by older adults vary widely depending on the population sampled and definitions of use. In one survey of primary care office practice rolls, the prevalence of risky drinking in patients aged 65 years and older was 15% for men and 12% for women. The prevalence of current problem drinking after age 85 years is very low. Because older adults with AUDs also have high rates of comorbid medical disorders, they are represented much more commonly in clinical settings than in community surveys. Reports of elderly clinical cohorts show rates of current AUDs that can vary from 4% to 23%, depending on the setting in which they are studied. Community prevalence rates for alcohol dependence are lower; in household surveys, only about 2% to 3% of elderly men and less than 1% of elderly women in the United States currently suffer from these disorders. The number of persons with lesser or potential alcohol-related problems far exceeds the clinical population who are alcohol dependent—those traditionally termed "alcoholic" patients.

Currently, older men are twice as likely to use alcohol as older women, and two to six times more likely than women to be problem drinkers. These patterns hold true across diverse ethnic and racial groups. Once alcohol dependence develops, it is more likely to persist in older men than in older women. Several factors contribute to the apparent decline in drinking and drinking problems with age, including premature deaths of early-onset alcoholics, moderation or cessation of drinking by surviving alcoholics and social drinkers as they grow older, reticence of older patients to report drinking accurately, under-recognition and under-reporting of cases by clinicians, cohort, and period effects. For many elderly individuals, drinking patterns established in early adulthood or middle age persist into old age.

Late-Onset Alcohol Problems

Retrospective studies of community-dwelling elderly have noted subsets of individuals who report increasing their alcohol consumption in later life, either for the first time or resumption of a fluctuating pattern established earlier. More recent household surveys and clinical reports demonstrate that onset of initial drinking problems at age 50 or older is not uncommon, although there are "intermittent" cases, in which persons with early-onset alcoholism achieve prolonged abstinence in middle life but relapse later; such a pattern can be mistaken for late-onset drinking. Studies show that an average of at least one third of older patients with AUDs have onset in the sixth decade or later. In treatment samples the proportion of patients with onset after age 60 years can vary from 15% to greater than 60%, depending on setting and demographic factors. The notion that late-onset alcohol dependence usually occurs secondary to a mood or cognitive disorder has not been upheld by recent systematic studies, although many persons with late-onset alcohol problems were risky or reactive drinkers earlier in their lives. Late-onset alcohol problems are typically milder and more circumscribed than those that begin earlier in life. Compared with early-onset cases, late-onset problem drinkers also tend to have less alcoholism among relatives, less psychopathology, and higher socioeconomic status; also these cases represent a larger proportion of alcoholic women. Although there is clinical evidence to support the view that late-onset drinking problems sometimes begin in reaction to life stress, it is not true that this group exhibits more reactive drinking than lifelong alcoholics, who are notorious for their tendency to drink more in response to any significant life event. Compared with alcoholism of long duration, late-onset drinkers tend to resolve problems more often without formal treatment, but there is little evidence to suggest that they respond more favorably to alcoholism treatment than early-onset patients.

Risk Factors

Risk factors for AUDs in the elderly population are listed in Table 26.1. A family history of alcoholism, a personal history of previous heavy or reactive consumption, or prior episodes of an AUD all increase the risk of a new episode of problem drinking. Frailty, dysfunction, and need for multiple prescription medications all increase the vulnerability of elderly patients to adverse alcohol effects, as do certain symptoms, such as insomnia, pain and depression, for which some elders take alcohol as self-medication. At the same time, in community surveys, alcohol consumption tends to be greater in older

Table 26.1. Risk Factors for Alcohol Use Disorders in the Elderly

Predisposing factors

Gender (male)
Family history of AUDs
Previous episode of an AUD
Previous pattern of alcohol consumption (individual and cohort effects)

Factors that may increase alcohol exposure and consumption level

Chronic illness associated with pain, insomnia, or anxiety
Life stress, loss, social isolation
Negative affects (depression, grief, demoralization, anger)
Family collusion and drinking partners
Discretionary time, money

Factors that may increase the effects or abuse potential of alcohol

Age-associated alcohol sensitivity (pharmacokinetics, pharmacodynamics)
Chronic medical illnesses
Other medications (alcohol-drug interactions)

adults who are physically fit and mobile, economically well off, and married. Response to a given alcohol load increases with age. Pharmacokinetics plays a role. In the fasting state, a nonalcoholic man in his 60s may have a peak blood alcohol level 20% to 25% higher than a man in his 30s after a standard alcohol load, and for women this difference is even greater. These changes are largely attributable to reduced volume of distribution for alcohol resulting from decline in lean body mass and body water with age, and also to reduced alcohol dehydrogenase activity in the gut wall, allowing absorption of a larger portion of ingested alcohol, especially in older women. However, even when one controls for blood alcohol level, performance is more impaired in an elderly person after a standard alcohol load, indicating an increasing neuropharmacodynamic effect of alcohol with age. This has been demonstrated on measures of subjective intoxication experience, memory, performance on divided-attention tasks, and measures of coordination—body sway and hand dexterity—after single alcohol doses.

SYMPTOMS, COMPLICATIONS, AND COURSE

Clinical Presentations

In an elderly individual, an alcohol-related problem may not be suspected because the presenting picture often does not correspond with stereotypes based on findings in younger patients. Severe primary alcohol dependence certainly is seen in older adults, but antisocial behavior and lower socioeconomic status are less common, and clinical manifestations are more variable. *Circumscribed* or *"focal" alcohol problems* most typically appear as biomedical symptoms or problems. Alcohol excess can cause, aggravate, or complicate the management of problems as diverse as hypertension, diabetes mellitus, osteoporosis, gastritis, macrocytic anemia, hypercholesterolemia, parkinsonism, and gout. A number of cancers (oral, esophageal, pharyngeal, laryngeal, hepatic, colorectal) are caused or aggravated by alcohol dependence. Breast cancer in one large survey was 1.3 times more common in women who currently drank than in nondrinkers. Alcohol-drug interactions can confound medical prescribing because acute alcohol intake reduces the action of many drugs, whereas, conversely, chronic high alcohol consumption may increase drug metabolism by inducing hepatic, microsomal, drug-metabolizing enzyme activity. Alcohol can potentiate the sedating effects of prescribed benzodiazepines and opioids, and some drugs (e.g., chlorpromazine and H_2 blockers), reduce alcohol dehydrogenase activity in the gut wall, permitting greater alcohol absorption and increasing susceptibility to intoxication when patients taking these drugs drink alcohol. Other commonly encountered circumscribed problems in older patients include repeated arrest for driving an automobile while under the influence of alcohol and recurrent family conflict associated with AUDs.

Older patients with *uncomplicated mild alcohol dependence*, including many daily risky drinkers, may have no specific complaints or findings. Tolerance may accompany this pattern. Because of risk of later medical or psychiatric sequelae of sustained heavy drinking, intervention is justified. *Medically complex dependence* is often the condition of aging persons with AUDs who are admitted to the emergency department or acute medical inpatient unit. The symptoms, although obvious, may be nonspecific and thus easily attributed to a cause other than alcohol abuse; indeed, alcohol may be just one of several factors contributing to the clinical picture. At time of presentation, features may include delirium, dementia, lack of self-care, dehydration, malnutrition, gastrointestinal complaints, bladder and/or bowel incontinence, muscle weakness or frank myopathy, gait disorder, recurring falls, burns, head trauma, or accidental hypothermia. Hypoglycemia, congestive heart failure, and aspiration pneumonia can also be caused or aggravated by alcohol dependence.

Psychiatrically complex dependence is seen in those patients who have an AUD associated with another major psychiatric disorder ("dual diagnoses"). The pattern of common psychiatric comorbidities in aging alcoholics differs from that seen among their younger counterparts. Drug-use disorders, which make up a large proportion of comorbid disorders in younger cohorts, are distinctly uncommon in older persons with an AUD. This difference often leads investigators to claim that dual diagnoses decline with age. However, if drug use disorders are not considered, the proportion of older persons with AUDs who also have comorbid psychiatric disorders is the same or higher than those found among younger alcoholics. Mood disorders—mainly depression (in about 25% of cases), cognitive disorders, and anxiety disorders (about 10% to 15% of cases in each)—are the three most common psychiatric comorbidities in this age group. Accurate differential diagnosis often requires repeated assessment over time.

Complications and Associated Features

Alcohol intoxication may occur at lower dose levels in older persons because of increased biological sensitivity. Although there is no evidence that alcohol withdrawal disorders (tremulousness syndrome, hallucinosis, seizures, and delirium tremens) occur at different rates in the elderly, alcohol withdrawal can be more severe and more difficult to treat in this age group and may be associated with greater mortality. Other central nervous system complications include reversible cognitive impairment; Wernicke-Korsakoff syndrome; dementia associated with alcohol dependence; and deterioration caused by another form of dementia, such as Alzheimer's disease. Alcohol-associated insomnia resembles the age-associated pattern of sleep disorganization: Both show frequent awakenings, especially from deep, slow-wave sleep, and reduced rapid eye movement (REM) sleep.

Medical complications have already been described. Psychosocial complications are diverse. Alcohol problems are found in 7% to 30% of older suicides, although the association of AUDs with suicide may actually be stronger in men of late middle age than in elderly men or women of any age. A 50-year longitudinal study of men has demonstrated that the strong association between poor social support and premature mortality is significantly mediated by alcohol abuse among several other variables. Case material has demonstrated problems of alcohol-related divorce and homelessness in late life, and also that alcohol intoxication may be a factor in geriatric pedophilia and other sexual misconduct, and in violent events (e.g., abuse or attacks by and on elderly individuals). Among substance-related comorbidities, active tobacco dependence—principally cigarette smoking—is highly prevalent in elderly alcoholics (about 50% to 70%), whereas active dependence on prescribed sedatives, anxiolytics, and opioid analgesics varies (from 2% to 14%) depending on the cohort studied. In most modern clinical settings, illicit drug abuse is uncommon, but it can be highly prevalent—as high as 25% of cases—in some culturally diverse urban patient groups.

Course

The span from onset of the first alcohol problem to recognition of current problems can be as long as 50 years, based on retrospective reports. Over this course, drinking may have been steady, progressive, or variable; in some cases, sober periods of 10 years or longer occur between problem drinking episodes. In one prospective 4-year repeated telephone survey of involving 1600 community-dwelling drinkers of late middle age and nondrinkers, 37% initially reported one or more current alcohol problems. Resolution of current problems within the next year occurred in 29% of the problem drinkers. Early-onset problem drinkers remitted less often than recent-onset problem drinkers (24% vs. 41%). Gains made at 1 year were sustained at the fourth year resurvey in 70% of the remitted problem group. Among nonproblem drinkers at baseline, 8% developed one or more alcohol-related problems in the next year. There is evidence that social drinkers tend to modify their consumption downward with age, whereas problem drinkers are more likely to choose to abstain. Mortality rates are very high when active drinking continues in the face of frank dementia or active, alcohol-related liver disease.

APPROACHES TO ASSESSMENT AND DIAGNOSIS

Diagnosis of AUDs and problem drinking requires alertness to the possibility of the problem in this age group, skillful interviewing (sometimes aided by screening tests and home visits), physical and neurological examination, and appropriate laboratory tests.

Interviews

As is true of younger patients, information elicited from interviews provides the foundation for accurate diagnosis. Sensitive inquiry about drinking practices is sometimes necessary to elicit this information, because denial of alcohol problems and defensiveness when asked about drinking are especially common in this age group. Reasons for this include alcohol-related amnesia for intoxication episodes, shame about reliance on alcohol, pessimism about recovery, and, often enough, of course, the desire to continue drinking. Comorbid depression or cognitive disorder can also influence veracity. Collaterals may shield the problem from detection. For these reasons, careful building of rapport through repeated contacts; thorough inquiry of relatives, caregivers, and others in the social network; reviews of medical records; and home visitation are especially useful assessment methods for elderly persons with suspected AUDs.

Screening Instruments

The CAGE (*C*ut down, *A*nnoyed, *G*uilty, *E*ye-opener) test and the geriatric version of the Michigan Alcoholism Screening Test (MAST-G) (short form displayed in Table 26.2) have both shown promise as preliminary screens for alcohol problems in older clinical populations, although not all studies find these measures to be sufficiently

---

Table 26.2.   Short Michigan Alcoholism Screening Test— Geriatric Version [SMAST-G]*

In the past year:

1. When talking with others, do you underestimate how much you actually drink?
2. After a few drinks, have you sometimes not eaten or have been able to skip a meal because you didn't feel hungry?
3. Does having a few drinks help decrease your shakiness or tremors?
4. Does alcohol sometimes make it hard for you to remember parts of the day or night?

In the past year:

5. Do you usually take a drink to relax or calm your nerves?
6. Do you drink to take your mind off your problems?
7. Have you ever increased your drinking after experiencing a loss in your life?
8. Has a doctor or nurse ever said they were worried or concerned about your drinking?
9. Have you ever made rules to manage your drinking?
10. When you feel lonely, does having a drink help?

Three or more positive responses is indicative of a recent or current alcohol use problem.

---

*From Blow FC: Michigan Alcoholism Screening Test—Geriatric Version (MAST-G). University of Michigan Alcohol Research Center, Ann Arbor, Michigan, 1991.

sensitive in elderly patients. In one study, among risky drinkers aged 65 years and older, only about 40% were CAGE positive. A positive result on either measure does not make the diagnosis of an AUD, but these tests can help identify patients who need more detailed assessment.

Physical and Laboratory Findings

Physical stigmata of alcoholic liver disease, peripheral polyneuropathy, and cerebellar ataxia are among physical findings that may help confirm a diagnosis, but these are often absent. Laboratory data may be helpful, especially in cases of mild dependence or in differential diagnosis of complex cases. Findings from one large group of older alcoholic patients are compared with findings in younger patients in Table 26.3. Macrocytic red blood cells, with or without anemia, and liver transferase enzyme elevations are the most typical findings. Toxicological examination of blood or breath samples for alcohol may help establish a diagnosis of severe alcohol intoxication in the moribund patient. In the ambulatory patient, a high blood alcohol level (greater than 150 mg/100 mL) in the presence of a relatively normal mental and neurological examination is strong evidence for tolerance and physical dependence.

Table 26.3.   Frequency of Laboratory Abnormalities in Elderly and Younger Inpatients with Alcoholism*

	Results[†]			
	Patients $\geq$65 years[‡]		Younger patients[‡]	
Blood tests	Number[§]	Percent	Number[§]	Percent
MCH increased	213	71	123	57[‖]
AST increased	234	56	123	42[#]
GGT increased	123	55	101	48
MCV increased	213	44	124	17[‖]
Glucose increased	206	32	124	36
Uric acid increased	201	21	123	<1[‖]
Albumin decreased	186	17	115	3[‖]
Alkaline phosphatase increased	213	11	123	15
Triglycerides increased	191	16	122	15
Phosphorus increased	198	9	124	1

*Adapted from Hurt RD, Finlayson RE, Morse RM, Davis LJ: Alcoholism in elderly persons: medical aspects and prognosis of 216 inpatients. Mayo Clin Proc 63: 753–760, 1988.
[†]MCH = mean corpuscular hemoglobin; AST = aspartate aminotransferase; GGT = gamma-glutamyltransferase; MCV = mean corpuscular volume.
[‡]Older patients: N=216; mean age 69.6 years; age range 65 to 83 years; younger patients: N=125; mean age 44.3 years; age range 19 to 64 years.
[§]Number = number of patients tested in each age group; Percent = percent of patients tested in the age group who had an abnormal value.
[‖]$p < 0.01$ using Wilcoxon two-sample rank sum test to compare age groups for proportion having an abnormal value.
[#]$p < 0.05$; for others, $p > 0.3$.

Table 26.4. Aging-Related Problems That Require Assessment During Alcohol Treatment

- Loss—people, vocation, status, independence
- Social isolation and loneliness
- Financial problems, poverty
- Dislocation of habitat
- Family conflict and estrangement
- Burden of time management (boredom)
- Physiologic changes affecting alcohol and drug effects
- Complex medical problems
- Multiple medications
- Sensory deficits
- Reduced mobility
- Cognitive impairment, loss
- Impaired self-care
- Reliance on caregivers
- Loss of physical attractiveness
- Reduced self-regard, demoralization

Diagnostic Criteria

DSM-IV criteria for diagnosing alcohol dependence are generally satisfactory when applied to aging persons, but this is less true of criteria for alcohol abuse. Criteria for alcohol abuse should—but at present do not—include recurrent use as a cause or aggravation of physical or psychiatric symptoms or illness, or interaction with other medications to cause adverse reactions; these are, in fact, among the most common manifestations of alcohol abuse in later life.

Assessment of Other Age-Associated Problems

Although not unique to the elderly, a number of problems that affect illness severity, participation in treatment, and prognosis are seen much more commonly in aging persons with AUDs. These problems are listed in Table 26.4. It is essential that screening and assessment be employed for these potential problems to ensure that patients are properly engaged in treatment and effectively managed for relapse risk..

DIFFERENTIAL DIAGNOSIS OF COEXISTING PSYCHIATRIC SYMPTOMS

Depression

As in younger patients, subjective depressive symptoms are present in more than half of older alcoholic patients who enter treatment after recent heavy drinking. More often than not, such depressive symptoms appear to be induced by alcohol, even in cases that meet criteria for major depression, because in a majority of cases scores on depression measures usually fall to normal levels without specific antidepressant treatment after 2 to 4 weeks' sobriety. However, there is also a strong comorbid association between true (nonalcohol-induced) major depression and alcohol dependence across the lifespan, including older adults. Although there is no convincing evidence that depression causes alcoholism in persons not predisposed

Table 26.5.   Alcohol-induced Depression Versus Comorbid Depression*†

Feature	Alcohol-Induced Depression	Comorbid (Persistent) Depression
May meet criteria for major depression	+	+
Prior episodes occurred while drinking	+	+
Begins to improve after just a few days' sobriety	+	−
May take 2–3 weeks to resolve if untreated	+	−
Tends to persist more than 3 weeks if untreated	−	+
First episode may have predated alcohol problems	−	+
Prior episodes occurred during abstinent periods	−	+
Family history of depression/suicide more likely	−	+
Current major life problems/stressors more likely	−	+

*The two conditions may co-occur.
†Table based on Atkinson R: Depression, alcoholism and ageing: a brief review. Int J Geriatr Psychiatry 14:905–910, 1999; and Brown SA, Inaba RK, Gillin JC, Schuckit MA, Stewart MA, Irwin MR: Alcoholism and affective disorder: clinical course of depressive symptoms. Am J Psychiatry 152:45–52, 1995.

to an AUD, once a pattern of excessive alcohol use has been established, negative emotional states associated with depression (e.g., sadness, boredom, anger, tension) may trigger repeated drinking episodes in older patients. Although such alcohol use may afford brief respite from emotional distress (self-medication), it can, over time, further aggravate a comorbid depressive condition. Factors that may help differentiate between alcohol-induced and true comorbid depression in this age group are listed in Table 26.5.

Recently drinking patients judged to suffer from true acute comorbid depression should, of course, be treated promptly and vigorously with antidepressants, as should any other patient suffering severely from depressive symptoms or found to be seriously suicidal, irrespective of the role of alcohol in inducing symptoms. Over the longer term, effective treatment of coexisting depression can result in reduced alcohol consumption, as demonstrated in some studies of mixed-age alcoholic patients, and heavy-drinking elderly depressed patients. However, in cases of mild-to-moderate depression in recently drinking alcoholic patients—cases in which it is unclear whether depressive symptoms are simply alcohol-induced—antidepressant medication should be withheld for up to 2 to 3 weeks if possible, so that remission is not falsely attributed to medication and an unjustified diagnosis of (nonalcohol-induced) depressive disorder can be avoided.

Cognitive Impairment and Dementia

In early sobriety, recovering alcoholic patients often show defects in memory, visual-spatial skills, abstraction, and problem solving that increase with age in frequency, severity, and duration. Such deficits may not fulfill criteria for dementia yet may resolve only over a protracted course of months to years in older patients. In mild cases, residual deficits after a few weeks of sobriety can be

Table 26.6a.   DSM-IV Diagnostic Criteria for Alcohol-Induced Persisting Dementia

A. The development of multiple deficits manifested by both:
  (1) memory impairment (impaired ability to learn new information or to recall previously learned information); and
  (2) one or more of the following cognitive disturbances:
    (a) aphasia (language disturbance);
    (b) apraxia (impaired ability to carry out motor activities despite intact motor function);
    (c) agnosia (failure to recognize or identify objects despite intact sensory function); and/or
    (d) disturbance in executive functioning (i.e., planning, organization, sequencing, abstracting).
B. The cognitive deficits in criteria A1 and A2 each cause significant impairment in social or occupational functioning and represent a significant decline from a previous level of functioning.
C. The deficits do not occur exclusively during the course of a delirium and persist beyond the usual duration of alcohol intoxication or withdrawal.
D. There is evidence from the history, physical examination, or laboratory findings that the deficits are etiologically related to the persisting effects of alcohol use.

sufficiently subtle that a coarse screen for dementia such as the Mini-Mental State Examination will not indicate them. Frank dementia is also commonly associated with alcohol excess (Table 26.6a). In a British community epidemiological survey of the elderly, men with a history of very heavy drinking were 4.6 times more likely to have current dementia than other men. In dementia registries, more than 20% of patients may have a history of alcoholism or heavy drinking.

Neuropsychological and neuroimaging studies point to wide-spread damage to the central nervous system (CNS) in chronic alcoholic patients. Age rather than duration of alcoholism tends to be the most critical factor in the extent of CNS damage. Cortical atrophy reflects loss of both gray and white matter, occurs in older alcoholic individuals beginning at about the fifth decade, and is over and above the changes associated with normal aging. Morphological changes are especially evident in frontal areas, and many of the deficits in cognitive performance also suggest the prominence of frontal lobe dysfunction in chronic alcoholic patients. Compromised metabolism in frontal and prefrontal areas in older chronic alcoholic patients ("hypofrontality") is also suggested by positron emission tomo-graphic studies and studies of regional cerebral blood flow and event-related potentials.

Differential diagnosis between dementia associated with alcohol-ism and Alzheimer's dementia can be difficult; some findings that are potentially useful in differentiating these conditions are offered in Table 26.6b. Alcohol may also be a risk factor, like hypertension, that increases vulnerability to various forms of dementia. Apart from the neurotoxic effects of alcohol and associated vitamin deficiency states, alcoholics are known to be at high risk for repeated head

Table 26.6b.   Features That May Distinguish Between Alcohol-Related and Alzheimer's Dementias*†

Feature	Alcohol-Induced Persisting Dementia	Alzheimer's Dementia
Meets criteria for dementia	+	+
Cortical atrophy on MRI	+	+
Long history of heavy drinking	+	−
Ataxia may be present	+	−
Peripheral polyneuropathy may be present	+	−
Cerebellar atrophy may be present on MRI	+	−
Abstinence halts cognitive decline	+	−
Cortical atrophy can be reversed	+	−
Anomia/dyanomia prominent	−	+
Cognitive decline continues despite abstinence	−	+
CSF tsu protein may be elevated	−	+

*Symbols "+" and "−" mean that the finding is more (+) or less (−) likely to be associated with this form of dementia: MRI = magnetic resonance imaging of the brain; CSF = cerebrospinal fluid.
†Based on Morikawa Y, Arai H, Matsushita S, Kato M, Higuchi S, Miura M, Kawakami H, Higuchi M, Okamura N, Tashiro M, Matsui T, Sasaki H: Cerebrospinal fluid tau protein levels in demented and nondemented alcoholics. Alcohol Clin Exp Res 23:575–577, 1999; Oslin D, Atkinson RM, Smith DM, Hendrie H: Alcohol related dementia: proposed clinical criteria. Int J Geriatr Psychiatry 13:203–212, 1998.

trauma and infectious diseases that could also predispose to dementia. In addition, heavy drinking aggravates cardiovascular diseases and thus can contribute indirectly to a vascular presentation of dementia.

TREATMENT, PROGNOSIS, AND OUTCOME

"Brief Intervention" for Risky Drinkers

Brief intervention is based on two principles: that simple advice can influence drinking behavior, and that the public health model of harm reduction (by reducing alcohol consumption) is a valid goal that may be more attainable than abstinence for patients who do not have severe alcohol dependence. This approach is effective in reducing alcohol intake in aging heavy drinkers who do not yet have significant alcohol-related problems, and also in mild cases of alcohol dependence and circumscribed problem drinking. Typically, it is a primary care physician who conducts this intervention, although any clinician can do so. Studies are currently under way in which geriatric caseworkers are trained to conduct brief interventions. In one randomized controlled trial in which 146 risky drinking elderly outpatients in 24 primary care practice sites were assigned to receive either a brief intervention or a control intervention (in which generalized health promotion advice was given), drinking was reduced by 36% in patients receiving advice to cut down, compared with no change in controls. Another multisite trial found comparable results, using home visitation by a psychologist or social worker to deliver a similar intervention.

General Issues in the Treatment of Geriatric AUDs

It is important to present information thoroughly and objectively to the patient and key collaterals (in the elderly age group this may be a professional caregiver, friend, or adult child rather than a spouse). It is helpful to emphasize that older persons with drinking problems actually tend to fare as well as, or better than, younger persons in a variety of treatment settings. Treatment has three aims: (1) reduce or cease alcohol use; (2) treat medical and psychiatric comorbidities; and (3) engender psychosocial and other changes to reduce the risk of relapse. Persons with more severe or complicated alcohol dependence should receive treatment in a specialized outpatient alcoholism program that begins with an intensive phase lasting up to several months. Ambulatory, gradual detoxification is often achieved without resorting to medications or hospital admission. Medications to reduce craving, such as naltrexone, may be helpful. For evaluation, consultation, and management of comorbid conditions, a program must have effective links to community social service agencies for the elderly and to general physicians and psychiatrists who are knowledgeable about geriatric problems.

In the most serious cases, including patients who have not been helped by outpatient treatment, such patients should be referred to an inpatient chemical dependency treatment unit— ideally, one where the staff is experienced in treating older adults. If severe medical or psychiatric complications are present or major withdrawal is anticipated or already occurring, initial treatment should take place in an acute inpatient medical or psychiatric unit, followed by transfer to a chemical dependency unit after stabilization. Intractable heavy drinking in the presence of dementia or other coexisting major mental disorder may force placement of the patient in long-term residential care, where, unfortunately, alcoholic patients are not always welcomed. In a few locales, alcohol-free foster homes and other residential facilities have been established, staffed by personnel trained to care for recovering alcoholic patients in an accepting manner.

Setting a Proper Tone for Treatment of the Older Alcoholic

In all interactions with elderly alcoholics, treatment staff should strive to be emotionally supportive, practical, and straightforward. Attention must be given to simple, clear communications paced to the older patient's slower tempo of information processing. Confrontational and "psychologizing" strategies should be avoided or used very judiciously and only for selected patients. Aging patients are often distressed by discussions they view as critical of parents, spouse, or other family members, or approaches that seek to provoke strong emotional displays. Profanity and accounts by younger patients of antisocial behavior in connection with substance abuse are often repugnant to older patients. Simple social amenities should always be observed. For example, the pseudointimacy (or, worse yet, infantilization) implied when calling patients by their first names is especially inappropriate for this age group. In both group therapies and individual case management, the mental health model of supportive treatment and problem-solving is a more useful paradigm for this age group than more conventional substance abuse treatment models intended for younger adults, which challenge the patient to be more honest and self-reliant. Gentle rather than tough love is in order for aging alcoholics. The ideal staff for work with elders are professionals who are comfortable with this age group and who have some training and experience in social gerontology and mental health, as well as substance abuse.

Psychosocial Treatments

Motivational counseling has generally displaced more confrontational crisis-precipitation techniques as the preferred approach to the older alcoholic patient who initially resists advice to enter treatment. Whenever it is possible to aggregate several older patients in the same treatment program, *age-specific group treatment* is indicated, because such arrangements foster peer bonding, shared reminiscence, longer retention in treatment, and improved drinking outcomes. When this is not possible, *individual case management* is the best approach, ideally using nursing personnel or other clinical personnel trained in social gerontology and addictions. Case management is also required for many patients in elder-specific, group-based treatment programs. *Family engagement* in the program tends to enhance treatment retention and efficacy. *Cognitive-behavioral* psychotherapeutic and educational methods, using specific, manual-assisted techniques, have also proved useful with older adult alcoholics. Participation in *Alcoholics Anonymous* is often beneficial, particularly when meetings are organized specifically for this age group.

Pharmacological Treatments

Use of the deterrent drug disulfiram can be hazardous in older patients because of the risk of a cardiovascular crisis precipitated by acetaldehyde toxicity if the patient drinks while taking disulfiram, and because of disulfiram hepatotoxicity. Naltrexone appears to be safe in geriatric usage and has shown some promise for reducing the extent of drinking lapses. Reports are lacking on the safety and efficacy of acamprosate in elderly persons, but it could prove equal to naltrexone in reducing craving and severe drinking lapses in this population. Although antidepressant drugs appear to reduce drinking in alcoholic elders who have current comorbid depression (see discussion earlier), there is no evidence that these agents deter drinking in older nondepressed patients.

Treatment Adherence and Outcome: The Evidence Base

As a group, older alcoholic patients seem to respond to alcoholism treatment as well as, or better than, younger alcoholic patients. Older patients are more likely to continue in longer term outpatient treatment than younger patients. Court-supervised older drinking drivers and married elders whose spouses participate in treatment are more likely to continue in treatment than their same-age peers who lack such third-party involvement. In a study comparing 1-year drinking outcomes of older alcoholics randomly assigned either to an age-specific inpatient alcoholism treatment unit (ATU) or to an age-heterogeneous ATU in the same facility, patients treated in the age-specific program were more likely to be abstinent a year later. In Project MATCH (Matching Alcoholism Treatments to Client Heterogeneity), the large, multisite, outpatient alcoholism treatment study, patients aged 60 years and older (7% of the sample) fared well. Their

12-month post-treatment drinking outcomes were highly favorable—as successful as those of younger patients—and equally successful for each of the three treatment conditions compared in the study: a cognitive-behavioral condition; motivational counseling; and a 12-step counseling model adapted from Alcoholics Anonymous (each modality was randomly assigned and individually administered in weekly sessions for 3 months).

ALCOHOL AND HEALTH MAINTENANCE

Does Moderate Drinking Help to Maintain Good Health?

The use of small amounts of beverage alcohol has been advocated as a safe social adjuvant in elder residential care facilities, but more comprehensive management of the facility milieu may better ensure optimal socialization. Alcohol has also long been touted as an appetite stimulant. In healthy elderly persons, caloric intake and blood levels of some micronutrients may increase with alcohol intake, although other micronutrient levels may decrease. Use of alcohol to aid sleep is problematic because regular alcohol late in the evening is apt to disorganize sleep. If moderate drinking is advised, several cautions apply. The list of potentially hazardous interactions of alcohol with chronic medical disorders and medications is lengthy (see prior discussion). Clinicians who advise outpatients to use alcohol should recall that in the residential studies quantity was carefully regulated and use within a social context was ensured. The National Institute on Alcohol Abuse and Alcoholism advises that *healthy* elderly persons should limit themselves to no more than one standard drink daily, or seven standard drinks per week, and no more than two drinks per drinking occasion.

Does Moderate Alcohol Use Prevent Coronary Heart Disease (CHD)?

An intriguing aspect of the alcohol and health maintenance debate is the well-validated association of regular but moderate alcohol use (one to two drinks/day) with lower morbidity and mortality from CHD, especially in men, compared with heavy alcohol users *and abstainers*. Why do teetotalers have higher rates of severe CHD than moderate drinkers do? One possible explanation is that the heterogeneous abstainer group might include subgroups at high risk for CHD (e.g., former alcoholics and others in poor health). Indeed, this tends to be the case. A past history of alcohol dependence also nullifies health-protective effects of current light or moderate alcohol use. In one large study, older persons who had experienced adverse health events or who demonstrated fewer adaptive coping skills were more commonly represented among abstainers than among moderate drinkers. Unfortunately, a number of studies have not controlled for such variables, including the two studies to date that report a "protective" effect of alcohol against CHD, which have focused exclusively on samples of elderly patients.

More recent mixed-age studies have provided such controls and still demonstrated a protective effect of alcohol in CHD. Studies suggest a number of biological mechanisms that may help explain the protective effects of alcohol in CHD, including alcohol-induced increase in an antiatherogenic fraction of circulating high-density lipoprotein cholesterol; anticoagulant effects; antioxidant effects;

decreases in circulating fasting insulin and fasting insulin resistance index values; and increased activation of epsilon protein kinase C in cardiac muscle.

Does Moderate Drinking Protect Against Other Late-Life Health Problems?

A smaller, more general apparent protective effect of moderate drinking on mortality from all causes has been demonstrated in several studies. Much of this overall effect is attributable to reduced mortality from cardiovascular diseases. Aggregated all-cause mortality rates obscure the fact that several important causes either have no association with alcohol consumption (e.g., deaths caused by colorectal cancer, hemorrhagic stroke, pneumonia and respiratory diseases) or a linear relationship in which any level of consumption is more likely to be associated with mortality than not drinking at all (e.g., deaths caused by alcoholism, accidents, and liver cirrhosis). Several reports suggest that moderate alcohol intake may have a beneficial effect on cognitive status, and even a possible protective effect against development of age-related retinal macular degeneration. These phenomena require further study.

SUGGESTED READINGS

Atkinson RM: Substance abuse. In: Coffey CE, Cummings JL (eds.), Textbook of Geriatric Neuropsychiatry, 2nd Edition. Washington, D.C.: American Psychiatric Press, 2000, pp. 367–400.

Barry KL, Oslin DW, Blow FC: Alcohol Problems in Older Adults: Prevention and Management. New York: Springer, 2001.

Beresford TP, Gomberg ESL (eds.): Alcohol and Aging. New York: Oxford University Press, 1995.

Center for Substance Abuse Treatment: Substance Abuse Among Older Adults: Treatment Improvement Protocol #26, DHHS Publication No. (SMA) 98–3179. Rockville, MD: U. S. Department of Health and Human Services, Public Health Service, Substance Abuse and Mental Health Services Administration, 1998.

Gurnack AM (ed.): Special issue: Drugs and the elderly: use and misuse of drugs, medicines, alcohol, and tobacco. Int J Addict 30:1685–2027, 1995.

Gurnack AM, Atkinson R, Osgood NJ (eds.): Treating Alcohol and Drug Abuse in the Elderly. New York: Springer, 2002.

ALCOHOL PROBLEMS IN WOMEN

Sheila B. Blume

Alcohol problems in women are hardly a recent phenomenon. The first book of Solomon in the Hebrew Bible tells the story of Hannah, a childless woman who prays at the temple of Shiloh to become pregnant. As she prays, moving her mouth soundlessly, she is observed by the priest Eli, who assumes she is drunk. His response to her may be the first recorded attempt at alcoholism treatment for a woman. He says, "How long will you make yourself a drunken spectacle? Throw off your wine from you." This approach of social pressure and shaming (here combined with a recommendation of total abstinence) has been commonly used for centuries with not very promising results.

Throughout history, societies that have allowed the use of alcohol have adopted different rules for its use by men and women. The earliest known example is the Code of Hammurabi, dating from ancient Babylonia in the 18th century BCE. In this first codification of laws, priestesses (but not priests) are forbidden to enter or own a wine shop. In the early days of ancient Rome, before the republic was established, the Law of Romulus forbade all alcohol use by women in the same sentence that forbade adultery by women.

SOCIETAL BELIEF, STEREOTYPE, AND STIGMA

It is logical to assume that both formal and informal rules for acceptable drinking in each culture are based on that society's beliefs about the differential effects of alcohol on the two sexes. The most important belief in Western society regarding drinking by women is that alcohol stimulates women's sexual desire and responsiveness. The Talmud counsels moderation for women, stating that drinking more than one cup of wine induces a woman to be immoral. The ancient Romans explained that women were not allowed to drink because alcohol stimulates women to lust. Cases of Roman women having been put to death for this offense by stoning or by starvation were recorded.

This idea persisted in Western thought. Chaucer, in the Wife of Bath's Prologue in his *Canterbury Tales*, written in the 14th century, has this uninhibited woman tell the story of a Roman husband who beat his wife to death for drinking. The Wife of Bath states that if she had been that woman, her husband would not have stopped her. She enjoys drinking because it always makes her "think of Venus." She comments, "A woman in her cups has no defense, as lechers know from long experience." As the poet Ogden Nash put it even more succinctly 600 years later, "Candy is dandy, but liquor is quicker."

Studies of sexual arousal and orgasm in adult women have shown that this societal stereotype is incorrect. Alcohol is a depressant of both sexual arousal and orgasmic intensity. In addition, alcohol delays the onset of orgasm. Furthermore, alcohol depresses sexual responsiveness in a dose-response relationship: The higher the blood alcohol level, the greater the effect.

In spite of the reality of alcohol's depressant effect, research in the general population finds the idea that alcohol is a sexual stimulant for women is also a part of American culture. Two groups of undergraduates were shown videotapes of a young woman being interviewed, which were identical in every respect except that in one version she had an unopened container of beer on the table and in the other an unopened container of soda. The students responded to the version with the beer as an indication that the young woman was more likely to indulge in sexual behavior than the one who had the can of soda beside her. In another study, a group of sexually active university women were asked to keep a 90-day diary of their activities and everything they ate or drank. When these diaries were returned to the researchers, the subjects were told that one of the objectives of the study was to examine the relationship between drinking and sexual behavior. They were asked what they thought their diaries would show. Most said that they thought the record would show that drinking stimulated them sexually. When they were analyzed, the diaries showed no relationship between drinking and sexual arousal, pleasure, or orgasm. Initiation of sexual contact was inversely related to drinking. This study illustrates the power of cultural beliefs on the women's expectations, even in the face of data carefully collected by the subjects themselves.

As our society believes that women who drink desire sex, a woman's drunkenness is accepted as an excuse for sexual assault. When a woman who has been drinking says "no", it is assumed that she really means "yes". In a study of attitudes about rape, young adults were asked to rate rape scenarios that differed only in whether the victim, perpetrator, neither, or both were depicted as intoxicated. Both men and women rated the perpetrator less responsible for the crime if he was intoxicated, whereas the victim was rated more to blame if she had been drinking.

Western culture stigmatizes the alcoholic woman in three ways. She shares the general stigma applied to problem drinkers as a self-indulgent person lacking in will power. To this is added the expectation that women, as bearers of culture to the next generation, should adhere to a higher standard of behavior ("putting women on a pedestal"), so that women are more severely criticized if their actions are found wanting. Finally, the expectation that drinking makes women "think of Venus" renders them fair game for sexual assault, including date rape.

A variety of studies show that women who drink are more likely to be victimized in a wide variety of ways. In a survey of domestic homicide, women who used alcohol were 1.4 times more likely to be killed in their own homes than women who were abstinent. Another study of partner femicide (killing one's wife) found diagnosable alcohol abuse or dependence in 10.5% of the victims of femicide or attempted femicide, compared with 7.6% of victims of domestic violence whose lives were not threatened and 1.9% of a matched control group. Alcohol use disorders were found in 49.6% of the femicide perpetrators, compared with 32.3% of the batterers who did not threaten death and 6.9% of control partners. In a series of surveys comparing women aged 18 to 54 years recruited from Alcoholics Anonymous (AA) and alcoholism treatment with matched community controls, spousal violence of all kinds (verbal, slapping, kicking, beating, threatening life) was found significantly more prevalent against the alcoholic women than against the controls. Likewise, these women were more likely to report being the victim of violent crime by other than a spouse or partner (61% compared with 20% of controls), including rape (33% compared with 8%.)

In addition to promoting violence against women who drink, the societal stereotype of the alcoholic woman as a sexually promiscuous "fallen woman" and its resulting stigma also increases denial in the alcoholic woman, her family, and the professionals who might be able to help her. When a woman is having problems related to drinking, she tends to blame them on depression, insomnia, stress, or environmental factors. The alcoholic woman compared with the alcoholic man is more likely to look for help from her primary care physician or a mental health facility than the alcoholism treatment system. She reasons that because she is nothing like our society's concept of an alcoholic woman, the problem must be something other than alcoholism. Family members reason similarly and are more likely to dissuade a female than a male alcoholic from seeking specific treatment. A study from Johns Hopkins University Hospital screened all patients admitted to the hospital for alcohol problems and then examined records to see how many were recognized and how often alcoholism treatment was recommended. The problem drinkers least likely to be identified and treated were those who were of higher socioeconomic status, had more education, had private insurance, and who were women. Thus, those who least matched the societal stereotype of a skid row derelict or fallen woman were seldom recognized. The middle-class professional woman must often be in the late stages of alcoholism before her clinician even considers the diagnosis.

Stigma is closely linked to shame, one of the factors that dictates the tendency of alcoholic women to drink alone, often at home, and to defer treatment, even if they are aware of an alcohol problem and desire to stop drinking. Because alcoholic women are often separated or divorced and are therefore single parents, women who hide their drinking at home may be observed only by minor children who are in no position to intervene. In contrast to women, who fight the disease on their own, the more exposed drinking of men presents greater opportunities for intervention..

ALCOHOLISM: A MAN'S DISEASE

Anthropological and epidemiological studies of male and female drinking patterns in cultures throughout the world find that men drink more than women in nearly all cultural groups, but that in no culture do women drink more than men. The relative extent of male-female differences in alcohol intake varies widely in different parts of the world. In general, men drink more frequently than women and consume more per drinking occasion. Women are more likely than men to be abstainers at all ages. In the United States, the average drinking woman consumes only about half as much as the average drinking man. The U.S. Department of Agriculture Dietary Guidelines recommends that for those adults who have no contraindications (e.g., pregnancy, history of alcoholism) and choose to drink, an acceptable level is defined as no more than one drink on any given day for a woman and two for a man.

Studies of alcohol use disorders also find that more males than females suffer from alcohol abuse and dependence, with a ratio of males to females of about 2.2 to 2.5:1, depending on the study. The National Comorbidity Study, a general population study of persons aged 15 to 54 years of age, found a male:female ratio of 2.2:1 for lifetime prevalence of alcohol abuse or dependence and 2.7:1 for 12-month prevalence. This may explain why, traditionally, alcoholism was considered a disease of men, and alcoholic women were considered aberrant cases. It is interesting that two studies of populations of Jewish alcoholics in the United States found male:female ratios close to 1:1, suggesting that ratios may vary by subgroup. Among adolescent populations in the United States, the intake of girls is closer to the intake of boys than among adults, and the rates of alcohol problems among those who drink are more similar.

Until the 1980s, nearly all research into the physiology and effects of alcohol as well as alcohol problems and alcohol-related diseases was done with male populations. In those studies that contained both sexes, the data were seldom analyzed separately; therefore, sex-related differences were not recognized. Although research was done on male populations, the results were assumed to apply to females as well. Treatment programs were designed for men. The women's movement of the 1970s raised the consciousness of both clinicians and policy makers about the importance of alcohol problems in women and the need to study these problems. The description of the fetal alcohol syndrome in 1972 further highlighted the need to understand alcoholism in women. When appropriate research was carried out, it was discovered that male-female differences occur in a wide variety of areas, ranging from the absorption and metabolism of alcohol to the clinical presentation and progression of alcohol dependence. It became clear that women have different treatment needs that were not always met by male-oriented programs.

AA, which was founded by two alcoholic men in 1935, began to admit women in the 1940s. The presence of female alcoholics in AA was controversial, and, at meetings, men and women often sat on opposite sides of the room. At some meetings, women met with the wives of male AA members rather than with the members themselves. Although the 12 steps were formulated by the earliest AA members, most of whom were men, the program has helped many thousands of women achieve and maintain sobriety. All-female meetings are available in many areas, and female sponsorship has helped make AA more comfortable for new women members. A 1998 survey of more than 6000 members of AA found a male:female ratio of 2:1, which had remained unchanged for the 10 years.

PHYSIOLOGICAL FACTORS AND MEDICAL COMPLICATIONS

Women are more sensitive to the physical effects of alcohol than men. Given a standard dose of alcohol, women experience higher blood alcohol levels. Because the alcohol that is absorbed into the bloodstream is distributed in the total body water, women's smaller size and lower proportion of body water explain part of this effect. However, even when the dose is corrected for weight and body water, women absorb more of the alcohol they drink. The alcohol-metabolizing enzyme, alcohol dehydrogenase, present in the gastric mucosa, breaks down some of the alcohol consumed while it is still in the stomach. Normal females have significantly less of this enzyme than males. Alcoholic women have even less of the enzyme and absorb essentially all of the alcohol they drink. This difference is thought to explain, in part, the fact that women experience liver damage due to alcohol at lower levels of drinking than men. Estrogens are also thought to contribute to this higher incidence of liver disease. Alcoholic women have also been observed to experience cardiomyopathy more readily and to develop greater loss of brain volume than men with comparable drinking histories.

In addition to the greater propensity of women to develop medical complications from excessive alcohol use, the course of these medical complications (including fatty liver, hypertension, anemia, malnutrition, and gastrointestinal hemorrhage) and the alcohol dependence itself differs with sex. Disease progresses more rapidly in women, a phenomenon known as the "telescoping effect" (the course of the disease is collapsed like a telescope). Although physiological causes have been postulated for this sex difference, there may also be psychosocial factors involved, because a similar telescoping effect has been described in female pathological gamblers compared with their male counterparts.

Research on genetic factors in the etiology of alcohol dependence has included both male and female subjects. Although the role of genetics in alcoholism is yet to be understood, there are no current studies that find sex differences in genetic susceptibility. A large study of female twin pairs found a genetic influence of about 50% to 60%.

The female reproductive system is affected by drinking in many ways. Even nonabusive drinking has been linked to a higher risk of breast cancer, although the effect has been found to be small in some studies. Heavy drinking is associated with an increased incidence of sexually transmitted diseases (STDs). Among young women, the use of a condom during intercourse is less likely if there is heavy alcohol use, making the drinker more at risk for unwanted pregnancy, HIV infection, and other STDs.

Although single doses of alcohol have little effect on sex hormone levels, regular drinking by prepubertal girls is thought to delay and interfere with menarche. In older girls and women, long-term heavy drinking is associated with a wide variety of sexual dysfunctions. Irregular menses and infertility are frequent. Other complaints of alcoholic women include a loss of interest in sex, anorgasmia, vaginismus (spasm of the vagina), painful intercourse, luteal phase dysfunction, and early menopause. The relationship between drinking and sexual dysfunction in women is complex. Some types of dysfunction may precede heavy drinking but become worse as a result of alcohol intake. As explained earlier, there is a cultural belief that alcohol is a sexual stimulant for women, even though the truth is quite the opposite. It has been shown that many alcoholic women in treatment are reluctant or afraid to have sexual intercourse after they stop drinking because of the mistaken idea that drinking has helped their sex life. Such women can be reassured that a study of married women entering treatment for alcoholism found remarkable increases in sexual desire, capacity, and responsiveness once abstinence from alcohol was established.

Among heavy drinkers who do become pregnant, the risk for birth defects is greatly increased. Both fetal alcohol syndrome and other alcohol-related birth defects are a major cause of disability. A 1992 study of in-hospital live births found that 19% of women reported alcohol use during pregnancy. About 5% admitted to drinking 14 or more drinks per week during this period. Taken together, the greater sensitivity to alcohol among women and the risk of alcohol-related birth defects indicate that early intervention and vigorous treatment of women with drinking problems should be a major societal goal.

SOCIOCULTURAL FACTORS

In addition to the influence of genetic predisposition, cultural values, norms, and rules play an important part in women's alcohol problems. The cultural expectation that women drink less than men do and only on special occasions in mixed company (whereas men drink on more frequent occasions and in all-male groups as well as mixed-sex groups) protects women from heavy drinking. Factors that break down social protections, such as leaving home for college or work or entering nontraditional settings (e.g., medical school, military service), tend to increase women's drinking. Advertisements for alcoholic beverages have aimed at the female market, aware that women often purchase the beverages for both members of a couple, and that women consume far less alcohol than men. These advertisements have tried to link drinking with empowerment and to encourage the violation of cultural expectations, for example, by showing women drinking with other women and on other-than-special occasions. If women are ever convinced to drink as much as men, their greater sensitivity to alcohol will result in more problems among women than among their male counterparts.

PSYCHOLOGICAL FACTORS

The greater prevalence of comorbid psychiatric illness is a particularly robust finding in research on alcoholic women. Whether the data are derived from clinical or general population samples, women show greater rates of most Axis I disorders than men in the American Psychiatric Association's classification of psychiatric disorders. The only exception is pathological gambling. Antisocial personality disorder (an Axis II diagnosis) is also more common in alcoholic men. However, among women who do have antisocial personality disorder, the rate of alcoholism is greatly increased.

In addition, women and adolescent girls are more likely to have experienced the onset of the psychiatric disorder before their alcohol-use disorder was manifest (i.e., the psychiatric disorder is primary). This is true for major depression and anxiety disorders, including post-traumatic stress disorder. In treating alcoholic women, establishing the temporal order of onset of comorbid disorders is of the greatest importance. Depressed alcoholic women who experience the onset of major depression before their alcoholism are less likely to recover from depression as a result of stopping drinking and more likely to require specific depression treatment. Data from populations in treatment for both alcoholism and depression show better outcomes if the comorbid disorder is successfully treated. These dually diagnosed patients must also be educated to be aware of early signs of recurrent depression, because vigorous treatment of these recurrences helps the patient avoid a relapse into alcohol dependence.

Research into psychological factors that contribute to problem drinking in women shows that in college-age women, low self-esteem and the use of alcohol as a way to feel better on dates predict later problems. Major depression has been found to increase the risk for later development of alcohol abuse or dependence in women by 2.6 to 4.1 times. Sexual abuse in childhood is a strong risk factor for both alcohol and drug problems in adult life. A large general population study found the risk increased by a factor of three for alcohol dependence and four for other drug dependence in women with a history of sexual assault, whereas a large twin study found four times the risk for alcohol dependence and 5.7 times the risk for dependence on other drugs.

CASEFINDING

When patients in alcoholism treatment are asked what problems prompted them to seek help, men and women give different replies. In men, problems on the job and with the law are most common. Women most frequently mention problems with health and family. Current programs to identify and refer problem drinkers tend to concentrate on workplace and the justice system (e.g., employee assistance and drinking driver programs). This may help explain why women are under-represented in alcoholism treatment.

Screening women for alcohol problems in health settings yields far higher rates of alcohol problems than are found in the general population. For example, 11% to 17% of medical and surgical outpatients and 12.5% of obstetrics-gynecology inpatients have screened positive in various studies. Either standard screening tools such as the CAGE (*C*ut down, *A*nnoyed, *G*uilty, *E*ye-opener) or AUDIT (Alcohol Use Disorders Identification Test) may be used, or special screening tools, such as the TWEAK, designed for women.

CLINICAL FEATURES OF ALCOHOLISM IN WOMEN AND ADOLESCENT GIRLS

Women begin to experience drinking problems at later ages than men but reach treatment at a similar age and similar level of severity (an illustration of the telescoping effect). They are more likely to relate the onset of their heavy drinking to a stressful event such as divorce, illness, or death of someone close to them. They drink significantly less than alcoholic men, both as a result of their greater sensitivity to alcohol and the fact that their drinking is more often accompanied by the abuse of sedatives, usually iatrogenic in origin. The morning (and/or afternoon) drink for a male alcoholic may be substituted by a dose of diazepam (Valium) for an alcoholic woman, and she may not begin to drink until evening.

Alcoholic women are more likely than men to have diagnoses of comorbid psychiatric disorders, as mentioned earlier, including eating disorders (particularly bulimia) and posttraumatic stress disorder, as well as major depression and other anxiety disorders. They are more likely to make suicidal attempts than men are, although men are more likely to complete suicide. Finally, alcoholic women have a very high mortality rate compared with the general population of women and with alcoholic men. For example, in one Swedish study of 4000 male alcoholics and 1000 female alcoholics who were followed for 2 to 22 years, the mortality rate for males was 3 times the expected rate, whereas for females it was 5.2 times the age-corrected expected rate for Swedish women.

PRINCIPLES OF TREATMENT FOR ALCOHOLIC WOMEN AND ADOLESCENT GIRLS

Based on the findings outlined in the preceding section, there is first a need for systematic screening for alcohol (and other drug) problems in obstetric and other medical-surgical populations, as well as in the family service, justice, and employment assistance systems. Once positive screening identifies a female problem drinker, intervention must be sensitive to stigma and the resulting shame universal among these women and girls. Assessment should include careful attention to physical and psychiatric comorbidity as well as the abuse of other drugs, usually prescribed benzodiazepines, other sedatives, or analgesics. Pregnancy testing and screening for STDs are recommended. When there are comorbid psychiatric disorders, an attempt should be made, as a guide to treatment, to determine which disorder is primary (that is, of earlier onset). Sensitivity is also required in eliciting a possible history of physical and/or sexual abuse. Alcoholic women who are living with current domestic violence may need temporary safe housing before treatment can begin.

The detoxification phase of treatment should include attention to the possibility of added sedative withdrawal. Treatment of comorbid affective and anxiety disorders should avoid the use of any medication with abuse potential.

Family assessment and involvement is especially necessary in treating alcoholic women. Their children should be assessed for fetal alcohol effects if the patients have a history of drinking during pregnancy, and help should be offered that is designed for children of alcoholic mothers. The patient's parenting skills, often weak because the patient herself came from an alcoholic or disrupted family, can be improved through counseling or special programs. Other special services include deep relaxation training, especially useful for those with anxiety disorders and insomnia, education on sexual functioning and pregnancy issues, and vocational rehabilitation. All of these can be added to the basic rehabilitation counseling at the appropriate time.

Much has been written about whether women do better in all-female programs than in those serving both sexes. There is little in the published literature to offer guidance. Often, the structure of the treatment setting is dictated by economic and social necessity. At the halfway house or recovery home level, separation of the sexes seems to be more practical and to make more sense than in detoxification, hospital, or outpatient clinic settings. In mixed settings, where group therapy is the primary modality, an all-female group can be helpful, especially for women and girls with sexual abuse issues. This can be either the primary therapy group or an additional group specifically focused on women's needs. If single-sex groups are not available, additional individual therapy may be added to give female patients a chance to explore these difficult areas. Women should be helped to understand and participate in self-help groups such as AA or Women for Sobriety (an all-women self-help group available in some areas).

BARRIERS TO TREATMENT

Several large studies of problem drinkers in the community have shown that women are less likely to seek and receive appropriate treatment than men are. Women are more likely to be unemployed or underemployed (e.g., in part-time jobs or service jobs) and therefore to lack health insurance. They are more likely to be single parents without resources and in need of child care services in order to take part in treatment. Programs that serve the needs of both the alcoholic woman and her children are successful and highly desirable but nearly nonexistent in most areas of the country. Child abuse/neglect regulations in many states penalize a woman who requests help from the child protective service system by automatically defining her as a child neglecter and putting her at risk of losing custody. In some states, pregnant alcoholics and addicts risk involuntary commitment or even criminal prosecution for "prenatal child abuse." Political and social action is clearly required to reduce these barriers.

PREVENTION OF ALCOHOL PROBLEMS IN GIRLS AND WOMEN

Little information specific to girls and women is included in the alcoholism prevention programs currently offered. Education about drinking in pregnancy is spotty, and screening in health and human service agencies is seldom a routine practice. Aid given to women who are undergoing stressful life events—such as leaving home, giving care to a chronically ill family member, dealing with physical or sexual victimization, or undergoing separation, divorce, or bereavement—would be useful, especially if preventing drinking as an effort to deal with distress is specifically included. Other measures to prevent alcoholism and its toll on women would include changes in social attitudes and removal of the stigma, which would require intense public education. Our society has a long way to go before the insights of science and clinical medicine are understood and applied to the prevention and treatment of alcoholism in women.

SUGGESTED READINGS

Blume SB: Women: clinical aspects. In: Lowinson JR, Millman RP, Langrod RB (eds.), Substance Abuse: A Comprehensive Textbook, 3rd Edition. Baltimore: Williams & Wilkins, 1997, pp. 645–654.

Blume SB: Understanding addictive diseases in women. In: Graham AW, Schultz TK (eds.): Principles of Addiction Medicine. Chevy Chase, MD: American Society of Addiction Medicine, 1998, pp. 1173–1190.

Blume SB: Addiction in women. In: Galanter M, Kleber HD (eds.), Textbook of Substance Abuse Treatment, 2nd Edition. Washington, D.C.: American Psychiatric Press, 1999, pp. 485–490.

Greenfield SF, O'Leary G: Sex differences in substance use disorders. In: Lewis-Hall F, Williams TS, Panetta JA, Herrera JM (eds.), Psychiatric Illness in Women: Emerging Treatments and Research. Washington, D.C.: American Psychiatric Press, 2002, pp. 467–533.

Russell M, Martier SS, Sokol RJ, Mudar P, Jacobson S, Jacobson J: Detecting risk drinking during pregnancy: a comparison of four screening questionnaires. Am J Public Health 86:1435–1439, 1996.

Wilsnack RW, Wilsnack SC (eds.): Gender and Alcohol: Individual and Social Perspectives. New Brunswick, NJ: Rutgers Center for Alcohol Studies, 1997.

BRIEF BEHAVIORAL COMPLIANCE ENHANCEMENT TREATMENT (BBCET) MANUAL*

Bankole A. Johnson
Carlo C. DiClemente
Nassima Ait-Daoud
Suzette M. Stoks

Abstract

This manual describes a brief (15-minute to 30-minute) standardized treatment program to be used in conjunction with a pharmacological intervention for the treatment of alcohol dependence. The purpose of the treatment is to increase and enhance compliance with the medication and other aspects of the treatment regimen. The manual describes a typical 12-week medication program that could be adapted for varying periods of time depending on the medication and the optimal course of treatment. Each session addresses patient issues related to the experience and tolerability of side effects, issues of safety and effectiveness, personal barriers to compliance, and a focus on how medication can assist the patient to achieve goals related to the control of drinking. The treatment emphasizes the role of medication and a problem-solving approach to resolving any difficulties related to compliance and modification of drinking. Included are descriptions of typical cases and interactions with patients. Although designed for use with clinical trials of medication treatments, this treatment can be used in primary care settings and with a variety of adjunctive treatments. In addition, the treatment can be adapted for use with medication management of other drugs of abuse.

Introduction

This treatment was developed to be an adjunct to pharmacological treatment protocols that address alcohol dependence. Because many

* *Disclaimer:* This manual provides information on how to deliver a compliance enhancement treatment as an adjunct to pharmacotherapy for alcoholism. The reader should be aware that the accurate delivery of this standardized intervention requires training. This training, as well as updates and operationalized techniques for delivery of this manual-driven intervention, can be obtained by contacting the authors at the South Texas Addiction Research and Technology (START) Center. Telephone: 210-562-5404; web page: http://www.uthscsa.edu/STARTcenter/.

patients come to these treatments convinced that medication can be a useful aid to modifying their drinking, the treatment focuses on increasing the behavioral compliance with the medication regimen by enhancing the expectations of effectiveness of the medication. This compliance enhancement treatment emphasizes how the medication and compliance with the medication are the critical elements for changing the patient's drinking behavior. Compliance management is a brief or minimal intervention treatment. Brief interventions for alcohol problems (such as motivational interviewing, physician advice, and education) have been used in a variety of settings and are being increasingly studied in medical settings (Brady et al., 2002; Smith et al., 2003; Chang et al., 1999; Wright et al., 1998; Fleming, 1993). Current research indicates that the use of brief interventions for alcohol problems is gaining acceptance among physicians and members of the medical community (Saitz et al., 2000; Graham et al., 2000; Carnegie et al., 1996). Results of Project TrEAT (Trial for Early Alcohol Treatment) (Fleming et al., 2002) showed that a brief physician advice intervention yielded positive changes that were maintained over the 48-month follow-up period. The benefit-cost analysis suggested that for every $10,000 invested in early intervention, there was a $43,000 reduction in future health care costs. Minimal interventions, such as the brief advice of Edwards et al. (1977), have proved to be active and effective treatments. The clinical management condition in the National Institute of Mental Health (NIMH) collaborative trial on depression was essentially a compliance management intervention and was found to be a rather significant intervention that compared well with other, more sophisticated psychotherapies (Imber et al., 1990). This Brief Behavioral Compliance Enhancement Treatment (BBCET) for alcohol dependence has been modeled after the clinical management condition in the NIMH collaborative trial (Fawcett et al., 1987).

Treatment Phases

BBCET can be conceptualized as having three phases: Phase One is focused on initiating treatment; Phase Two focuses on maintaining commitment to treatment, and Phase Three deals with phasing out the medication and terminating treatment.

In Phase One of this 12-week treatment, the health care providers engage the patient in a positive relationship and inspire confidence in the treatment by creating an atmosphere of warmth and trust. They convey a positive and optimistic attitude about the use of the medication and the patient's outcome. In each session, the provider communicates and discusses medication effects, side effects, and compliance barriers with the patient in understandable terms, and clearly conveys knowledge and experience with the pharmacotherapy of alcohol problems. Moreover, the providers anticipate problems with compliance and review past history of medication compliance with the patients.

In the first few sessions, the provider attempts to develop an accepting and supportive relationship with the patient and to convey hope and optimism regarding the efficacy of the medication and patient's outcome. A basic and easily understandable model of how and why the medication is effective is provided. Theoretical and practical aspects of the treatment rationale are presented in the patient's own language, and discussion of the patient's concerns and questions is facilitated. Any patient resistance to the idea of medication is explored and addressed. The patient has an opportunity to air prejudices, distortions, and fantasies regarding either the positive or negative effects of the medication. Misconceptions are corrected, and the provider offers further clarification and support, emphasizing that the medication will be closely monitored. At the end of the first session, a pamphlet and medication information sheet are provided, as well as emergency contact cards.

In these sessions, the patient is instructed about the importance of taking the prescribed dosage of study medication, and the concept of gradual response or progressive improvement is discussed so that patients do not unrealistically expect an "all or nothing" response. The possibility of the occurrence of side effects during treatment is discussed, and the patient is instructed that these side effects are not dangerous if reported and managed correctly. The patient is instructed that future visits will be devoted to reviewing the patient's general progress and to discussing questions and concerns. In each session, the patient is encouraged to continue the medication. Taking a problem-solving approach, the provider is responsive to the patient's complaints and needs while also maintaining control of the session. A special effort is made to reinforce the patient's continued hope and optimism regarding improvement. By assisting the patient in developing a positive set of hopeful expectations that link the relief of cravings with the medication's effects, the provider creates opportunities for ongoing discussions focused on those aspects of the treatment that are important to the patient.

In Phase Two, the emphasis is on maintaining compliance and avoiding early discontinuation of the medication. These sessions involve a systematic inquiry into the presence, intensity, and features of positive therapeutic gains and any side effects and continue the compliance enhancement approach. If there are minor side effects, especially in patients who are apprehensive about taking medication, further educative efforts regarding the "how" and "why" of medication use are employed. Over-the-counter medication may be advised, to help reduce the discomfort of some of the side effects—for example, acetaminophen for headaches. This may be necessary to avoid the patient's dropping out and noncompliance, particularly during the earlier stage of the treatment.

In Phase Three, the provider and the patient discuss plans regarding how to discontinue the medication, and a rationale is provided detailing how the medication has helped assist sobriety during the most difficult period of action and how the patient can now maintain these gains without assistance. It is expected that a significant provider-patient relationship has been developed during the study. In light of this, the issue of termination is discussed in this session.

Provider Role

The study medical provider (physician, nurse practitioner, nurse, etc.) should offer treatment similar to that offered by a primary care provider in a clinical setting. The study provider should act in a role that stresses patient care as the provider's primary responsibility. The study provider *should act not as a researcher* but as a primary care provider. It is essential that the study provider establish a relationship with the patient that conveys a trusting and committed role toward patient care.

Support Appropriate to BBCET

The health care provider is the patient's main connection to the treatment program. The following types of support are permitted in BBCET:

1. Empathy and concern for the patient's well-being.
2. Interpersonal support—providing reassurance for compliance and a positive outcome.
3. Communication of hope and optimism, especially under situations of lack of improvement or medication side effects.
4. Provision of information related to medication and education of the patient regarding its effects.
5. Giving nonspecific advice; troubleshooting medication compliance obstacles.
6. Allowing the patient to express frustrations.

Support Not Appropriate to BBCET

Under no circumstances should the provider engage in psychotherapy. BBCET is designed to be delivered by a doctor or nurse in a primary care setting (i.e., general practitioner's office). A trusting therapeutic relationship should be developed in the context of enhancing treatment compliance and retention. An example of this relationship would be that of a renal doctor encouraging a patient to participate in kidney dialysis and to comply with the medication program in order to experience any therapeutic benefit.

The following types of interactions are *not* permitted in BBCET:

1. Psychotherapy
2. Addressing interpersonal relationships
3. Addressing cognitive factors
4. Providing interpretation of feelings, cognition, or events
5. Addressing any psychological reasons for alcohol addiction
6. Applying problem-solving techniques to life areas other than medication compliance
7. Applying relapse prevention strategies

Treatment Sessions

The following pages contain the operationalized BBCET manual used in a 12-week study investigating the use of a study medication for the treatment of alcohol dependence. We use a model of 12 sessions plus one final end-of-study session. However, the model can easily be adapted to shorter or longer time frames as needed. The first section after each session heading outlines the tasks to be accomplished and then contains narrative text that provides a more comprehensive description of the session. Each session also has a checklist, which includes each of the major tasks of the session and a rating scale that the provider can use at the end of the session to rate confidence in the completion of the session goals. Some sessions have shared tasks; thus, some of the checklists can be used for multiple sessions and are labeled accordingly in this manual. BBCET can be adapted for use in any medication trial. The medication information sheet and side-effects evaluation sheet should be tailored to each medication.

SESSION 1

(20 to 30 minutes)

Outline

1. Establish a trusting, positive therapeutic relationship.
2. Convey an optimistic attitude regarding the ability of the medication to decrease alcohol consumption.
3. Provide a basic explanation of how the medication works (see Study Medication Information section in the back of this manual).
4. Provide a medication information sheet and emergency contact cards.
5. Discuss and establish "Target Symptoms."
6. Address medication side effects (*highlight the most common*).
7. Complete a baseline side-effects checklist.
8. Obtain a past and present history of medication use.
9. Instruct the patient on how to take the medication and on the importance of following the regimen.

Note: Be supportive and empathic, but remember not to provide any psychotherapy or psychological counseling.

In Session 1, the provider should establish a trusting, positive, therapeutic relationship with the patient. The provider should be empathic and convey optimism regarding the patient's treatment. *Remember not to provide any psychological counseling in the BBCET sessions.* Provide a brief explanation in lay terms of the study medication and how it works. (Do not use medical jargon or verbiage, which may be a source of confusion.) Stress gradual and progressive changes, and dispel "all-or-nothing" thinking regarding the effects of the medication. Next, provide an explanation of alcohol and its effects on the human body. Discuss the theoretical model of how the medication works to decrease the effects of alcohol in the brain. Address any concerns or prejudices about medication use with the patient, and provide additional rationale if necessary. Discuss the potential side effects of the study medication and highlight the most common side effects. Complete the side-effects checklist and discuss/establish Target Symptoms.

Establishing Target Symptoms is important for detecting any changes in patient status during future sessions. Explain to the patient that each week these Target Symptoms will be discussed to follow the patient's progress. Obtain a history including present usage of medications for alcoholism. Disclosure of any concurrent medication use or plans to start a medication regimen should be obtained. Provide the patient with a medication information sheet. Instruct the patient on how to take the medication and on the importance of following the treatment program. Stress the relationship between medication compliance and the likelihood of positive results.

SESSION 1 CHECKLIST
(Place a check mark after completing each component)

_____ 1. Establish the groundwork for a trusting, positive, therapeutic relationship.

_____ 2. Convey an optimistic attitude regarding the ability of the medication to decrease alcohol consumption.

_____ 3. Give a basic explanation of how the medication works (provide a medication sheet). Stress gradual and progressive improvement over time.

_____ 4. Address medication side effects (*highlight the common side effects*).

_____ 5. Discuss and establish Target Symptoms.

_____ 6. Complete the side-effects checklist.

_____ 7. Obtain past and present history of medication use.

_____ 8. Provide a medication packet. Instruct the patient on how to take the medication and emphasize its importance.

Confidence in Completion of Session 1 Goals (*circle one*)

1   2   3   4   5   6   7   8   9   10

No   Extreme

Any session scored below 5 needs to be addressed with the BBCET supervisor to discuss issues and plan solutions for improving future sessions.

SESSION 2
(15 to 30 minutes)

Outline

1. Continue to establish a trusting, positive, therapeutic relationship.
2. Discuss the Target Symptoms (note any change in symptoms on the Target Symptoms form).
3. Continue to provide encouragement on the efficacy of the medication and the importance of treatment compliance.
4. Complete the symptom side-effects checklist.
5. Assess any serious medical change in the patient's status.
6. Collect the unused portion of the medication packet (complete the returned medication sheet).
7. Dispense week 2 medication and provide instructions for how to use.

Note: Stress a positive outlook, gradual and progressive improvement, and continued compliance.

In Session 2, the goal is to continue establishing a positive therapeutic relationship with the patient. A discussion of the patient's Target Symptoms is initiated, and any changes in status are noted on the Target Symptoms form. *It is crucial to explain that the medication requires time to achieve its therapeutic effect. Provide positive reinforcement for continued medication compliance and future improvement on alcohol reduction/abstinence.* Provide further explanation of how the study medication works to reduce drinking. Complete the side-effects checklist for week 2. Collect the unused portion of the medication packet and reinforce compliance with the medication regimen. Dispense week 2 medication and inquire about any difficulties with use.

SESSION 3

(15 to 30 minutes)

Outline

1. Continue cultivating and establishing a trusting, positive, therapeutic relationship.
2. Discuss the Target Symptoms (note any change in symptoms on the Target Symptoms form).
3. Continue to provide encouragement on the efficacy of the medication and the importance of treatment compliance.
4. Complete the symptom side-effects checklist.
5. Assess any serious medical change in the patient's status.
6. Collect the unused portion of the medication packet (complete the returned medication form).
7. Dispense week 3 medication and provide instructions for how to use.

Note: The patient may have experienced side effects after being on the medication for 14 days.

In Session 3, continue to provide a positive outlook regarding treatment and medication compliance. A discussion of the patient's Target Symptoms is initiated, and any changes in status are noted on the Target Symptoms form. If the patient has experienced any medical complications that may jeopardize the patient's health, contact the study P.I. *If the patient has unpleasant side effects, continue to provide support and positive reinforcement for continued medication compliance and future improvement leading to alcohol reduction/abstinence.* Discuss why the patient may be experiencing side effects and alleviate any unreasonable anxiety that the patient may be experiencing. Suggest some over-the-counter medications that may relieve unpleasant side effects. Provide further explanation of how the study medication works and how it may be helpful in reducing drinking. Complete the side-effects checklist for week 3 (note any changes). Collect the unused portion of the medication packet and reinforce the importance of continued compliance with the medication regimen. Dispense week 3 medication and inquire about any difficulties with use.

SESSION 4

(15 to 20 minutes)

Outline

1. Continue to provide a supportive and trusting therapeutic relationship.

2. Discuss the Target Symptoms (note any change in symptoms on the Target Symptoms form).
3. Continue to provide encouragement on the efficacy of the medication and the importance of treatment compliance.
4. Complete the symptom side-effects checklist.
5. Assess any serious medical change in the patient's status.
6. Collect the unused portion of the medication packet (complete the returned medication form).
7. Dispense week 4 medication and provide instructions for how to use.

Note: Subjects have been in treatment for 1 month. Improvement may be minimal in some patients, and they may become discouraged. Provide encouragement, empathy, and support, and stress the importance of the patient's continued participation, which will lead to progressive future improvement.

In Session 4, the goal is to continue establishing a positive therapeutic relationship with the patient. Discuss the effects of the study medication and how improvement or changes in drinking behavior will be gradual over time. A systematic inquiry regarding the patient's Target Symptoms is initiated, and any changes in status are noted on the Target Symptoms form. Continue to monitor the patient's health and address any serious medical complications. *Improvement may be minimal in some patients, and they may become discouraged. Provide encouragement, empathy, and support, and stress the importance of the patient's continued participation, which will lead to future improvement. Provide positive reinforcement for continued medication compliance and future improvement in alcohol reduction/abstinence.* Complete the side-effects checklist for week 4 (note any changes). Collect the unused portion of the medication packet, and reinforce the importance of compliance with the medication regimen. Dispense week 4 medication, and inquire about any difficulties with use.

SESSIONS 2, 3, AND 4 CHECKLIST
(Place a check mark after completing each component)

_____ 1. Continue to establish a trusting, positive, therapeutic relationship.

_____ 2. Discuss the Target Symptoms and list them on the form.

_____ 3. Convey an optimistic attitude regarding the ability of the medication to decrease alcohol consumption.

_____ 4. Provide reinforcement for continuation in the program and medication compliance.

_____ 5. Address medication side effects (*highlight the common side effects*).

_____ 6. Complete the side-effects checklist (note any serious medical complications).

_____ 7. Provide a medication packet. Instruct the patient on how to take the medication and emphasize its importance. Complete the returned medication form.

Confidence in Completion of Session Goals (*circle one*)

1 2 3 4 5 6 7 8 9 10

No   Extreme

Any session scored below 5 needs to be addressed with the BBCET supervisor to discuss issues and plan solutions for improving future sessions.

SESSION 5

(15 to 20 minutes)

Outline

1. Provide empathy, support, and encouragement on the continued use of the medication, which will lead to future improvement in decreasing drinking.
2. Discuss the Target Symptoms (note any change in symptoms on the Target Symptoms form).
3. Remind the patient that the medication needs to be taken for several weeks before any therapeutic effects can be seen.
4. Continue to provide encouragement on the efficacy of the medication and the importance of treatment compliance.
5. Complete the symptom side-effects checklist.
6. Assess any serious medical change in the patient's status.
7. Collect the unused portion of the medication packet (complete the returned medication form).
8. Dispense week 5 medication and provide instructions for how to use.

Note: The patient has successfully completed 4 weeks of the treatment. Stress the importance of completing the full 12 weeks.

In Session 5, the goal is to assess the patient's ability to remain in treatment and not to drop out. A discussion of the patient's Target Symptoms is initiated, and any changes in status are noted on the Target Symptoms form. *Remind the patient that the medication needs to be taken for several weeks and that therapeutic effects may be delayed. Provide positive reinforcement for continued medication compliance and future improvement in alcohol reduction/abstinence.* Discuss the medication and its effects on reducing drinking. Complete the side-effects checklist for week 5 (note any changes). Continue to monitor the patient's health and address any serious medical complications. Collect the unused portion of the medication packet and reinforce compliance with the medication regimen. Dispense week 6 medication and inquire about any difficulties with use.

SESSION 6

(15 to 20 minutes)

Outline

1. Continue providing empathy, support, and encouragement on the continued use of the medication, which will lead to future improvement in decreasing drinking.

2. Discuss the Target Symptoms (note any change in symptoms on the Target Symptoms form).
3. Continue to provide encouragement on the efficacy of the medication and the importance of treatment compliance.
4. Complete the symptom side-effects checklist.
5. Assess any serious medical change in the patient's status.
6. Collect the unused portion of the medication packet (complete the returned medication form).
7. Dispense week 6 medication and provide instructions for how to use.

Note: Stress the importance of completing the full 12-week course.

In Session 6, the goal is to assess the patient's ability to remain in treatment and to avoid dropping out. A discussion of the patient's Target Symptoms is initiated, and any changes in status are noted on the Target Symptoms form. *Provide positive reinforcement for continued medication compliance and future improvement in alcohol reduction/abstinence.* Discuss the medication and its effects on reducing drinking. Complete the side-effects checklist for week 6 (note any changes). Continue to monitor the patient's health and address any serious medical complications. Collect the unused portion of the medication packet and reinforce compliance with the medication regimen. Dispense week 6 medication and inquire about any difficulties with use.

SESSIONS 5 AND 6 CHECKLIST
(Place a check mark after completing each component)

_____ 1. Assess the patient's ability to remain in treatment. Continue to establish a trusting, positive relationship.

_____ 2. Discuss Target Symptoms and list them on the form.

_____ 3. Discuss the possible delayed therapeutic effects of the medication. Highlight any positive changes in drinking behavior or compliance related to treatment.

_____ 4. Provide reinforcement for continuation in the program and medication compliance.

_____ 5. Address medication side effects (*highlight the common side effects*).

_____ 6. Complete the side-effects checklist (note any serious medical complications).

_____ 7. Provide a medication packet. Instruct the patient on how to take the medication and emphasize its importance. Complete the returned medication form.

Confidence in Completion of Session Goals (*circle one*)

1 2 3 4 5 6 7 8 9 10
No   Extreme

Any session scored below 5 needs to be addressed with the BBCET supervisor to discuss issues and plan solutions for improving future sessions.

SESSION 7
(15 to 20 minutes)

Outline
1. Stress the fact that half of the treatment has been completed. Spend a majority of the session focusing on the success of completing 6 weeks. Encourage continued participation, which will lead to a reduction in drinking and an increase in well-being.
2. Discuss the Target Symptoms (note any change in symptoms on the Target Symptoms form).
3. Continue to provide encouragement on the efficacy of the medication and the importance of treatment compliance.
4. Complete the symptom side-effects checklist.
5. Assess any serious medical changes in the patient's status.
6. Collect the unused portion of the medication packet (complete the returned medication form).
7. Dispense week 7 medication and provide instructions for how to use.

> *Note: Reinforce the successful completion of half of the treatment program. Provide encouragement for participation and maintain a positive outlook toward continued participation.*

In Session 7, the goal is to provide encouragement for continued participation and completion of the 12-week treatment program. Focus on the success of completing 6 weeks of treatment. A discussion of the patient's Target Symptoms is initiated, and any changes in status are noted on the Target Symptoms form. *Some patients may not be experiencing any positive changes. In these circumstances, a trusting therapeutic relationship can be effective for encouraging patient compliance and continuation in treatment. Provide positive reinforcement for continued medication compliance and future improvement in alcohol reduction/abstinence.* Stress positive points and changes (e.g., completion of 6 weeks of the program). Provide further explanation of how the study medication works and how it may be helpful in reducing drinking. Complete the side-effects checklist for week 7 (note any changes). Continue to monitor the patient's health and address any serious medical complications. Collect the unused portion of the medication packet and reinforce compliance with the medication regimen. Dispense week 7 medication and inquire about any difficulties with use.

SESSION 8
(15 to 20 minutes)

Outline
1. Encourage continued participation. Continue to highlight any positive results.
2. Discuss the Target Symptoms (note any change in symptoms on the Target Symptoms form).
3. Continue to provide encouragement on the efficacy of the medication and the importance of treatment compliance.
4. Complete the symptom side-effects checklist.
5. Assess any serious medical changes in the patient's status.

6. Collect the unused portion of the medication packet (complete the returned medication form).
7. Dispense week 8 medication and provide instructions for how to use.

Note: Continued support is essential for ensuring compliance!

In Session 8, the goal is to help the patient maintain a positive outlook and attitude toward the progress being made. A discussion of the patient's Target Symptoms is initiated, and any changes in status are noted on the Target Symptoms form. *Provide positive reinforcement for continued medication compliance and future improvement in alcohol reduction/abstinence.* Complete the side-effects checklist for week 8 (note any changes). Continue to monitor the patient's health and address any serious medical complications. Collect the unused portion of the medication packet and reinforce compliance with the medication regimen. Dispense week 8 medication and inquire about any difficulties with use.

SESSION 9
(15 to 20 minutes)

Outline
1. Continue encouraging the patient and provide support.
2. Discuss the Target Symptoms (note any change in symptoms on the Target Symptoms form).
3. Continue to provide encouragement on the efficacy of medication and the importance of treatment compliance.
4. Complete the symptom side-effects checklist.
5. Assess any serious medical changes in the patient's status.
6. Collect the unused portion of the medication packet.
7. Dispense week 9 medication and provide instructions for how to use.

Note: Highlight the patient's compliance for the past 8 weeks and maintain a positive outlook.

In Session 9, the goal is to reinforce progressive improvement, which may be gradual over time. A discussion of the patient's Target Symptoms is initiated, and any changes in status are noted on the Target Symptoms form. Provide positive reinforcement for continued medication compliance and future improvement in alcohol reduction/abstinence. Complete the side-effects checklist for week 9 (note any changes). Continue to monitor the patient's health and address any serious medical complications. Collect the unused portion of the medication packet and reinforce compliance with the medication regimen. Dispense week 9 medication and inquire about any difficulties with use.

SESSION 10
(15 to 20 minutes)

Outline
1. Reinforce the patient's participation and address how this will aid in achieving a positive outcome.

2. Discuss the Target Symptoms (note any change in symptoms on the Target Symptoms form).
3. Review any changes from the baseline.
4. Continue to provide encouragement on the efficacy of the medication and the importance of treatment compliance.
5. Complete the symptom side-effects checklist.
6. Assess any serious medical changes in the patient's status.
7. Collect the unused portion of the medication packet (complete the returned medication form).
8. Dispense week 10 medication and provide instructions for how to use.

Note: Provide praise and reinforcement to the patient for completing 9 weeks of the program.

In Session 10, the goal is to discuss the patient's progress and highlight any positive results. If the patient is not experiencing any positive results, provide encouragement to help the patient develop a more positive outlook. *Remember that staying in the treatment program for the past 9 weeks is an excellent outcome and should be commended.* A discussion of the patient's Target Symptoms is initiated, and any changes in status are noted on the Target Symptoms form. Provide positive reinforcement for continued medication compliance and future improvement in alcohol reduction/abstinence. Complete the side-effects checklist for week 10 (note any changes). Continue to monitor the patient's health and address any serious medical complications. Collect the unused portion of the medication packet and reinforce compliance with the medication regimen. Dispense week 10 medication and inquire about any difficulties with use.

SESSIONS 7, 8, 9, AND 10 CHECKLIST
(Place a check mark after completing each component)

_____ 1. Highlight the positive outcome and completion of ____ weeks of treatment.

_____ 2. Discuss the Target Symptoms and list them on the form.

_____ 3. Convey an optimistic attitude regarding the ability of the medication to decrease alcohol consumption.

_____ 4. Provide reinforcement for continuation in the program and medication compliance.

_____ 5. Address medication side effects.

_____ 6. Complete the side-effects checklist *(note any serious medical complications).*

_____ 7. Provide a medication packet. Instruct the patient on how to take the medication and emphasize its importance. Complete the returned medication form.

Confidence in Completion of Session Goals (*circle one*)

1 2 3 4 5 6 7 8 9 10

No   Extreme

Any session scored below 5 needs to be addressed with the BBCET supervisor to discuss issues and plan solutions for improving future sessions.

SESSION 11

(15 to 20 minutes)

Outline

1. Encourage treatment completion.
2. Discuss the Target Symptoms (note any change in symptoms on the Target Symptoms form).
3. Continue to provide encouragement on the efficacy of the medication and the importance of treatment compliance.
4. Complete the symptom side-effects checklist.
5. Begin discussing termination.
6. Assess any serious medical changes in the patient's status.
7. Collect the unused portion of the medication packet (complete the returned medication form).
8. Dispense week 11 medication and provide instructions for how to use.

Note: Begin to address termination of treatment and future plans.

In Session 11, the goals are to encourage completion of treatment and to begin discussing the patient's future plans. A discussion of the patient's Target Symptoms is initiated, and any changes in status are noted on the Target Symptoms form. *Provide positive reinforcement for continued medication compliance and future improvement in alcohol reduction/abstinence.* Complete the side-effects checklist for week 11 (note any changes). Continue to monitor the patient's health and address any serious medical complications. Collect the unused portion of the medication packet and reinforce compliance with the medication regimen. Dispense week 11 medication and inquire about any difficulties with use.

SESSION 12

(15 to 20 minutes)

Outline

1. Discuss the Target Symptoms (note any change in symptoms on the Target Symptoms form).
2. Discuss termination and review progress over the past 11 weeks.
3. Continue to provide encouragement on the efficacy of medication and the importance of treatment compliance.
4. Complete the symptom side-effects checklist.
5. Assess any serious medical changes in the patient's status.
6. Collect the unused portion of the medication packet.
7. Dispense week 12 medication and provide instructions for how to use.

Note: Stress completion of the treatment program. Highlight the successful completion of the program to date.

In Session 12, the goal is to stress completion of treatment and to highlight positive events. Discuss termination and completion of the treatment. A discussion of the patient's Target Symptoms is initiated, and any changes in status are noted on the Target Symptoms form. *Provide positive reinforcement for continued medication compliance and future improvement in alcohol reduction/abstinence.* Complete the side-effects checklist for week 12 (note any changes). Continue to monitor the patient's health and address any serious medical complications. Collect the unused portion of the medication packet and reinforce compliance with the medication regimen. Dispense week 12 medication and inquire about any difficulties with use.

SESSIONS 11 AND 12 CHECKLIST
(Place a check mark after completing each component)

_____ 1. Discuss positive events and provide support for the patient's successful participation in the treatment.

_____ 2. Discuss termination and future plans.

_____ 3. Discuss Target Symptoms and list them on the form.

_____ 4. Provide reinforcement for continuation in the program and medication compliance.

_____ 5. Address medication side effects.

_____ 6. Complete the side-effects checklist (note any serious medical complications).

_____ 7. Provide a medication packet. Instruct the patient on how to take the medication and emphasize its importance. Complete the returned medication form.

Confidence in Completion of Session Goals (*circle one*)

$$1 \quad 2 \quad 3 \quad 4 \quad 5 \quad 6 \quad 7 \quad 8 \quad 9 \quad 10$$
No   Extreme

Any session scored below 5 needs to be addressed with the BBCET supervisor to discuss issues and to plan solutions for improving future sessions.

FINAL SESSION
(30 minutes)

Outline
1. Discuss termination issues. Address the patient's thoughts about being in the study, future plans, and medication termination.
2. Discuss the Target Symptoms (note any change in symptoms on the Target Symptoms form).
3. Complete the symptom side-effects checklist.
4. Assess any serious medical complications.
5. Collect the unused portion of the medication packet (complete the returned medication form).
6. Assess the patient's progress and provide an appropriate referral for further treatment if necessary.

Note: A trusting relationship has been developed and termination needs to be addressed.

In the Final Session, treatment termination issues need to be addressed. Discuss the patient's thoughts about the treatment program and about future plans. A discussion of the patient's Target Symptoms is initiated, and any changes in status are noted on the Target Symptoms form. Complete the side-effects checklist for the end-of-study visit (note any changes). Collect the unused portion of the medication packet and provide praise to the patient for completing the treatment. Assess the patient's current clinical status and provide appropriate referrals. Complete the end-of-study forms and assessments.

FINAL SESSION CHECKLIST
(Place a check mark after completing each component)

_____ 1. Complete the termination discussion.

_____ 2. Discuss Target Symptoms and list them on the form.

_____ 3. Provide praise for successful compliance and completion.

_____ 4. Address medication issues and side effects.

_____ 5. Complete the side-effects checklist (note any serious medical complications).

_____ 6. Collect the unused portion of the medication packet (complete the returned medication form).

_____ 7. Assess the patient's status and provide a referral if necessary.

_____ 8. Complete the end-of-study forms and assessments.

Confidence in Completion of Final Session Goals (*circle one*)

1   2   3   4   5   6   7   8   9   10

No   Extreme

Any session scored below 5 needs to be addressed with the BBCET supervisor to discuss issues.

Common Problems and Solutions

The following are some issues commonly encountered in compliance enhancement treatment, along with suggested ways of dealing with each problem.

Forgetting to Take Medications
- Associate study medications with other medications, vitamins, etc.
- Place the study medications in sight, associated with other daily activities (e.g., toothbrush).
- Place post-it note reminders (on bathroom mirror, refrigerator, car dashboard, etc.).
- Set the alarm on a watch, pager, or cell phone.

Experiencing Medication Side Effects

- Evaluate/educate about other factors that may exacerbate the experience (e.g., fatigue as a perceived drug effect when the patient is still drinking, possible poor nutritional intake, etc.).
- Assess safety issues related to side effects (e.g., drowsiness while driving).
- Ask the patient how intrusive/bothersome the side effects are; be supportive.
- Change the timing of the doses if timing of onset is an issue for intrusive side effects.
- Recommend over-the-counter/nonpharmacological treatment if appropriate (e.g., laxative or increased fiber intake for constipation).
- At the first visit, discuss the most common side effects, the usual intensity/duration of these effects, and what the patient can do to cope with the effects.
- Encourage open discussion with a partner for sexual side effects (i.e., if this has not previously been a problem, the difficulty is most likely due to the medication and will resolve at the end of the study—and ask the patient: Isn't it worth some short-term discomfort or inconvenience when you are making such good progress with your drinking?)

Not Getting an "Adequate" Drug Effect (Believing That a Placebo Is Being Given)

- At the first visit, inform the patient that the medication effect is not immediate. State that this is research so we are still learning how the medication works in different people. Some people feel the effects quickly, but it is more likely that you'll feel increasing effects over several days or weeks.
- Emphasize that the study is blinded—clinic staff also do not know whether the patient is taking a placebo. There's a little man up on a mountain doing the randomization with a computer, so we do not know whether you are taking the active medication.
- Remind the patient that not having side effects does not mean that a placebo is being given; side effects are not a requirement. We hope that you won't have any!
- Remind the patient that taking the medications as prescribed is how to get the most benefit from them. Each time you take a pill is a little reminder for you to keep working on your drinking.
- Reflect on any positive changes. If you haven't had this kind of success in the past, you may be experiencing the effect of the drug —or, if you are taking the placebo, all the better for you in the long run. These medicines are not like insulin—you don't want to be taking pills for the rest of your life—but for the length of the study, they seem to be helping you (or at least not causing you any significant distress).
- Medication is just a part of alcohol recovery; it's important that you do things to live your life differently to change these behavior patterns, particularly for long-term success. Encourage participation in support groups if the patient is receptive. *Caution:* Remember not to engage in problem-solving related to anything other than medication compliance.

Drinking While on Medication

- Explain that medication may exacerbate effects of alcohol such as drowsiness.
- Instruct the patient not to skip medication doses just because he or she has been drinking.
- Clarify the study medication effects vs. those of disulfiram.

Feeling Down Because of Poor Progress in Recovery

- Provide lots of positive reinforcement, even for continued attendance at study visits.
- Remind the patient that continuous drinking and/or slips are not uncommon—the most important thing is to continue to try. Even cutting down on quantity/frequency is a step in the right direction.
- If the patient has a bad week, discuss any positive changes compared with baseline rather than with the previous week. You've been in the program for only ___ weeks. I'm sure that drinking has been a problem for you for much longer than that.

REFERENCES

Brady M, Sibthorpe B, Bailie R, Ball S, Sumnerdodd P: The feasibility and acceptability of introducing brief intervention for alcohol misuse in an urban Aboriginal medical service. Drug Alcohol Rev 21:375–380, 2002.

Carnegie MA, Gomel MK, Saunders JB, Britt H, Burns L: General practice receptionists' attitudes and beliefs towards preventive medicine before and after training and support interventions. Fam Pract 13:504–510, 1996.

Chang G, Wilkins-Haug L, Berman S, Goetz MA: Brief intervention for alcohol use in pregnancy: a randomized trial. Addiction 94:1499–1508, 1999.

Edwards G, Orford J, Egert S, Guthrie S, Hawker A, Hensman C, Mitcheson M, Oppenheimer E, Taylor C: Alcoholism: a controlled trial of "treatment" and "advice". J Stud Alcohol 38:1004–1031, 1977.

Fawcett J, Epstein P, Fiester SJ, Elkin I, Autry JH: Clinical management—imipramine/placebo administration manual: NIMH Treatment of Depression Collaborative Research Program. Psychopharmacol Bull 23:309–324, 1987.

Fleming MF: Screening and brief intervention for alcohol disorders. J Fam Pract 37:231–234, 1993.

Fleming MF, Mundt MP, French MT, Manwell LB, Stauffacher EA, Barry KL: Brief physician advice for problem drinkers: long-term efficacy and benefit-cost analysis. Alcohol Clin Exp Res 26:36–43, 2002.

Graham DM, Maio RF, Blow FC, Hill EM: Emergency physician attitudes concerning intervention for alcohol abuse/dependence delivered in the emergency department: a brief report. J Addict Dis 19:45–53, 2000.

Imber SD, Pilkonis PA, Sotsky SM, Elkin I, Watkins JT, Collins JF, Shea MT, Leber WR, Glass DR: Mode-specific effects among three treatments for depression. J Consult Clin Psychol 58:352–359, 1990.

Saitz R, Sullivan LM, Samet JH: Training community-based clinicians in screening and brief intervention for substance abuse problems: translating evidence into practice. Subst Abuse 21:21–31, 2000.

Smith AJ, Hodgson RJ, Bridgeman K, Shepherd JP: A randomized controlled trial of a brief intervention after alcohol-related facial injury. Addiction 98:43–52, 2003.

Wright S, Moran L, Meyrick M, O'Connor R, Touquet R. Intervention by an alcohol health worker in an accident and emergency department. Alcohol Alcohol 33:651–656, 1998.

Study Medication Information

[Using lay terminology, insert a general description of the study medication.]

ALCOHOL'S EFFECTS ON THE BODY

[Insert a brief description of alcohol's effects in the brain as it relates to the chosen study medication(s).]

STUDY MEDICATION EFFECTS

[Insert a list of potential study medication effects on drinking behavior.]

The study medication must be taken according to the prescribed methods. Daily oral dosing is required to achieve the proper therapeutic blood levels. The beneficial effects of the study medication on alcohol drinking may not be seen for several weeks. However, every person's body reacts differently, and some positive effects may be felt within 1 or 2 weeks. The study medication should be taken and not stopped unless you are directed to do so by a physician. It is important to take the medication, even though you may not be experiencing a reduction in drinking or related behaviors such as craving, because the medication may not have achieved therapeutic levels.

Side Effects Evaluation

The most common side effects of the study medication include:

[List the 10 most common side effects of the study medication.]

[Include a disclaimer, if appropriate, on the use of the study medication in women with childbearing potential and children.]

[Include a specific checklist of the medication's exclusion criteria.]

Notify the study physician or provider before taking any medications in order to avoid any possible adverse medication reactions.

Weekly Target Symptoms

SESSION _____   DATE: __/__/__

Participant ID#_____

INTERVIEWER: _____

1. TARGET SYMPTOMS (e.g., drinking excessively, becoming intoxicated, social consequences):

_____

_____

_____

_____

2. COMPLIANCE AND TREATMENT PROBLEMS:

_____

_____

_____

_____

2. CRAVING AND ALCOHOL USAGE:

_____

_____

_____

_____

Index

Note: Page numbers followed by f indicate figures; page numbers followed by t indicate tables.